SCHIZOPHRENIA

A LOOK THROUGH INDIAN CULTURE

SCHIZOPHRENIA

A LOOK THROUGH INDIAN CULTURE

P.K. Chattopadhyay
Formerly Professor, Department of Psychology
Calcutta University, Kolkata
in collaboration with
Barna Chattopadhyay

PUBLISHING FOR ONE WORLD

NEW AGE INTERNATIONAL (P) LIMITED, PUBLISHERS

New Delhi • Bangalore • Chennai • Cochin • Guwahati • Hyderabad
Jalandhar • Kolkata • Lucknow • Mumbai • Ranchi
Visit us at **www.newagepublishers.com**

Published by New Age International (P) Ltd., Publishers
First Edition: 2009

Branches:

- 36, Malikarjuna Temple Street, Opp. ICWA, Basavanagudi, **Bangalore**. ✆ (080) 26677815
- 26, Damodaran Street, T. Nagar, **Chennai**. ✆ (044) 24353401
- Hemsen Complex, Mohd. Shah Road, Paltan Bazar, Near Starline Hotel, **Guwahati**. ✆ (0361) 2543669
- No. 105, 1st Floor, Madhiray Kaveri Tower, 3-2-19, Azam Jahi Road, Nimboliadda, **Hyderabad**. ✆ (040) 24652456
- RDB Chambers (Formerly Lotus Cinema) 106A, Ist Floor, S.N. Banerjee Road, **Kolkata**. ✆ (033) 22275247
- 18, Madan Mohan Malviya Marg, **Lucknow**. ✆ (0522) 2209578
- 142C, Victor House, Ground Floor, N.M. Joshi Marg, Lower Parel, **Mumbai**. ✆ (022) 24927869
- 22, Golden House, Daryaganj, **New Delhi**. ✆ (011) 23262368, 23262370

ISBN : 978-81-224-2380-8

Rs. 395.00

C-08-06-2655

Printed in India at Glorious Printers, Delhi
Typeset at Subham Composers, Delhi

PUBLISHING FOR ONE WORLD

NEW AGE INTERNATIONAL (P) LIMITED, PUBLISHERS
4835/24, Ansari Road, Daryaganj, New Delhi - 110002
Visit us at **www.newagepublishers.com**

Dedicated to
Our Beloved Parents

PREFACE

Producing a book on schizophrenia merits specific justification, more so when it is concerned with culture and symptomatology. On the basis of our own and several other colleagues' teaching and clinical experiences, we believe that there is an increasing need for a text which can inform the upper-level undergraduate, graduate, medical students, postgraduate students and research fellows of our culture the importance of this culture in understanding schizophrenia - both from its etiology and therapeutic points of view. This book intends to meet that need.

While preparing this manuscript, we had a feeling that presently available literature, by and large, have failed to provide a more objective and comprehensive overview of the diverse factors contributing to schizophrenic illness. We recognised that the current state of understanding about psychopathology was still in a relative state of flux. We also have experienced a severe shortfall in understanding schizophrenia in context to our culture because of lack of adequate text and research reports highlighting the role of our culture in etiology and treatment, particularly psychotherapy and rehabilitation (with emphasis on psychosocial rehabilitation). Therefore, we attempted to survey such factors as genetic, familial, sociocultural, neuropsychological, psychophysiological, and psychological. We tried to present a more balanced approach regarding the possible origins of psychopathology. Also, we have given a pragmatic and empirical discussion regarding the possible dynamics and treatment thereupon. We have recognised that a single theoretical or therapeutic set of models could not explain or alter pathology. Therefore we have focussed on the necessity to have an integrated approach in understanding schizophrenia.

Modern research trends have been taken into account in the preparation of the chapters; to give a clear idea to the students about the changes noted over time in certain concepts, hypotheses, and theories, sometimes an historical account has been given of those views and theories. That is why, some very old references have also been incorporated, but the chapters have been updated through recent literatures available in India and abroad.

It aims to produce a scholarly and balanced compendium that might serve as an important source for the current state of the field. Accordingly, its emphasis has been on issues of contemporary controversies. Among these are–issues related to the applicability of diagnostic classification (DSM/ICD) in relation to our culture, the worth of applying Western model of the disease in understanding psychopathology of Indian patients, the efficacy of traditional psychotherapies, validity and ethical issues of the Western healing methods for the patients of our culture, and the future of the community mental health concept in India, etc. Of course this book might not have been able to offer easy solutions to these ponderous problems, it does deal with all of them in a way, that is likely to sensitise students and research scholars to these burning issues; the present write-up would be used as a pointer by the students/research scholars to find easy solutions to those problems in near future.

We hope that the book will be a comprehensive source of information, stimulation, and challenge to those who are interested to know psychopathology of schizophrenia and its methods of amelioration in context to Indian culture.

The book has been present in twelve chapters. The first chapter is devoted to a brief survey of the historical development of the concept of schizophrenia. Such conceptual frames of reference are needed to achieve an effective comprehension of the complex and variegated array of-behaviours manifested by such patients which force the attention of clinicians and mental health professionals.

Instead of becoming traditional in presentation of other chapters, the text includes chapter contents that are often overlooked in books on this topic - namely chapter on hidden symptoms of schizophrenia; role of Indian culture in developing hallucinations and delusions, background culture and symptoms in migrated patients, psychotherapy: Indian scenario which also concerns family transactions in Indian systems and its impact in management of such patients.

Some problems, in relation to Indian culture, in the acceptance of the diagnostic subclassification of schizophrenia, given by the American Psychiatric Association have been focussed. The chapter on symptoms (Chapter IV), may appear unconventional. This is because instead of listing the diagnostic nomenclature given by DSM and/or ICD, this chapter has focussed on the importance of symptoms which are present in individuals in disguised form, and later get manifested as schizophrenia. Such delay in detection obviously cause treatment hazards and poor prognosis. Later in this chapter some of the key symptoms mostly found in patients with schizophrenia have been explained with special reference to the impact of our culture in developing such symptoms. Therefore the order of presentation has not been conventional, especially when it has seemed best to assist the students/researchers in organising their learning tasks.

A comprehensive account of several treatment procedures/therapeutic measures usually employed on such patients has been provided keeping in view the need for certain revisions which are demanded out of advances made in scientific research and changes in social attitude. Also the community mental health movement and the human relations training approaches are discussed elaborately, as because these emphasise altogether a different philosophy of treatment. The human relations training techniques such as, that for the sensitivity group, namely, psychoeducation, family therapy, family training, in interpersonal interaction/communication, and also for implementation of relapsed prevention treatment strategies have been discussed. A major addition in this regard is the introduction of a section on need for an integrated approach in the treatment/management of patients with schizophrenia.

All bibliographies have been updated, retaining from the past only those writings of primary seminal or historical importance. Preference in selection of articles have been to outstanding review articles or other relevant articles published in English particularly, though article published in any local language have been scanned through. More emphasis has been given to those articles which enable cross cultural comparison in relation to symptom manifestation. Indian research reports have been scanned as far as practicable. However, no review is free from limitation. Therefore, if any research articles has been left out, the omission is inadvertent.

– **Authors**

ACKNOWLEDGEMENT

The support and encouragement received from the publishers, in particular John Wiley & Sons. Inc., Hoboken, NJ 07030-5774 and Springer Publishing Company, New York are appreciated. We acknowledge with thanks their kind permission to reuse some of the important materials from their publications and also to quote some of the excerpts particularly in relation to cross-cultural findings.

We are indebted to the patients and their family members who helped us enormously to enrich our knowledge about schizophrenia in context to Indian culture.

We are also thankful to the students for their inquisitiveness to know about cultural impact in symptomatology, which inspired us for the present effort.

Again, we are indebted to our beloved parents whose passion for learning motivated us to write-up this book.

– **Authors**

CONTENTS

1
CHAPTER

Nosology and Evolution of the Concept

History of the evolution of the concept of schizophrenia is usually traced to Benedict – Augustin Morel (1809-1873), a Belgian Psychiatrist, who in the 1850s called it "Dementia (Démence Précoce) Praecox", a type of stupidité (Lewis, 1960). Morel used this term while describing a case of a boy of 13 or 14 years, who previously had always been very brilliant, active and smart but became gloomy, reserved, with a tendency to solitude (Morel, 1957). This state deteriorated further and Morel interpreted this disorganisation of personality as an arrest of development of the different faculties of the organism, *viz*., intellectual, physical, and moral. Morel considered this to be a hopeless case of "hereditary insanity".

The next step in the history of dementia praecox was Heckev's (1871) detailed description of hebephrenia, a term which had been used previously by Kahlbaum. Heckev considered hebephrenia to be a progressive diseases of puberty and adolescence.

Somewhat later, in 1874, Kahlbaum gave description of Catatonia. Kahlbaum called it "tension insanity" and assumed that Catatonia was the symptom of a structural brain disease.

Another step in the development of the concept of dementia praecox was in 1887, when Emil Kraepelin (1856-1926), a German Psychiatrist wrote book on this topic. During Kraepelin's time, the term *dementia praecox* was used to refer to schizophrenia, where dementia means deterioration and praecox refers to the early age of onset. Kraepelin opined that a common denominator exists among apparently unrelated syndrome such as the hebephrenia of Heckev, and the Catatonia of Kahlbaum, and many paranoid psychoses. Features, according to him, these clinical syndromes had in common are – a beginning in adolescence or early adulthood and dementia following progressive deterioration. Therefore Kraepelin is credited with first grouping the schizophrenic disorders together. The causes of the various clinical features, he believed, might be either a degenerative disease of the brain, or metabolic disturbances that produced auto-intoxication. He also believed that injury to the germplasma might be a significant factor in its development, resulting in weakening of emotional and volitional reactions and a loss of harmonious relations among emotional, volitional and intellectual reactions of the individual. However, he was very critical of any attempt to interpret the behaviour of the patient on a psychological basis.

Still later, in the 1896 version of his text book, Kraepelin distinguished three major types of schizophrenia – Hebephrenia, Catatonia and Paranoia. However, his classification, with a few modern additions, is being used even today.

The next significant contribution in the history of the development of the concept dementia praecox was made by Adolf Meyer (1906) (published in 1910). He was of the opinion that the interest should be not so much in a classificatory diagnosis. This is because he emphasized the clinical picture of schizophrenia not as an autonomous disease entity, but as a form of habit disorganisation, "Habit disorganisation, as Meyer viewed it, results from a progressive maladaptation in terms of the patient's experiences and life history. In such progressive maladaptation there takes place "insufficient and faulty attempts" to avoid difficulties rather than to meet them by decisive action."

Meyer advocated that the failure to find any physiological or structural changes in nervous system excludes an organic etiology, but he believed that an inferior constitution as well as some other pathologic conditions of a physical nature may be contributory in manifestation of symptoms.

Another most important landmark in the history of Dementia Praecox was the introduction of the term "Schizophrenia" by Eugene Bleuler, another famed German Psychiatrist, in 1911. He believed that the disease was not one of de-mentia, a state of diminished mind, but rather a disharmonious state of mind in which contradictory tendencies, thoughts and feelings exist together so much so that the harmony of the personality is split. To designate such a state of the personality, Bleuler used the term schizophrenia, (*Schizin*, to divide or split, and *phran*, the mind (Greek)), which means a disharmony or "split" of the psychobiological expression of the organism. He also added a fourth form of this disorder, known as the *Simple type.*

As already mentioned before, prior to Bleuler's time there was a firm and prevailing belief that all mental disorders, be it psychosis or neurosis, were of somatic origin. Bleuler too was initially influenced by such prevailing belief and hesitated to conclude that schizophrenia itself was of functional in nature and as such could be understood psychologically. He therefore, opined that symptoms of schizophrenia could be primary and secondary. The former he considered were the direct manifestations of a hypothetical somatic morbid process such as, loosening of the associational links in thought process, a morbid ambivalence that dominates the affective life of the patient, and a tendency to replace reality by fantasy, etc. The latter *i.e.*, (secondary symptoms), he believed were of psychic origin and these included delusions, and a part of the hallucinations explainable by the patient's frustration, conflicts, and hopes, the mannerisms, the catatonic musculature symptoms and a large part of the complicated attitudes that others have designated as dementia or deterioration. Later in 1897, Bleuler became acquainted with Freud, developed a great interest in psychoanalysis and concluded that schizophrenic symptoms could be understood employing the same symbolization that Freud had discovered in dreams and in the development of neurotic disorders. Bleuler has been criticized in the sense that he has assumed an unwarranted dualism of mind and body in his conception of schizophrenia (Meyer). Nevertheless, Bleuler's monograph on schizophrenia is regarded as one of the classics in psychiatry. Of course, the concept of schizophrenia advocated by Kraepelin, Meyer and Freud also are subject to criticisms, as there exist recently a number of working hypotheses, which will be discussed later in this book in the chapter on etiology.

2

CHAPTER

The Classification of Schizophrenia: An Account of a Century (1899–1999)

(CONTRADICTIONS, CONFUSIONS, AND NEED FOR CULTURE BOUND MODIFICATION)

It has been just mentioned in the previous chapter that in 1899, Kraepelin classified schizophrenia into three groups, *viz.*, hebephrenia, catatonia, and paranoid, and latter in 1911 Bleuler added a fourth variety to it, which he called simple schizophrenia. However, clinicians would agree that the boundaries between these groups may not always be hard and fast, so that the clinical features in any given case may change rapidly in the acute shifts of the illness, and also that during the course of the illness over years the symptomatology may change and the illness may have to be re-classified.

Childhood Schizophrenia

It is controversial as to whether childhood schizophrenia is the same as adult schizophrenia in symptom manifestation. There is a wide variety of clinical pictures in childhood schizophrenia. These ranges from regressive, retarded, inhibited, withdrawn (loss of contact and affect) to overfast development with exaggerated intellectual, brilliance, precautious in language development and excessively abstract in their thinking (Kleinmuntz, 1974). The older the child, the more the clinical picture resembles that seen in adults. Hallucinations and delusions do not occur before 8 years of age (Kolb, 1973). Some patients become aggressive, and destructive, while some others show brooding or obsessive rumination. Self-mutilation may also be present in them.

Diagnostically these children show impairment in ego functioning. Their ability to conceive clearly time and space, and also the development of a clear body image, and sexual identity is impaired. They show a tendency to use preferably the sensory information available from the contact receptors, such as, touch/taste and smell rather than distance receptors, *i.e.*, hearing and vision (Kolb, 1973). In this way, their ability to find a personal identity and capacities for anticipation and generalisation become limited. A good proportion of such children may be considered to be suffering from personality disorders associated with organic brain damage. Consequently, many diagnostic nomenclature have been used to describe them. Some of these are – atypical child, infantile autism, infantile symbiotic psychosis, anaclitic depression, etc. (Suinn, 1975).

Childhood schizophrenia must be differentiated from mental deficiencies, other chronic brain disorders in early years, and familial dysautonomia, etc. Case history, physical and mental status of the patient, neuroimaging and responses to psychological testing usually can discriminate the various conditions. It should be recalled that the overlap between autistic and schizophrenic children is great, and many clinicians feel that differentiation can not be made between these two disorders, except on the basis of some etiological information (*e.g.*, parental characteristics etc.). Contrary to this, some professionals feel that at least for future research purposes, it is wise to differentiate between these two conditions. The field is too vast to review here. However, some of the most pertinent literature will be mentioned.

Effects of the separation of children from parents and later difficulties in developing attachment has been depicted well by Bowlby (1980). Excessive stimulation and its negative consequences (Weil, 1989a,b), the damaging impact of deprivation of empathic care have been studied in large number of children. Likewise, inhibition of normal development of autonomy (Mahler, Pine and Bergmann, 1975) and the effects of early parental death (Altschul, 1988) in problem behaviour have been studied extensively. Longitudinal studies are available (*e.g.*, Wallerstein and Blakeslee, 1989) on the effects of broken home environment in causing lack of trust in such children, which is perhaps the reason for their preference capsuled life interaction.

In sum : Parental care and style of interaction have been reported to be significant cause of such disorder, of which cool parents, *viz.,* 'freezing' mother and emotionally 'frizid' father (Cameron *et al.*, 1998) and their interaction pattern have been pointed out by most of the researchers. In many ways however, treatment procedures used with schizophrenic children are similar to those used with the autistic children (O'Leary and Wilson, 1975) (for treatment of such children, see Chapter VIII).

Paranoid Schizophrenia

Of all types of schizophrenia, the Paranoid type is found to be most homogenous and least variable. Primary delusions followed by Secondary delusional interpretations, and hallucinations are the leading symptoms. The delusions are often the persecutory variety with the patient believing that he is the centre of a carefully devised plot. He might complain that his food is being poisoned, or he is being followed, talked about, or being controlled by sophisticated scientific instruments, like "automatic electric cosmic-ray machine" (Suinn, 1975). He might also possess delusion of grandeur. Hallucinations in these patients are mostly auditory : vivid voices speak to him, command him, or curse him. Such a patient may be destructive/homicidal in response to his hallucinations or delusions. State of fear, rage, wish, or feeling of overwhelming well-being and vigour or the opposite are experienced in acute cases. Affective disorders if occur, very mild, and are not prominent. 'Paranoid schizophrenics' orientation and intellect are preserved. He is on the average, brighter than other schizophrenics and in spite of his suspiciousness, he is relatively in better contact with his environment than that of other schizophrenic types. Disturbances of thinking, feelings, and volition, *i.e.*, those symptoms which lead to gross deterioration of personality, may be absent or inconspicuous in this group. Only under special circumstances, these may be revealed. According to the Western Literature, the average age of onset of this illness is late. Thus, *e.g.*, Kallman (1930) reported that the age of onset of paranoid type was 35, and for all other types it was on an average 30 years. Wyrson (1942) observed that onset of this illness in majority of his cases was at the age of 30 and as late as 50, though some of the patients showed symptoms of this illness within the third decade. However, in Indian set up some of the patients are found to develop paranoid symptoms as early as 24 years or so. Since paranoid symptoms are prominent in other psychoses and attempts have been made by clinicians to differentiate paranoid schizophrenia from paranoid states, and so on, a separate chapter will be devoted to paranoid psychoses later in this book.

Catatonic Schizophrenia

In this the disturbance is exhibited primarily in motor symptoms. Delusions, hallucinations, disorders of thought and affect are usually present to some degree, but motor symptoms dominate much more than these. Speech may be affected by catatonia as a mere part; in general, its effects are prominent on motor behaviour. Speech disorders like, Verbigeration, Neologisms, Eholalia, Word Salad, or Iteration may occur. A detailed description of all these has been given later in this chapter. However, without mentioning the physical abnormalities, the clinical picture of catatonia appears to remain incomplete. Some of these are – shallow colour and greasiness of the skin, especially of the face; blue and mottled extremities which are always cool, a peculiar odour of the patient's sweat which is rather difficult to describe, excessive salivation, low pulse rate and blood pressure, shallow respirations interrupted by sighs, and relatively low body weight. Usually this illness tends/occur in adolescence and early adult life, but occasionally it is found to occur in the fourth decade or even later. Most frequently it is acute in onset and is precipitated or preceded by an emotionally disturbing experience. The patient may evidence a stuporous condition, or he may display excitement, or in some cases the two may alternate. The prognosis for a recovery from the first attack of catatonia is more favourable than in other types of schizophrenia. If however, the illness is progressive, there is likelihood for the catatonic type to pass over into states approaching hebephrenia or paranoid, with permanent personality disorganisation.

Catatonic Stupor

This is often preceded by discontent, depression, or emotional fermentation. Stupor varies in degree from a transient blocking of some movement to that of immobilization of the whole body of the patient in a fixed posture. The patient appears to be as if, in a state of physical suspension. He is usually mute and his behaviour reflects in attention, preoccupation, having emotional poverty and dreaminess. He is unresponsive to even uncomfortable stimulation. With mask like faces, these patients may occasionally keep their eyes closed, but more frequently they stare fixedly and blankly downward. He may spend the whole day standing immobile, or sitting on the edge of a chair, or pouncing on floor. The patient may have to be tube fed, and assisted with bladder and bowel movements. Occasionally if the patient thinks he is unobserved, he will eat greedily. Saliva dribbles out of the mouth as the patient does not swallow it. The immobility may take the form of retention of a fixed position (Catalepsy) (Suinn, 1975), or the retention of any posture in which the patient is placed by someone else (waxy flexibility), or the patient may be found to carry out any verbal instructions regardless of their absurd or even dangerous nature (automatic obedience) (Suinn, 1975). Except for his odd posturing, the catatonic patient resembles a deeply depressed patient. However, a distinguishing diagnostic feature for the catatonic is his waxy flexibility. Gestures, grimacing, and grimming are common in the catatonic. The patient may go on repeating everything he hears (echolalia), or the opposite behaviour may occur (negativism). Occasionally the physical manifestations of catatonia show some similarity to Parkinsonian akinesis and rigidity. However, a detailed description of the motor abnormalities and abnormalities of speech and behaviour has been given later in this chapter. There are evidences (Suinn, 1975) that during the stuporous condition the catatonic may be highly aware of the surroundings rather than inattentive. Thus, *e.g.*, some patients after emerging from such a phase report that they hear with extreme acuity although they had failed earlier (during the stuporous condition) to show any outward evidence of their alertness. This inability to respond is, as some patients report, because of the fact that they were convinced that responding to would cause something catastrophic in them. The stupor may be thought of (Kolb, 1973) as a protective withdrawal from contact with the environment that seem threatening. In this sense, stupor may be compared to a retreat into an intense, trance – like preoccupation (reverie). According to some clinicians stupor may be regarded as a profound regression, a dramatization of death. Arieti (1955) suggested that the immobility of the catatonics originates from family transactions, where criticisms are directed toward action tendencies of the growing child and is accepted by the complaint child. Catalapsy, thus, is an expression of compliance to the demands of others. It may symbolize an ambivalent negativism, and be used to discharge aggression and hostility in a passive way.

Catatonic Excitement

This is characterized by unorganised and aggressive motor behaviour. Since it is not influenced by external stimuli, it seems apparently purposeless and stereotyped. Thus, without any apparent cause or even warning the patients may suddenly attack someone, or break a window glass and so on. He disregards all excretory cleanliness, destroys his cloths and remains nude. Mannerisms, stereotypes, grimaces, and negativism are markedly present (Kolb, 1973). The flow of speech may vary from mutism to that of flight of ideas. The patient may react to terrifying or joyous visual or auditory hallucinations. Mystical experiences are not uncommon in these patients. Hostility and feelings of resentment are also common. There is refusal of food and a rapid loss of weight; the patient becomes aggressive and even assaultive. Such an acute catatonic excitement is probably the same as that reaction which Kumpf termed "acute homosexual panic" (cited by Kolb, 1973, p.334).

Despite the seemingly severe state, stupor or excitement either, catatonic schizophrenia has a relatedly better outlook for recovery than any other type of schizophrenia.

Hebephrenic Schizophrenia

An insidious onset is typical, especially if it starts between the ages fifteen to twenty-five. Initially there may be only some degree of difficulty of concentration in mental work. But such a difficulty may not be apparent in persons engaged in manual work or unskilled labour, but it is definitely evident in a student. A formerly promising student may pass after several attempts or with much help and cramming which earlier he was not in need of. Such a deterioration in performance is usually attributed by the guardians or physicians to unbalanced development in puberty, or overwork in school and so on. Hypochondriacal ideas may colour the picture and these are often centered around masturbation, menstruation or fear of severe illness, such as cancer or insanity. All normal/commonly occurring problems of pubescence provide the content of the oncoming psychosis – hence its name (Mayer-Gross, Slater and Roth, 1974).

The disorders of affect and abstract thinking are the outstanding clinical features. Affective reactions, of such patients, may be described as shallow and inappropriate, and memory of them are silly and childish in behaviour. Giggling, incongruous or inappropriate smiling and laughter are common. Silliness is, sometimes found to be combined with 'vorbeireden'. In 'vorbeireden', also known as 'paralogia' (Kolb, 1973) the patient's replies to the questions though are wrong, responses bear obvious relation to the questions asked. The patient understand the meaning of the question, but his answers are not to the point (approximation in reply is marked). The patient sometimes complaints that his thoughts are broadcast to others known to him. At times thoughts race through his mind as if under pressure, in contrast to other times of complete emptiness. Hallucinations, especially auditory are present and these are often pornographic in nature. Vague and diffused thinking makes planning and anticipation of future impossible by the patient and thus the patient becomes in aimless drifter in real life. Sense of values in life is lost and the patient appears to be as if, in a 'permanent state' of dreaminess (Mayer-Gross, Slater and Roth, 1974). Feelings and instincts gain the upper hand and rule their behaviour. A flare-up of sexual appetite is not uncommon. This may lead to excessive masturbation or promiscuity. Associative processes are loose, incoherent speech and neologisms are common. Posturing and mannerisms are also frequently noted. Unless supervised and directed at every step, these patients are unable to do any work themselves. They show interest in pseudo-philosophical and pseudo-scientific ideas and consider themselves capable of great discoveries but all without activity and real attempts. The majority of such patients lose their drive and volition early in the illness. Mild apathy is often found to proceed the thought disturbances. However, at the present stage of knowledge it appears difficult to say as to which of the two symptoms, thought disorder or passivity is more responsible for their inadequacy.

Some authors (Suinn, 1975) have suggested that mood variations represent different subgroups of hebephrenia – *viz.*, the silly and giggling variety, a depressed type, an apathetic variety, and an autistic excitable sub-group. Depending upon the sub-group, the patient is likely to show childish behaviour, complaining hypochondriacal concerns, apathetic detachment, or excited paranoid belief (grandiose).

Of all the types of schizophrenia, an overall disintegration of personality and habits is perhaps the greatest in hebephrenia. Regressive features to the extent of wetting and soiling are prominent, and the patient eats in a ravenous, unmannerly fashion. The patient becomes highly autistic, bafflingly inaccessible, greatly introverted and severely withdrawn. Kraepelin (1919) called this variety of schizophrenia "Silly dementia" and this term perhaps, sums up the clinical picture very well.

Often depressive reactions are the first sign in young hebephrenics but clinicians, initially explain this depression as a reaction to conflicts at the critical and problematic time of adolescence. Since this is also an age of exaggerated emotional response and inadequate expression of feeling, it becomes really difficult for the clinicians to recognise the depressive reaction as the initial sign of a schizophrenic illness. Diagnosis in such cases, however, has often to be postponed till the persistence monotony, lack of modulation of the affect, or incongruity, the flatness, or stiffness of its expression confirm, and disturbances of thought confirm the suspicion of a schizophrenic illness. Likewise, the occurrences of depersonalisation and derealization in early cases may be considered for sometime as indication of the progressive personality changes, until it takes a final quasi-delusional character, or till the other features of the schizophrenic illness become apparent.

Simple Schizophrenia

In 1903, Diem described a simple dementing form of schizophrenia and a little later Bleuler (1911) used the term 'Simple Schizophrenia'. The disorder takes place in a gradual insidious fashion, a starting as early as adolescence (Kleinmuntz, 1974). The patient goes downhill socially so slowly that sometimes it is difficult to determine the exact point of onset. Since the symptoms are not dramatic in nature, many such patients can live without being suspected of their illness for quite sometimes, though they are instead accused of being shiftness, lazy, unassertive, obstinate, eccentric, moody, irritable, and indolent. The most marked disturbances in it are of interest, activity, and emotion. Reduction of external attachments, apathy and indifference, impoverishment of interpersonal relation, inattentiveness to school of work commitments, failure to complete required period of training in preparation for a profession, callousness, and an overall lowered level of adjustment and functioning than those noted in the individual prior to its onset are evident. He becomes so much seclusive and aloof that would prefer confinement in his own room, or in his quest for seclusion may wander off to strange places or even spend nights sleeping in abandoned places, and being questioned of his aimless wandering or lack of ambition, he appears to be vague, evasive, monosyllabic and even perplexed about his condition. He seems to have difficulty in focusing or sustaining his attention on activities, and though intellectually unimpaired, capable of performing only some simple routine task and that too under supervision. The patient may refuse to bathe or comb his hair, dresses unsystematically and performs with such little concern that he may mistakenly be considered mentally retarded (Kleinmuntz, 1974). Psychological tests and other examinations help ruling out the possibilities of brain damage and confirming the diagnosis of schizophrenia. Appreciation of aesthetic and moral value is lost. His goals are no longer realistic, and is found unable to complete the transition from adolescence to maturity with adult heterosexual adjustment. Many become irresponsible, idlers, vagrants, delinquents, and prostitutes. In fact, these are some of the prominent factors which call them to medical attention. There are no delusions, ideas of reference, or catatonic symptoms (Mayer-Gross, Slater and Roth, 1974; Kleinmuntz, 1974). Though disorder may occur, but is often difficult to detect (Mayer-Gross *et al.*, 1974), and not that prominent. However, disorder of forms of thought is likely to be present. Again, Mayer-Gross *et al.* (1974) and others reported there is absence of hallucinations, whereas some that other authors, like Kleinmuntz (1974), and Kolb (1973) are of the opinion that hallucinations though rare, are auditory in nature and manifest themselves as a "buzzing", or "ringing" in the ears.

Vague hypochondriacal complaints sometimes bring some of these schizophrenics for consultations. Likewise, some of these patients are difficult to distinguish from schizoid personalities who have never had a schizophrenia. However, (a) in majority of the patients, a break in the life-history around adolescence can easily be demonstrated; (b) insensibility which is already in childhood is found to remain as a prominent character trait of the affected individual even when he grows up; (c) educational and penal measures, such as child guidance, special schooling, *etc.* are of no avail to the affected individuals (Mueser and Bellack, 1989). He appears to be a 'born criminal' (Lombroso, 1911) and as if, destined for an asocial life. The term 'delinquente nato' coined by Lombrosso may be used to describe the behaviour of such patients. However, differential diagnoses will be discussed in detail elsewhere.

In sum, the four groups of schizophrenics so far discussed may succiently be narrated as; the simple schizophrenic is apathetic to the environment, the hebephrenic appears to ignore all but his own peculiar environment, the catatonic prefers to inhibit his spontaneous reactions to the environment, while the paranoid grips and unslothfully inspects it in his delusions.

Based on the behaviouristic concepts, Cameron (1947) had classified schizophrenia into three main groups and later divided each of the groups into sub-groups, the terms for which are self-explanatory. The three main groups are : the aggressive, the submissive, and the detached. The aggressive group is sub-divided into persecuted, grandiose, and self-punitive. The submissive group into complaint, dedicated, and transformed, and the detached group into avoidant and adient. The word 'adience' signifies making use of an approach to others. However, Cameron's classification does not seem to have added much to our understanding of schizophrenia. Also, he seems to have dispensed with simple schizophrenia and has renamed paranoid, catatonic, and hebephrenic using terms aggressive, submissive, and detached respectively.

Schneider (1942) described three symptom-complexes in schizophrenia and claimed that those symptom-complexes could occur alone or in combination either. The three syndromes are (a) the thought withdrawal syndrome, (b) the desultory syndrome, and (c) the drivelling syndrome. Thought withdrawal is associated with a fragmentation of thought, verbal derailment, and blocking. Also, these patients have cosmic or religious experiences, and sudden delusional ideas. The later appears to come from natural sources. Again, these patients experience that their own actions are being made or forced upon from outside. Perplexity is the outstanding affective disorder in this syndrome.

The desultory syndrome, as the name implies, is characterized by desultory thinking. That is, thought makes jumps and thus proceeds in an irregular way. These patients show lack of inner drive and are unable to react promptly and adequately to environmental changes. These patients feel changed in themselves and complain of bodily hallucinations. They are unable to feel happy or sad, *i.e.* affect is flattened, but they may pass into states of anger, anxiety, or despair.

The outstanding features of the drivelling syndrome is the vague drivelling thinking. There appears to have no grammatical disorder and speech and thinking are though superficially integrated, the content is drivel. Primary delusional experiences are also reported by these patients. Inadequate affect is noted, and a lack of interest in real things and values is evident.

Based on Schneider's explanation, it appears that each of these syndromes is characterized by a special variety of experience. Thus, the experience of alienation of one's own acts is associated with thought withdrawal syndrome, whereas, disorders of social feeling, and bodily hallucinations are found to be associated with desultory syndrome. Drivelling syndrome is associated with primary delusions.

According to Kleist (1923, 1960) schizophrenia is disease of the nervous system which may be confined to one neurological system or which may affect many different systems within the central nervous system. The first group of system illnesses, he called 'typical schizophrenia', while those due to disorders of many different neurological systems, were designed 'atypical schizophrenia'. Kleist further added that the disorders of the nervous system in these atypical schizophrenia may be caused by hormones.

Kleist classified schizophrenia into four major groups : paranoid, catatonic, hebephrenic, and confused. The term 'Confused' used to designate a clinical picture in which there is severe disorder of speech or thought which gives rise to grossly muddles behavioural expressions. In 'hebephrenia' the outstanding symptom is a disorder of affect without any severe catatonic symptoms, and paranoid symptoms, if present, only miled or transient. Kleist had divided each of the paranoid and catatonic groups into seven typical and one atypical form. Confused group has been divided into three typical and two atypical, and hebephrenic group into four typical forms. This sub-classification of Kleist gives an impression that the hebephrenic group is relatively more homogenous than the rest other varieties. However, Kleist believed that (a) the symptomatology in the atypical forms is much more variable than in the typical forms; (b) the courses of the illnesses is more episodic in the atypical form; (c) marked remissions are much more commonly noted in the atypical forms than the typical, (d) typical variety of schizophrenia tends to have a more insidious onset; (e) typical forms show a more sleedily progressive course than the atypical one; (f) genetic loading is found to be much greater in the atypical variety than the typical one.

Leonhard (1936, 1960, 1961) had classified chronic schizophrenia into systematic and non-systematic types, which however seem to correspond well to Kleist's typical and atypical forms. Like Kleist, Leonhard also has separated from schizophrenia a group of non-affective functional psychoses, which he called 'Cycloyd psychoses'. These are anxiety-elation psychosis, excited–inhibited confused psychosis, and hyperkinetic – akinetic motility psychosis. According to Leonhard, all these have a favourable outcomes. Leonhard (1959) believed that the non-systematic types of schizophrenia are more closely related to the Cycloyd psychoses than to the systematic schizophrenia. However, a brief description of the Leonhard sub-types of schizophrenia (also see Hamilton, 1976) will now be given since it has a significant clinical importance.

Non-Systematic Schizophrenias

(*a*) **Affect-laden Paraphrenia.** The clinical picture at the onset of the illness is that of anxiety with ideas of reference. But sometimes the patient appears to be irritable and aggressive. At the onset severe affective swings into anxiety and ecstasy often occurs (Hamilton, 1976). Such affective swings may continue as the illness progresses. These affective changes however, are found to be always associated with the formation of delusional ideas. In anxiety, ideas of self-reference, and auditory hallucinations occur, while in ecstasy, ideas of happiness in association with visual and auditory hallucinations occur. In affect – laden paraphrenia, the abnormal body sensations have a completely hallucinatory character since they are connected with outside influences. In anxiety elation psychosis, on the contrary, these sensations arise from the abnormal affective state.

In the systematic paranoid schizophrenias, delusions have very little affective loading and therefore the patient often does not become upset if someone laughs at his delusions, or even if he is upset, these passes away soon. But in affect – laden schizophrenia the patient talks about delusions with enthusiasm, and if his delusions are denied of, he becomes upset so much so that he may even shout, scold and threaten with a feeling that his beliefs are being treated discourteously (Hamilton, 1976). So the most distinguishing feature of affect – laden paraphrenia is affective–loading of the paranoid delusions.

The degree of systematisation of delusions varies quite well from one case to the other, in that sometimes it may be so well systematized that the clinical picture is that of paranoia. Because of the bipolar nature of the affect, delusions of persecution and happiness may be found to occur together. Delusions become progressively more illogical finally leading to a fantastic delusional system in which there are extravagant grandiose ideas, misinterpretation of people, absurd ideas, memory falsifications, and hallucinations in all sensory fields. Catatonic and schizophrenic symptoms may be found in affect – laden paraphrenia (Hamilton, 1976).

(*b*) **Schizophasia.** This was described as a variety of schizophrenia by Kraepelin (1913). Gross confusion of speech was reported to be the predominant features of it. Confusion in its extreme form makes the patient's speech completely unintelligible. But is contrast to such a gross confusion of speech, the patient's behaviour otherwise appears to be fairly well ordered, having his ability to work and make social contact fairly preserved.

Leonhard claimed a relationship between schizophasia and confusion psychoses, but reported that the morbid phenomena are more pronounced in schizophasia. He described of two forms of this disorder, one being the Kraepelinian variety and the other consisting of disorder of speech but tends to be associated with catatonic symptoms. In the former, a marked pressure of speech with severe confusion, many grammatical mistakes, few neologisms are evident, while in the latter very little drive, and neologisms are common. Severe confusion is found to be restricted here. Leonhard believed that these two forms are not genetically distinct (also see Hamilton, 1976).

(*c*) **Periodic Catatonia.** This illness can be said to be a catatonia. There is an admixture of hyperkinetic and akinetic symptoms in it (Hamilton, 1976). The hyperkinesis acquires a certain degree of rigidity because of the admixture of akinetic symptoms. Therefore, movements tend to proceed in a stiff, jerky manner and their natural grace is found to be absent. Reactive and expressive movements appear to be meaningless. Gestures are found to be vague, and facial expressions become grimaces. Excitements which occur in them are parakinetic because of this modification of the natural course of the motor acts. When these patients are akinetic they show an aimless movement of an extremity which however, generally becomes uniform and may be a stereotype or iteration. Therefore, despite the general postural rigidity and the rigidity of the mimic expression, stereotype (postural) occurs (Hamilton, 1976).

In this illness there are remissions after the acute shifts, but permanent defect is likely to occur more after attacks of akinesia than after hyperkinesias. These defects could be mild, moderate, and severe, which Leonhard designated as states of psychic lameness, dullness, and stupidity respectively. In stupidity, there is a degree of deterioration which is reminiscent of organic-disease. In the dull state, there is an impoverishment of drive. The mild state may resemble a motility psychosis both in the symptomatology and the course of the illness (Hamilton, 1976). At some stage of the illness, symptoms of schizophrenia or affect – laden paraphrenia may be found to occur.

Systematic Schizophrenia

(*a*) **Systematic Catatonia.** Leonhard has described the following six sub-groups of Catatonia : (i) Parakinetic Catatonia, (ii) Manneristic Catatonia, (iii) Proskintic Catatonia, (iv) Negativistic Catatonia, (v) Speech-Prompt Catatonia, and (vi) Speech Inactive Catatonia. Each of these varieties (also see Hamilton, 1976) may briefly be described as follows :

(*i*) *Parakinetic Catatonia.* Voluntary actions are carried out in an unnatural, awkward way. It appears, as though, the motor activity is broken down into its constituent movements and thus, the smooth transition from one individual movement to the next is absent. Jerk choreiform involuntary movements occur. Particularly, facial movements are significantly affected and these patients often grimace. Speech is found to be affected in which the patient speaks in short, sharp utterances. Words that the patient uses appear to be chopped up, and the sentences are short and agrammatical. Regarding content of speech, it is noted that sometimes these patients make remarks which are to the point, though at times fortuitous and irrelevant remarks are not uncommon. As the disease progresses, parakinetic movements become more obvious (Hamilton, 1976). However, parakinesis in itself may not be diagnostic of this condition as because it may occur on the background of general motor excitement in periodic catatonia.

(*ii*) *Manneristic Catatonia.* At the onset of the illness mannerisms occur, and with the progress of the illness all involuntary movements gradually become less and less, finally leading to a condition in which posture and movement become stiff. As the impoverishment of movement become more pronounced, mannerisms of commissions are found to be replaced by mannerisms of omission. The patient shows stereotyped attitudes, stiff facial expression, mannerisms of food refusal, refusal to go to toilet, and so on.

(*iii*) *Proskinetic Catatonia.* Since these patients appear to be as if, ready to turn towards the examiner when spoken to, this was originally called 'prosectic'. But Leonhard opined that the term 'proskinetic' should replace the term prosectic, since in these patients an abnormal readiness to begin automatic movements in response to external stimuli is markedly noted. Interwining movements, are observed. Marked affective flattening and typical prosectic speech disorder are evident in these patients (Hamilton, 1976). In the acute stage, severe excitements occur in which the patient shows aggressive and restless behaviour.

(*iv*) *Negativistic Catatonia.* As the name implies, negativism is the prominent feature in it. But in the beginning it is not that severe, rather it appears to be as if, the patient fails to carry out instructions or to answer questions. When the examiner approaches the patient in a friendly manner, ambitendency may occur. If however, attempts are made to overcome their negativism by force, then these patients show severe excitement (Hamilton, 1976). Their basic drives are preserved as this is seen in greediness and erotic tendencies.

(*v*) *Speech–Prompt Catatonia.* In this when spoken to, the patient turns towards the examiner with an empty, meaningless facial expression and answers questions with the immediate impression comes to his mind regardless of its suitability as an answer to the questions.

(*vi*) *Speech-inactive Catatonia.* In the early stage of the illness, these patients may answer questions slowly, but as the illness progresses they do not answer at all. During interview, they show loss of eye–contact, look here and there and often make whispering noises. Auditory hallucination, and fantastic confabulations are present (Hamilton, 1976). While responding to hallucinatory voices these patients are found to scream and gesticulate and become very excited. Since they are distracted by hallucinations, difficulty to attend to stimuli around, as well as slow motor reactions are evident.

(*b*) **The Hebephrenias.** Leonhard classified these into : (*i*) Silly Hebephrenia; (*ii*) Eccentric Hebephrenia; (*iii*) Shallow Hebephrenia, and (*iv*) Autistic Hebephrenia.

(*i*) *Silly Hebephrenia.* Severe affective and ethical blunting is marked. A characteristic smile or giggling is noted. In the early stage of the illness they tend to play silly, childish tricks on others. These tricks are often found to be spiteful and malicious (Hamilton, 1976). At times they may become ill–humoured and irritable. In the acute state however, mood states of all kinds may occur. Sometimes they may become inactive so much so that they give the impression of a catatonic illness. But their postures and movements are not typical of catatonia. The silly smiling is indicative of this diagnosis.

(*ii*) *Eccentric Hebephrenia.* Mannerisms and a general querulous attitude are the characteristic features. It often begins with obsessive, compulsive symptoms. Uniform and monotonous manner of speaking together with the repeated querulous complaints and demands suggests the manneristic quality of the illness. The mannerisms however, are most unlike those of manneristic catatonia, since these patients often do not talk about them and try to keep them secret (Hamilton, 1976). The evidence of their existence comes from the reports of the nurses or relatives. In eccentric hebephrenia collecting is a very common mannerism. Sometimes mannerism appears in the guise of senseless stealing. In the initial stages of the illness ill-humoured mood states are present, and irritated excitements are evident. Affective blunting being associated with ethical blunting often leads to anti-social behaviour, like beggary, prostitution. Impoverished thinking is noted in these patients. Performance on intellectual tasks may not be too bad. Paralogia does not occur (Hamilton, 1976).

(*iii*) *Shallow Hebephrenia.* These patients have a very marked flattening of affect. But in contrast to this, they may be readily accessible to a conversation and may carry on the same in a factual way. The mood state may be described as one of the indifferent satisfaction. Sometimes this mood state is interrupted by states of ill humour, in which the patient may be anxious, irritated, or euphoric. The latter occurs very rarely. In these mood states hallucinations and ideas of reference occur (Hamilton, 1976) which may make the patients excited and aggressive. The hallucinations may occur in all sensory fields but most common is auditory form. During excitement though these patients are found to shout at hallucinatory voices, they have a clear understanding of the morbid nature of these voices as and when the excitement subsides. This therefore, has been described by Leonhard as Pseudo-hallucinations (Hamilton, 1976). Though there is a general lack of initiative in these patients, they may take part in day-to-day activity in the hospital without requiring a very close supervision.

(*iv*) *Autistic Hebephrenia.* Autism and marked affective blunting are the predominant features in it. The facial expression of the patient is stiff and impenetralate like that of a speech-prompt catatonia. Ill-humoured mood states occur in which the patient appears to be irritated, starts shouting, threatening and even may attack someone in the environment. Since here the aggression of the patient is directed against a specific person only, these mood states differ from those of shallow hebephrenia (Hamilton, 1976). The mood, which is reminiscent of eccentric hebephrenia, is one of rejection mixed with discontent. Therefore, it is in marked contrast to indifferent satisfaction found in the silly and shallow hebephrenics. If motivated, their answers to the items of the intelligence tests are not indicative of a very great defect in intelligence but may usually give short off-putting answers to such questions. In general, they show a tendency to avoid others and lack of initiative, but examiner may be able to train them to carryout work requiring some independence of action. They show a relatively better efficiency in doing their works rather than communication. They have a tendency to speak the absolute minimum required, if spoken to. (Hamilton, 1976).

(*c*) **The Systematic Paraphrenias.** The term 'paraphrenia' was used by Leonhard to designate all the paranoid schizophrenias (see Hamilton, 1976). These are characterised by delusional ideas and sense deception. But thought disorder is also present. Anxiety, and ideas of reference may occur : perplexity is not uncommon. On the whole, only paranoid symptoms occur in predominate in systematic paraphrenias, and catatonic and hebephrenic symptoms are very rarely present. Severe affective disorders are unusual and its onset is usually insidious. According to Leonhard (see Hamilton, 1976) the following are the sub-forms of systematic paranoid schizophrenias : (*i*) Hypochondriacal paraphrenia (*ii*) Phonemic paraphrenia, (*iii*) Incoherent paraphrenia, (*iv*) Fantastic paraphrenia, (*v*) Confabulatory paraphrenia, and (*vi*) Expansive paraphrenia.

(*i*) *Hypochondriacal Paraphrenia.* Bodily hallucinations are prominent in this and these are usually referred to internal organs. To describe these sensations the patient may produce technical neologisms. In the early stages frightening visual hallucinations are occasionally present. The patient is more distressed by the occurrence of frightening voices, rather than its content. As the disease progresses gradually such hallucinations fade away and then the occurrence of marked visual hallucinations may even contraindicate the diagnosis (Hamilton, 1976). Hallucinations of smell and taste may occur but these are not characteristic. The patient frequently attributes all these voices and sensations to devices which he thinks, affect him from a distance. Very rarely these are attributed to his people in the environment. The mood of such patients can be described as permanently morose and dissatisfied, but this often develops into irritation. Their affectivity appears to be fairly well preserved since they show interest in their home and family and also that become excited when contradicted (Hamilton, 1976). During conversation they are found to be inclined to verbal derailments, *i.e.*, wander from the points, and talk about subjects loosely related to the topic in discussion or task in hand. Therefore, their thought disorder is designated by Leonhard as 'unconcentrated thinking'. In sum, bodily hallucinations, hallucinatory voices, and a certain mood state must all occur for the confirmation of the diagnosis of this sub-type.

(*ii*) *Phonemic Paraphrenia.* Hallucinatory voices are the outstanding features in this sub-group. However, bodily hallucinations as well as hallucinations of taste and smell do not occur in it (Hamilton, 1976). The voices the patient hears often contradict or confirm what the patient is thinking. These also appear to be very closely related to the patient's thinking so much so that the patient treats them as real people with whom conversation is possible. This is thus, incontrast to hypochondriacal paraphrenia where (a) The hallucinatory voices are only partly connected with what the patient thinks, and (b) these do not fit in with his thoughts content he is on at that moment, and (c) patients never seen talking to their voices, they merely complain about the voices (Hamilton, 1976).

The patient thinks that the whole world knows what he thinks. Voices the patient hears, talk about unpleasant things, but the voices are not abusive. Voices are often thought of coming from wireless, or from close or distant people, or from some invisible beings, such as, spirits, or witches, only occasionally they appear to emerge from within the body or from some apparatus. At times visual hallucinations also occur. Unlike hypochondriacal paraphrenics, these patients appear to become habituated to his hallucinations in the later stage of the illness and complains of hallucinations calmly. The mood state is usually well-balanced with the exception that in the early stage of the illness when the patient talks of unpleasant hallucinatory voices, becomes somewhat angry. Regarding their affect, it is difficult to say in one word that it is well preserved throughout. This is because at times some degree of affective blunting does occur in them since they are found to tolerate their apparently unpleasant symptoms with patience rather (Hamilton, 1976). At the same time, in hospital set-up, these patients are found capable of carrying out responsibilities assigned to them which in turn makes them suitable for 'parole'. In Indian set-up, parole system is found to work more in South Indian Mental Hospital than in the North or Eastern parts of India. However, where there is no parole system, in those hospitals, these patients after their treatment when sent back home, relatively a less number of patients require hospital admission again. From this it may be said that their affective responsiveness is well preserved. Little disorder of thinking is evident in them through general conversation, but in problem solving they talk about the problem indecisively and are found unable to orientate themselves towards the objective of the thought. This variety of thought disorder has been described by Leonhard as 'woolly thinking' (cited by Hamilton, 1976). However, these patients are often found successful in simple problem solving.

(*iii*) *Incoherent Paraphrenia.* Auditory hallucinations are prominent throughout the illness. Even during conversation the patient appears to be hallucinating and is often seen whispering or talking quietly to the phonemes. Also, sometimes the patient appears to be excited and starts talking loudly or shouting sentences like, "you are a great liar" (cited by Hamilton, 1976), etc. In no other form of paraphrenia this type of hallucinatory aversion and continuous hallucinosis to the extent of disturbing conversation is found. During conversation either they fail to look at the examiner or may look at with a peculiar rigid gaze. Incoherent expressions are prominent so much so that only occasionally one can separate confabulatory remarks from among such expressions. Contaminations is also found to be associated with incoherence. Short, and superficial and mechanical replies and that too in a low voice are the characteristics. Thought disorder becomes marked when auditory hallucinations become very severe. In the early stage of the illness bodily hallucinations are commonly reported, but as the disease progresses they are not present. In everyday life, lack of initiative and interest is noted (Hamilton, 1976). Often they remain dirty and incontinences of urine and feces are also observed in them.

(*iv*) *Fantastic Paraphrenia.* Hallucinations and delusions have equal parts to play in this. Bodily hallucinations are marked and the description of bodily sensations resembles that of hypochondriacal form of paraphrenia. However, hallucinatory voices are less importunate, while visual sense deceptions play an important role here. Scenic hallucination is the characteristic in which scenes are visualised and accompanied by auditory and somatopsychic experiences. The content of such scenes is mostly horrible tortures and mass murders (Hamilton, 1976). These patients have absurd, grandiose ideas to the extent of calling themselves God. Gross illogicality also occurs in these patients in their misidentification of people in the environment, *i.e.*, they consider that people in contact with them are all different from those they say they are (Hamilton, 1976). Their affect is shallow to the extent that they do not object being treated as mental patients. Of course sometimes they are found to flareup somewhat if their ideas are laughed at, but the affect quickly dies away. In general they show interest in their family. The main feature of the formal thought disorder in this sub-form of paraphrenia is that of derailment.

(*v*) *Confabulatory Paraphrenia.* Falsification of memory and perceptual falsification are the outstanding features in it. The patient produces plastic, detailed description of alleged events. In some cases, the confabulations may clearly be noted at the onset of the illness, while, in some others, in the early stage, there may be dream like experiences which appear to be precursors of the late confabulations. The confabulations generally have a fantastic quality and are found to be concerned with the other world, including the moon, and stars etc. In perceptual falsifications, the object especially people in the environment continually appears to be different to the patient so much so that the size, shape, and general appearance of objects change from day to day. According to Leonhard this is abnormal concretisation of memory images (Hamilton, 1976). That is, when an individual is perceived by the patient today, he is contrasted with the detailed memory image of his appearance in the patient had on the day before. Interestingly enough, in such a contrast in memory images, general similarity of the features of the individual is over looked by the patient, while the different features of his present appearance are emphasized by the patient. Grandiose ideas are present in these patients which make them often extravagant. In favour of grandiose delusions, these patients have an elevated mood. Leonhard opined that in these patients the transition from concrete to abstract thought is disturbed. Therefore, they may be able to maintain a critical judgement in concrete thinking, a failure to carry out abstract talks may be evident (Hamilton, 1976). Accordingly, in everyday life though they are found well ordered, in intelligence test performance they show a peculiar pictorial form of thinking.

(*vi*) *Expansive Paraphrenia.* In the early stage of this illness sense deceptions occur but later on these are entirely absent. So, in the later stages this illness is almost entirely delusional in nature. The delusions are expansive and are not associated with persecutory delusions : grandiose ideas are within reasonable limits. The grandiose delusions do not cause any apparent inconsistent behaviour, the patient behaves as if he is highly placed. This is in contrast to the fantastic and confabulatory paraphrenics in whom grandiose delusions lead to some inconsistent behaviour. Again, in the fantastic and confabulatory paraphrenias richness of ideas is noted while in the expansive paraphrenia the patients repeat same ideas and attitudes without much variation, and thus the expansive behaviour of the patient shows a monotonous character (Hamilton, 1976). While speaking about their grandiose ideas expansive paraphrenics tend to become garrulous and also exercise a great deal of prolixity to bring forward their requests and complaints. A general deficiency of initiative is noted in their behaviour, even though they are found to carry out their expansive behaviour with some amount of eagerness. Their affect is found to be gradually become blunted so much so that in the final stages even if they are laughed at they are not irritated. Thought disorder is markedly present mainly affecting verbal thinking and thus mistakes in grammar and word formation frequently occur. According to Leonhard concepts are not absent in these patients but these are found to be very inexact and devoid of finer details. This variety of thought disorder is called "Coarsening of thinking" by Leonhard (see Hamilton, 1976).

Summing up: In the non-systematic schizophrenias because of the diversity of symptoms it is difficult to outline the clinical pictures very sharply. In the systematic schizophrenia, on the other hand, because of clear-cut symptomatology clinical picture is unequivocal. Leonhard was of the opinion that in each sub-form of systematic schizophrenias a definite higher function of the nervous system is involved (Hamilton, 1976). Hence, investigations of the systematic schizophrenias, according to Leonhard, should lead to an understanding of the higher functions of the nervous system. However, such sharply delimited clinical pictures of these disorders are generally seen in the end states, and therefore, in the early stages of the illness, it may be difficult to classify because of intermixture of symptoms. Despite such difficulties, it is much easier to classify the illness once the clinician has learned to recognise the typical end states. In general, however, in the systematic group the onset of the illness is gradual, whereas, in the non-systematic group an acute stormy onset is more likely.

Leonhard claimed that his sub-groups do not overlap. So, Leonhard's sub-groups may be considered as syndromes (Hamilton, 1976). He also believed that those relatively rare cases which do not fit into one of his sub-groups may be due to combinations of some of two different sub-groups or so. However, despite the presence of some atypical symptoms it seems best to classify chronic schizophrenics according to the most prominent symptoms they manifest. Compared to Kleist, Leonhard's scheme for the classification of chronic schizophrenia appears to be more satisfactory (Astrup 1957) and Fish (1958).

Using the concepts of Carl Schneider, (1942) Astrup, (1957) classified acute clinical pictures into the following four main groups, *viz*., hebephrenic and hebephrenic-paranoid psychoses, catatonic and mixed catatonic psychoses, paranoid psychoses dominated by projection symptoms, and paranoid psychoses with systematized delusions. Astrup designated 'hebephrenic' as one with severe schizophrenic affective disorder, and his hebephrenic group showed marked affective blunting, autism, and the desultory syndrome (Hamilton, 1976). His catatonic group also showed desultory syndrome along with marked catatonic symptoms. Thought withdrawal syndrome and projection symptoms were prominent in his paranoid psychosis group dominated by projection symptoms, while in the paranoid psychoses, with systematized delusions drivelling syndrome was predominant.

Based on the severity of the average clinical picture, Astrup has also ranked the sub-groups in each of Leonhard's major groups. Severity of the clinical picture he estimated on the basis of the level of social integration. Thus he considered that the hebephrenias ranges from the mildest to the most severe as follows: autistic, eccentric, shallow, and silly. He ranked the paranoid group from mildest to the most severe as affect – laden paraphrenia, schizophasia, phonemic paraphrenia, hypochondriacal paraphrenia, expansive and confabulatory paraphrenia, fantastic paraphrenia, and incoherent paraphrenia.

In the end, Leonhard's scheme appears to be a useful research tool in understanding schizophrenia. This is because research on schizophrenia has come to a point where further research should be guided by and based on clinical phenomena and their differentiation. A similar viewpoint regarding usefulness of Leonhard's scheme has also been propounded by Astrup (1957), and Fish (1958) long before and thereafter by Hamilton (1976).

In addition to the preceding categories of schizophrenia there are some more, of which the most widely accepted categories will now be mentioned briefly.

Process and Reactive Schizophrenia

Though this distinction was first noted by Bleuler in 1911, it was not followed up by him. Later Kantor, Wallner, and Winder (1953) on the basis of their study, emphasized the importance of differentiating between these two categories. In process schizophrenia the patient has a life history of psychological difficulties, withdrawal from environment, ineffectuality, and also an unfavourable prognosis for recovery. In reactive schizophrenia, incontrast, the patient has a history of better social adjustment and competence. Also in the latter, a more sudden onset of symptoms, a lesser degree of thought disturbance, and a more favourable prognosis for remission are noted (Phillips, 1966). Kantor *et al.* (1953) have given a detailed description of some of the differentiating characteristics of these two categories, such as in process schizophrenia, birth till adulthood, the patient has a life history of psychological difficulties throughout. The history reveals early childhood trauma, prolonged and/or severe physical illness, sibling rivalry, difficulty in school adjustment. Their family interaction is grossly unsatisfactory with "over protective" or "rejecting" mother or rejecting father. These patients show difficulty in adjustment with persons of opposite sex. Their premorbid personality show inner aggression to the extent of its sudden violent physical experiences, presence of somatic delusion and suspiciousness, and poor response to treatment. Patients with reactive schizophrenia, on the other hand, show relatively better history of adequate social, physical, and mental functioning though they show verbal aggression and minor paranoid trends in their premorbid personality, show good response to treatment and better prognosis than their process counterpart.

From the above, it is clear that based on clinical studies these two groups are found to differ, but a note of caution should be exercised while interpreting some of the case history items mentioned above since these have not been supported by many subsequent research evidences. Thus, *e.g.*, Kleinmunts, (1974) reported that "early psychological trauma", "physical illness", "family troubles", and "overprotective or rejecting mother", or a "rejecting father", are not necessarily a part of the background of schizophrenica, though Kantor *et al.* (1953) believed so. Likewise, earlier formulation held that the first process disorders were of genetic and constitutional origin, and reactive disorders were of psychogenic origin. But more recent theories tend to discard this view, and instead, proposed that they are two end-points on a continuum of greater (process) to lesser (reactive) psychopathology (Kleinmuntz, 1974). Again, distinctions are sometimes made that refer to the process-reactive continuum as points on a malignant-benign, or on a chronic-acute scale. However, these demarcations are of interest since they point to differences that may have etiological and prognostic significance.

Schizo-affective Schizophrenia

This may be regarded as a cross between a schizophrenic disorder and an affective disorder. These patients appear to have the same features of schizophrenia but that instead of showing a general blunting of emotions, they show pronounced and exaggerated mood similar to that noted in the patients with manic depressive psychosis. Mood shows a mixed picture of elation and depression (with frequent changes from one to the oher). Bizarre thoughts and hallucinations are present. Their feelings of guilt and dejection do interact with disturbances of reality contact. However, with the progress of this disorder the schizophrenic features are found to become increasingly dominant, while the manic-depressive aspects decline. If one considers that psychiatric disorders exist on a continuum starting from mental health and passing through psychoneurosis and conduct disorder to manic-depressive psychosis and ultimately terminating in schizophrenia, then schizo-affective psychosis appears to be the transitional point in the patient's progression through the manic-depressive condition to the schizophrenic disorder (Bellak, 1958). But this viewpoint of Bellak fails to account for the pseudo-neurotic schizophrenics and pseudo-psychopathic schizophrenics, though these two groups appear to be on the way from a neurotic or personality disorder condition directly to the schizophrenic state, apparently bypassing the manic depressive stage. Again, one may argue that schizo-affective diagnosis is an artefact of misdiagnosis (Suinn, 1975). This is because a close scrutiny and evaluation of the patient would identify him as schizophrenic or manic-depressive either, and therefore, the classification of schizo-affective psychosis has no real value (Suinn, 1975). However, Clark and Mallen (1963) on the basis of their data did refute this argument and reported that at least from the point of view of prognosis differences exist between them. They claim that the prognosis for the psychotic depression is good, while the presence of schizophrenia makes it unfavourable. The diagnosis of schizo-affective psychosis may be considered as a mixed condition and accordingly in prognosis it tends to be a midway between that for schizophrenia and that for depression. Kallmann (1953) in this context has suggested with evidences that the two disorders, *viz.*, schizophrenia and manic depressive psychosis are genetically distinct and tend to be mutually exclusive, while the schizo-affective psychosis appears to be an exception. The prepsychotic personality of such patients may have been strongly schizoid in some cases, while in some others outgoing and well-socialised. But clinical pictures in this may be quite at variance with the early personality pattern.

Summing up: Some authors are of the opinion that at least from genetic and prognostic points of views schizo-affective psychosis appears to have some distinctive features than those of schizophrenia and manic-depressive psychosis.

Borderline or Pseudoneurotic Type of Schizophrenia

Applying the term "Pseudoneurotic Schizophrenia", Hoch and Polatin (1949) have described a clinical condition in which the dynamics are psychotic in character, although the symptom picture, at least in the early stages, appears neurotic. Likewise, both Bleuler and Adolf Meyer were of the opinion that in this type of illness the onset of the schizophrenic reaction is often concealed by symptom formation considered as neurotic. In pseudoneurotic schizophrenia the obsessive–compulsive hysterical facades are most commonly recognised. But usually an admixture of anxiety and of pobic, obsessive, depressive and hypochondriacal symptoms is seen (Hamilton, 1976). Hoch and Polatin described this symptomatology as a pan–neurosis. A diffuse anxiety pervades all over the patients life experiences (Mayer-Gross *et al.*, 1974). Although the patient tries to force pleasurable experiences, he finally fails to derive pleasure from anything. The neurotic manifestations constantly shift but are never found to be completely absent. Now, question remains as to how to differentiate this from neurosis? While describing symptoms to the clinician true neurotic is usually anxious to describe these in minute details, and secondly he presses his clinician with his explanations. The pseudoneurotic schizophrenic's explanations, on the other hand, are vague, indistinct, and even contradictory. Secondly, these patients repeat information to the clinician in a stereotyped manner without details. Thirdly, the organisation of the patient's sexuality is often chaotic. Next, some of these patients may have brief psychotic episodes. Finally, some of these patients may go on to a frank psychosis, but in that less regressive behaviour than that noted in the usual schizophrenic is seen. The borderline syndrome, in general may be said to have the following characteristics: (a) anger is the major affect; (b) transactions with other may be described as infantile, dependent or complementary, but only rarely reciprocal adult transactions; (c) unclear self-identity; (d) depression reflects a sense of loneliness rather than caused by guilt or shame. However analysing the borderline syndromes Grinker, Werble, and Drye (1988) have concluded that there exists four separate sub-groups in it differing in behaviour. (a) This group is most closely related to the psychotic behaviour. The patients have the least well developed ego functions; express their abnormality either in inappropriate or in negative affect toward others. They show immaturity in their sleeping, feeding, and grooming behaviours. Their spontaneity is found to be limited and occasional impulsive angry eruptions are evident in their verbal and non-verbal communications. (b) The second group is considered the "core" borderline category. They seem to have a reasonable personal identity, but do not always act consistently with that individuation. They display a pervasive negative affect. They are found to be depressed except when "Acting out", rebelling against, or participating in their environment. This group seems to be the same as that described by Hoch and Polatin as "pseudopsychopathic". (c) Individauls with blandly adaptive behaviour constitutes the third group. Positive affect – love or affection for others is missing here. Their self identity is uncertain. (d) This is the smallest sub-groups in which individuals exhibit positive affective behaviour toward others. But their feeling is mostly directed to females and their behaviour resembles with that of a child like clinging depression. In their affective life, anxiety and depression are found to be predominant. Lack of self esteem and confidence are marked in them.

In sum: In borderline cases the underlying schizophrenic disorder may be said to be hidden by a façade of neurotic manifestations.

Atypical Forms of Schizophrenia

Schulz and Leonhard (1940) made an attempt to break down Schizophrenia into clinical – genetical sub-groups, *viz.,* 'typical' (patients with progressively deteriorating disorders and 'atypical' (patients suffering from recurrent phasic disturbances). Related to them are the studies of Langfeldt (1937) who tried to differentiate the two groups in terms of features of the clinical profile and the outcome. However, atypical features, derived from personality or environment either, may colour the onset of any mental illness. These features, however, are submerged as and when more severe and characteristic symptoms become prominent.

Schizophrenia beginning around the age of puberty may take an unusual appearance, in which affective abnormalities dominate in the clinical picture. Apathy, moods of whimpering, sulkiness, obstinacy, impudence, and rude mischievousness are prominent. These are the typical qualities of the teenager, who has lost his balance, but in the early schizophrenia they lack the freshness and natural emotional colouring of normal children of this age. What looks like stubbornness may be considered a 'semi-stuporose state' (Mayer-Gross, *et al.*, 1974) and likewise, the contradictoriness of the feelings which the patient shows towards his people may be considered as sign of ambivalence of emotional response and the cooling-off of normal sympathy of the patient. Not only during early adolescence, in childhood as well atypical features of schizophrenia are evident but the latter will be dealt with in full, later in this chapter.

Schizophrenia in mental defectives is called 'Pfropf schizophrenia' (Mayer-Gross *et al.*, 1974), or 'grafted schizophrenia' (Hamilton, 1976) in which the atypical feature is the poverty of ideational content. Childish and silly conduct usually dominate the clinical picture. Also, there may be massive hallucinations of primitive and monotonous kind. In some cases, stereotyped hypochondriasis is also evident. However, they are not always shut in, and mostly unaggressive, which may sometimes make them relatively accessible too to the examiner.

Atypical forms of schizophrenia may be expected to occur at the time of menopause and involution (Mayer-Gross *et al.*, 1974). Some authors are of the opinion that atypical forms occurring during these stages of life may even constitute separate diagnostic entities, *viz.*, 'Presenile delusional psychosis', 'Late catatonia' (Kraepelin, 1909), 'Involutional paranoia' (Kleist, 1913). Involutional depressive of a certain rigid type (Mendow, 1922) may also be considered atypical schizophrenics. Paranoid and depressive symptoms are found to be common in all forms of mental illness occurring at a higher age and therefore, it is quite likely that schizophrenia occurring at a higher age would be coloured by such symptoms. So, such features alone should not be considered sufficient to justify a separation of the late paranoid psychosis from that of full-fledged schizophrenia. Particularly some personality features are found to be prevalent in these states. Thus, *e.g.* endogenous paranoid states commencing in middle age, such as, the delusional jealousy syndrome are often found to be characterised by marked sensitivity aggravated by inferiority feelings, a history of familial disruption or rejection and insecurity in childhood and lifelong tendencies, to a certain extent, of enviousness and jealousy. On the other hand, the delusional or near delusional ideas expressed by the patients with 'psychogenic' paranoid reactions are not always understandable to us any more than we can understand all the rituals of obsessive compulsive patients as a natural extension of the premorbid personality.

'Late catatonia', as described by Kraepelin, is a rare psychosis which begins with depression and hypocondriasis and shows a rapid progress into stupor and negativism. The latter conditions may even lead to death. The relation of this condition to schizophrenia is very doubtful (Mayer-Gross, Slater and Roth, 1960), and perhaps, it would be better to consider this as a special form of organic presenile dementia, a suggestion put forward by Grünthal (1936) long before.

Alcoholism may veil the symptoms of schizophrenia (Mayer-Gross *et al.*, 1974). Many schizophrenics with mild symptoms start taking drinks in order to overcome their increasing solitude. Again, among many chronic drunkards symptoms of schizophrenia are noted.

Of late, researchers have opined that chronic alcoholic psychoses, 'alcoholic hallucinosis' and 'alcoholic paranoia' have a genetical relationship to schizophrenia (Mayer-Gross *et al.*, 1974).

While discussing 'atypical' forms of schizophrenia mention should be made of 'mixed' schizophrenia, a diagnosis made by some clinicians. In clinical practice it is found that an admixture of the symptoms of affective psychoses may produce a clinical picture of a 'mixed' kind (Mayer-Gross *et al.*, 1974). Some of the affective disturbances found in such patients may be characterized as attacks of depression or elation, as well as those of unmotivated rage, desolation, panic, ecstasy etc. However, since blunting of affective response as well as positive anomalies of affect are among the primary symptoms of schizophrenia, it is of no wander that affective disturbances, as those mentioned above, occur in schizophrenics and thus, the presence of an endogenous mood change, either of depression or elation in a patient showing characteristic schizophrenic symptoms does not weaken the diagnosis of schizophrenia. Rather any attempt to segregate such patients from other schizophrenics would lead to a source of confusion only (Mayer-Gross *et al.*, 1974). Clinical experience claims that over a prolonged follow-up study, the outcome of these states does not differ from that of the generality of schizophrenia (Mayer-Gross, Slater, and Roth, 1974). Of course a depressive reaction may be found to be common in early schizophrenia but in such cases too, characteristic features of schizophrenia should be considered of a much greater diagnostic significance. However, in every such case, the quality of emotional changes takes place in the patient should be examined carefully.

With a view to avoid difficulty in distinguishing between schizophrenic and affective psychoses an intermediate class, *viz.*, periodic schizophrenic disorder has come into existence. Periodicity as a symptom is most commonly seen in affective disorders. However, about one-third of schizophrenics as well show some periodicity (Mayer-Gross, Slater and Roth, 1974), in having one or more remissions, and sometimes this periodicity is found to be very marked.

Kleist (1921) and Schroeder (1922) opined that all those cases which do not fit either into a schizophrenic nor into an affective classification may be brought under the heading 'degeneration psychoses'. This term was taken from the French psychiatry of Magnan, and adopted by German psychiatrists to cover a number of infrequent but distinctive syndromes (Mayer-Gross *et al.*, 1974).

Another group of atypical psychoses is called schizophrenic psychoses with clouding of consciousness (Mayer-Gross *et al.*, 1974). In this a peculiar dream – like state of consciousness is evident in the patients, *e.g.* in some early hebephrenics, and catatonics. Also mention should be made of the catatonic stupors which seem to have passed in a mental vacuum and leave no recollection behind. Likewise, one should not fail to mention in this heading the acute catatonic cases which begins with a subacute delirious picture, even in the absence of any toxic or ineffective bodily illness. Again, there are states with multiple scenic hallucinations, in which the patient loses all contacts with reality and acts like a dreamer ('Oneiroid States') (Mayer-Gross *et al.*, 1974; Hamilton, 1976). Such states may last for weeks or months. They show some resemblance to epileptic twilight states.

The content of their fantasy resembles that of the acute paranoid schizophrenia, but includes elements of a semi-realistic melodramatic kind such as, catastrophes, dangerous adventures etc. Such a dream like change of consciousness in psychotic states (called Oneiroid States / Oneirophrenia) was described by Mayer-Gross in 1924. Mayer-Gross believed that ecstatic states, marked wish-fulfilling delusional experiences, and severe hallucinosis are responsible for the oneiroid form of experience.

Latent Schizophrenia

This term was introduced by Bleuler (1911) to designate patients with deteriorated personalities. Such a deterioration, he believed, is due to a schizophrenic process which has not been acute and has ceased to be active. Some British and German psychiatrists regard latent schizophrenics as psychopathic personalities (Mayer-Gross *et al.*, 1974). However, this view appears to be debatable even now.

Symptomatic Schizophrenia

The very concept of symptomatic schizophrenia has been a topic for long dispute. This is because previously authors used to maintain a view that tough psychoses resembling schizophrenia could be found in some specific pathogenic process, such as, cerebral syphilis, should be distinguishable to the experienced clinician. These authors also maintained a view that such psychoses, be regarded as a momentary illusion of schizophrenia and in fact, pathological, physiological and psychological processes involved are common to both schizophrenia – like psychoses and nuclear schizophrenics (Mayer-Gross *et al.*, 1974). However, in recent years some authors are of the opinion that some disturbances of central nervous mechanisms may result, at least momentarily, in clinical pictures which appear to be indistinguishable from schizophrenic psychoses. The following are some examples of such symptomatic schizophrenia:

(*a*) **Amphetamine Psychoses.** Psychotic states accompanying amphetamine intoxication was first described by Connell (1958) and later by Bell (1965). This is claimed to be the best established of the schizophrenia – like psychoses. In this, subsequent to an intake of a single large dose of amphetamine acute hallucinations, perhaps with a delirious tinge, and impairment of contact with reality are evident. The state of consciousness may be completely lucid. Visual hallucinations and illusions are usually prominent but if these do not appear, its resemblance to a typical schizophrenic psychoses appears to be extremely close (Mayer-Gross *et al.*, 1974). Also, primarily delusional experiences, extreme emotional reactions to this in the form of fear and suspiciousness are prominent. If the state continues for sometimes, secondary systematisation and elaboration of delusions develop. If however, such psychoses arise due to chronic intoxication, resemblance to a schizophrenic illness becomes even more closer. The patient starts feeling that something strange is going on in him, as if, he is under supervision of gang, or that strangers on the street are talking about his sexual life. He becomes depressed, tense and anxious. Auditory hallucinations more commonly of a persecutory kind, hearing once's thoughts spoken aloud, feeling one's thoughts interfered with and other passivity feelings are typical. If the psychosis lasts, it may be entirely indistinguishable from schizophrenia, though in majority of cases there are exogenous features. Visual illusions and hallucinations are common. A demonstrable degree of confusion, and some impairment of memory for recent events may be found, although it is rarely found to be severe and sustained. The affective reaction is brisk and adequate.

For differential diagnosis, testing of urine for presence of amphetamine metabolites is the easiest thing to do (Mayer-Gross *et al.*, 1974). Other features which distinguish such a patient from the generality of schizophrenics are – a history of psychopathically deviant behaviour in the past, rapid onset, and rapid recovery once amphetamine is withdrawn. A fairly close parallel to chronic amphetamine psychosis is offered by chronic hallucinosis of alcoholic addiction, and at times the later also shows a close resemblance to schizophrenia. However, the clinical picture of alcoholic hallucinosis is dominated in a characteristic manner by the auditory hallucinations.

(*b*) **Gross Brain Lesions.** Schizophrenic symptomatology has been reported in association with brain tumour (Mayer-Gross *et al.*, 1974). Also the aural phenomena observed in temporal lobe lesions appear to be psychopathologically indistinguishable from schizophrenic experiences. However, in such cases schizophrenic symptoms pass off rapidly under the influence of treatment, and later sequelae resembles those of an organic personality change rather than those of post-schizophrenic state.

(*c*) **System Degenerations.** Off the different forms of system disorders known to be associated with schizophrenia form psychoses, the best known is Huntington's chorea. Panse (1942) reported 23 cases in which the original diagnosis was schizophrenia and recognition of organic pathology could be made only after many years. Paranoid hallucinatory type of psychosis was noted in this and catatonic states appeared but rarely. Based on clinical psychiatric approach it was difficult, as Panse reported, to differentiate this from genuine schizophrenia. However Panse's observation of such cases revealed that both the delusions and hallucinations noted in this were of a rather primitive kind, lacking the richness and complexity of schizophrenic symptomatology. Occurrence of paranoid psychoses of schizophrenic form in Huntington's chorea has also been confirmed by Streletzki (1961). However, schizophrenia like states usually gets off into an organic picture after a couple of years of suffering (Mayer-Gross *et al.*, 1974).

(*d*) **Aging.** Schizophrenia – like symptoms occurring in old age show much resemblance to long lasting schizophrenia (Kay and Roth, 1961). In this context late paraphrenia (Roth, 1955) is worth mentioning. This illness is relatively more common in female and that especially in widows or spinsters living alone (Roth, 1955). Some such patients complain of defect of sight or hearing. These patients also complain of being raped and gassed. Hallucinations of all kinds occur. There is a presence of a florid paranoid state, but no signs of dementia is noted. Intelligence and judgements on matters not concerned with the paranoid symptoms are extremely good. Due to their strong persecutory belief they eat very little and thereby develop a confusional state due to malnutrition. Clinically there does not appear to have any obvious difference between late paraphrenia and paraphrenia of earlier onset (Mayer-Gross *et al.*, 1974; Hamilton, 1976). Both are a syndrome of schizophrenia. Of course, schizophrenia can occur after age of 60 years but appears to be very uncommon.

Interim Summary on the Existing Classification Systems

Unlike the practice of other branches of medicine in which pathological entities are ordinarily demonstrable, psychiatry usually bases its attempt to classify disorders either on similarity of descriptive facts or on prognosis. Formerly based on this psychiatry endeavoured to classify personality disturbances, *i.e.*, similarity of descriptive facts and prognosis, as if these two are distinct entities. But in such an attempt one may easily err in mistaking reaction sets for different disease entities. It is more important to know the patient's intrapsychic processes and how they reflect themselves in the patient's behaviour and interpersonal interactions, instead of categorising the disease entities only to present a factual digest of the origin and types of reaction. Except in organic disorders or organic involvement in psychiatric cases, a classificatory diagnosis is less important than a psychodynamic understanding of the personality of the patient. Mental health professionals should be interested in the process, not in labels, an issue which has been raised by such professionals long before (Kolb, 1973). A particular pattern of behaviour may stem from widely varying psychological causes, and a diagnosis on a purely descriptive level, without regard to the patient's thought content, is no diagnosis at all. Even in such disorders, *e.g.*, General Paresis of Insane (GPI), in which undoubtedly organic pathology exists, a study of the earlier functioning of the personality is necessary to clear-up many points which can not be explained by neurohistology alone. This is because organic brain disease permits release of impulses that were formerly inhibited or repressed (Kolb, 1973).

One might argue that classifications are necessary for statistical and other purposes, namely research. Eysenck (1976), *e.g.*, advocated for dimensional classification instead of traditional symptomatic classification. But there too, at times a great disposition in psychiatry was noted whether its objective was attained when such a categorisation has been made. Nomenclatures used, *e.g.*, do not serve well for statistical classifications. Statistical complication of data is made to furnish quantitative data useful in providing answers in regard to groups of cases; the interest in individual occurrence is totally lost.

It does not mean that advantages of a good classification system is totally ignored. A diagnostic label enables the professionals, who work with disturbed individuals, to communicate information concisely and quickly to individuals, and also in deciding about the treatment strategies of the patients promptly. From this point of view diagnosis of schizophrenia indicates quite a few about the patient's behaviour. However, disadvantages arise, if one becomes totally dependent on diagnostic label. Labeling induces us to overlook the unique features of each case coming under the rubric of a given diagnosis (Smith, Nolen-Hoeksema, Fredrickson and Loftus, 2003), and thus expect the person to conform to the classification. Classification does not tell us the origin of (what causes it to continue) the behaviour thus, label for maladaptive behaviour is not an explanation of that behaviour.

The classification of mental disorders, mostly used by mental health professionals is the Diagnostic and Statistical Manual (DSM-IV) of the American Psychiatric Association (1994), which corresponds generally to the International System of the W.H.O. Once again, nomenclature shows quite a few differences between those even by the International Classification of the Diseases (ICD) and those by the DSM. Description of the major categories of illness given by DSM-IV, and ICD is beyond the scope of this book, but scanning of the recent classifications makes the older generations of mental health experts to wonder as to where to fit into the original terms neurosis and psychosis in the recent classification. Traditionally these terms denoted major diagnostic categories (unlike DSM-IV). There are several reasons for this departure from earlier classification systems, but the main one concerns precision of diagnosis. But such precision does not necessarily always suffice to cover all varieties of disorders seen in other cultures. Some of these disorders may have the same underlying causes as of certain disorders recognised by the DSM-IV, but are manifested by different symptoms in other cultures. Other disorders may be really unique to the cultures where these are manifested. The presence of such culture-bound syndromes suggests that "the disorders listed in DSM-IV represent only the disorders that occur in mainstream of American culture rather than a universal list of disorders to which all humans are susceptible" (p.531; Smith, Nolen-Hoeksema, Fredrickson and Loftus, 2003). This brings a support to those who argue that abnormality cannot be defined without reference to the culture the patients belongs to. Some culture-bound syndrome do exist. To name a few, ataque de nervios (uncontrollable shouting, crying, trembling with verbal and physical aggression, seizures, and fainting) found in Latin Americans; Ghost Sickness (loss of consciousness) in American Indians, Susto (a feeling that Soul has left the body) in Mexico and Central Americans and Taigin Kyofusho (intense feeling that one's body displaces, embrrases others) in Japanese (APA, 2000). Moreover, the classification system of developed countries have not been satisfactory in developing countries (Walker, 1981). In developing countries acute psychiatric symptoms may present difficulties of diagnosis; such difficulties we can overcome only when we consider important cultural factors and varying use of language (more so in India which is, perhaps, the best comprehensive laboratory for experimentation on different language related and religious issues) to describe emotion and behaviour (Kapur, 1987). Impact of culture in symptom manifestation has been updated later in this book (Chapter V and VI).

3

CHAPTER

Paranoid Psychoses

This disorder shows insidious development and is characterised by persistent, systematised (logically reasoned) delusions. Emotional and behavioural reactions of the patient including talk remain unaltered except that these seem to have been overshadowed by delusional beliefs of the patient. Delusional beliefs not only become the uppermost theme of the patient's life, such unalterable delusions also seriously impair direction and judgement of the patient. To designate such a striking mental state of the patient, Kahlbaum first used the term paranoia in 1863 (cited by Kolb, 1973; Hamilton, 1976).

The causes of this disorder are psychological in origin; causes have a wide spectrum, ranging from specific traumatic life experiences to failure to achieve overvalued goals, need for enhancing prestige or self-esteem. Feelings of insecurity, guilt, a need for defense of the personality against undesirable tendencies and repudiated impulses are also commonly noted. The family atmosphere of such patients is found to be very significant. Mostly they come from a family which is found to be severely authoritarian, harsh, and cruel. One of the parents (usually of the same sex) is reported to be hostile and controlling to the patient who rejects the patient since his childhood. Through indictment such a parent produces fear, anxiety, feelings of inadequacy, as well as a self-image of the "bad me" (child) in the patient which however the patient can not accept (Kolb, 1973). This in turn, causes hatred and aggression in the child which he tries to repress because of fear of his parent. In some cases an early over identification with the parent of the opposite sex has been reported (Kolb, 1973). Mostly parents of such patients are found to have uncongenial relationships with their parents. In some cases, child witnesses this and in some cases this is reported to the patient by his relatives and friends. On occasions, the patient may deny the act or even threaten the child insisting that he should hold it secret. Thus, the child learns the use of denial and rationalization. At the same time the child represses his own rage towards the parental figure. Such an atmosphere in the family make the child feel rejected and he withdraws from social contacts. This in turn is likely to stimulate resentment, finally leading to contribute a paranoid element in the growing personality. Role of sibling rivalry in developing paranoid element in the growing personality is also worth mentioning. Likewise, high expectations for outstanding achievement from parent may contribute a paranoid element in the growing personality (Artiss, 1966). Initially the child develops a secret longing to keep up the expectation of the parents for outstanding achievement in life (this gives him a chance to overcome his sense of rejection and also a chance to lead to a desired goal of gaining love and attention from parents) but because of his lack of confidence onto himself simultaneously he develops a tendency to be away from such longing (putting him in a dilemma) (Kolb, 1973). Thus, fantasies which the child restores as a means of maintaining respect with the family are frustrated. The child experiences of sudden and terrifying anxiety and depression within. As a compensatory measure he employs defensive internalisation and projections.

As a child, the future paranoid usually finds it difficult for him to participate with other children freely for more than a brief period. This is because, he can't take others in confidence to that extent necessary to go for exchanging perspectives. He is lonely, unhappy, brooding, stubborn, obstinate, morose and irritable (when crossed) suspicious and resentful to discipline. As the child approaches adulthood, he becomes increasingly sensitive so much so that he develops a tendency to "build mountain out of mole hills" (Kolb, 1973), in his attitude and behavioural interaction with others. Because of his basic inferiority, he needs to demonstrate superiority. If he gets a position of authority in life, he may be a cruel ruler. He is meticulous, precise and in some respect highly efficient but is jealous, and unadaptable. He is intolerant of accepting self criticism though readily criticizes and belittles others. In such patients repressed homosexual impulses are not very uncommon. Such paranoid personality characteristics become gradually and insidiously intensified until the patient lands clearly as paranoid psychotic. Thus, paranoid psychosis represents a progressive developing continuance of paranoid personality.

Such patient is found to be over aggressive. This is because he always sees an aggressor in everyone around him. He feels as if, the whole world has united against him and has declared war against him. He treats others (even his intimate friend) as projections of certain of his own unconscious trends, and as such, his manner and behaviour alienate friends and relatives and create enemies. As a result he is often rejected and isolated by others which adds a further fuel to the psychopathogenic fire.

The content of paranoid delusions varies widely. This is largely determined by the particular psychological needs the patient wishes to fulfil. Also it depends upon the type of rationalisation that will appeal to the beliefs and ideas prevail in the patient's environment.

At times delusions may take their origin in some actual fact. For example, patient's relatives and friends might have actually tried to victimise the patient but failed. Thus the patient develops a firm belief, extends it, and rationalises so plausibly that unknown persons can easily be convinced and accept his allegations (*i.e.*, some specific individuals and not the patient himself are responsible for his difficulties) as true. The patient's superior intellectual endowment may remain unimpaired. His judgement may be defective only in relation to his delusional system, which however ultimately becomes intricate and complex. The ideas of persecution, grandiose, or both are found to be main theme of his contention.

With the development of persecutory ideas, the patient becomes hostile and aggressive to others. In his efforts to control his hostile impulses, the patient projects them and experiences them as being directed against him. He believes that he is the victim of persecutors; he is the victim of a conspiracy. All events in his environment are interpreted wholly, regardless of their relevancy, with reference to his delusional content. Even incidents of the remote past receive a new interpretation and the patient fits them well into the framework of present persecution (known as retrospective falsification).

As the patient thinks that he is always "right," he may even initiate legal action against those whom he perceives as persecutors. But there too, he fails to see that he has not proved his case. Being dissatisfied he goes for taking a further legal action , and thus every litigation (Kolb, 1973) brings further controversies and new grievances (litigious form of paranoia). This attempt to put others in the "wrong" (Kolb, 1973), shows that the patients wants to prove his superiority (to meet the subconscious feelings of inferiority, to protect weak points of his personality). But ultimately he remains dissatisfied to prove his "rightness" as he extends his delusional system constantly. He feels overwhelmed by an environment with which he cannot cope; an environment which is beyond his control. As a result he may become depressed and suicidal.

Ideas of invention constitute grandiosity (exalted type of paranoia). Such patients neglect their usual method of livelihood and devote their time in the construction of models. But there too, the patient claims that the models are complete but enemies prevent him from securing a patent (Kolb, 1973). In some paranoid states the exalted beliefs are religious in nature.

At times paranoia assumes an erotic form. The patient believes that some women whom he causally saw or met is in love with him (one sided love) (Kolb, 1973). The patient starts writing affectionate letters and possesses that women in imagination.

Some clinicians are of the opinion that repressed homosexual impulses may act as dynamic agents in the genesis of paranoid delusions. But this view is subject to criticisms as because many instances of paranoid symptomatology do not necessarily always reflect a homosexual reference. Secondly, in some cases it is found that patients accept homosexual impulses overtly without conflict. However, psychoanalytically speaking manifest and latent homosexuality are dissimilar and they occupy different levels in the psychic apparatus and operate independently.

Perhaps clinicians would agree that from childhood interaction especially with parents the child perceives himself as weak, defective, or inadequate in meeting and exerting himself independently in his interaction with an adult of the opposite sex. (Inadequacy in role playing). In other words, the individual develops a fear of failing to exert 'power, (since he has a deep sense of shame or humiliation, a fear of rejection or lack of success in relating to members of the opposite sex), and thus prefers members of the same sex where he/she feels more competent and secured. Thus, "power anxiety" (Ovesey, 1962) may be regarded as the primary motivating force in the development of his pathological defences (Ovesey, 1962). Ovesey (1962) further added that such "power anxiety" may not be restricted to sexual interaction only. The individual may perceive himself inadequate no matter whether he evaluates his performance socially, vocationally or sexually. Such a feeling of inadequacy makes the individuals build up (Kolb, 1973) a structure of projective defence – the paranoid system.

A good number of paranoids do not marry while many others and their marital life ends in divorce. This may be partly because of their homosexual desires and partly because of their basic hostility and anger which make them undesirable as partners.

In general, in spite of having superior intellectual endowment the rate of constructive achievement in the life of paranoid patient is not proportionate. This is because their energy is largely expended in compensatory efforts (to enhance self-esteem though outcome is mostly nil). Superior intellectual endowment finds rationalisation and projection to be readily available and satisfactory defenses for them. With such defenses paranoids do not give up, rather sustain active struggle for enhancing self-esteem and for recognition. Such a striving is likely to lead to paranoia (Kolb, 1973). On the contrary, prompt and passive may to give up struggle is likely to result to approach the schizophrenic. The paranoid schizophrenic patient lacks the intensive desire for achievement which is usually seen in paranoia. From affect point of view, in paranoia there is a greater tendency to project and to rationalize one's affective component than is usually seen in manic episode (Hamilton, 1976).

Initially treatment should be as permissible as possible. The greater the overt hostility, the more imperative is commitment (removal from society). To start with, drug treatment would be helpful in getting the patient relieved from his tension and anxiety. But this has to be followed by psychotherapeutic approach which consistently would allow a deeper examination of reality finally leading to a satisfactory social adaptation.

4
CHAPTER

Symptoms and Their Diagnostic Implications : Search for Precursors

Many attempts have so far been made to find a single character which could be diagnostic of schizophrenia, but in vain. Jasper believed that the observer's 'intuition' of what is schizophrenic is the most important determinant. Failure to diagnose a case of schizophrenia, according to Jasper, may be, attributed to the observer's inability to feel with the patient and to understand him. However, in practice one might find such a quality of the observer in cases in whom organic factors are involved, or in understanding the reactions of a neurotic. Perhaps clinicians would appreciate that it is rather impossible to think and feel oneself into the role of the schizophrenic who experiences symptoms like primary delusions, passivity phenomena etc. (Mayer-Gross *et al.*, 1974). After all, application of such a criterion of 'intuition' as a determinant of schizophrenia is subjective, and hence, far from becoming a universal character. Schneider (1925) opined that the lack of personal rapport felt by the clinician in examining a schizophrenic patient may be considered as one of the most important determinants. Once again, such a determinant (symptom) is not free from the limitations of subjectivity. At the same time there is hardly any single test or anyone reliable or universal method available which could be taken with full confidence as an index of the diagnosis of schizophrenia. Even now clinicians are to depend on a totality of observations and impressions which might in some cases be proved to be misleading. However, in the majority of cases the diagnosis is not difficult, and even the followers of different psychiatric schools may come in agreement with regard to a typical case of schizophrenia. Some such typical symptoms of schizophrenia will be mentioned later in this chapter. Clinician however, come across problems with regard to early diagnosis of schizophrenia. Therefore, unlike traditional presentation of the typical clinical characteristics given by ICD-10 and/or DSM (APA), in a chapter on diagnosis, the present chapter focuses on some of the symptoms which might create confusion to the clinicians to reach an early diagnosis of schizophrenia. In the following pages, such disguised symptoms will be described first with an attempt to focus premorbid personality factors which could be taken as precursors for the diagnosis of schizophrenia later in life. For an elaborate descriptions of first rank symptoms, positive symptoms, negative symptoms, *etc.*, the reader is referred to DSM-IV-TR (APA, 2005). Specific symptoms in context to particular diagnostic sub-categories of schizophrenia have been dealt with separately under differential diagnosis (see chapter VII). Influence of Indian culture in the formation of clinical features of schizophrenia has been discussed elaborately in the Chapter VI and VII.

Disguised Symptoms

A variety of subjective experiences associated with excessive anxiety, fear of personal dissolution precede the onset of schizophrenia. Symptoms of different dimensions may occur one after another, in a given individual over time; these symptoms may wrongly be considered similar to, but not actually schizophrenia. From this point of view, a beginning schizophrenic illness may be disguised as one of the neurotic reactions. Thus for example, as is evident in our culture, mounting anxiety, sexual and aggressive fantasies, severe obsession over sexual matters and subsequent persistent guilt in an immature adolescent, long standing uncertainty in young adults, hysterical symptoms in an unhappy married woman, induced terrifying fear (*e.g.*, threat of robbery on a young cloth merchant) or panic states under the pressure of terrifying delusions, and hallucinations, and so on, may shed a different tinch of colour onto the total clinical picture of the case. No satisfactory evidence exists that these patients are schizophrenics rather than highly disturbed neurotics; but one has to be sure at this stage whether the patient is reacting with a malignant form of schizophrenic psychosis. Secondly, there is frequently no abrupt transition from the schizoid type of personality to the manifest schizophrenia. In adolescence, for example, there might have been a tendency to be highly sensitive, extreme jealousy, loneliness, and unhappiness (leading to depression). In young adults, hypocondria is occasionally met with among the disturbances of affect in schizophrenia (background information – detailed later in this chapter). The proper illness with its characteristic and full-fledged symptoms will suddenly appear one day. Such problems are well summed up in the following paragraphs quoted from Gillies (1949), which have been mentioned later (1974) by Mayer-Gross *et al.*

'In adolescence the growing-up process tends normally to excite a rebellious, questioning attitude towards parents and teachers, and the gonadal changes often give rise to shyness, perplexity, slight depression, anxiety, hypochondriacal preoccupations with the body, and shame over masturbation. It is also normal enough for the adolescent to brood over the meaning of life, religion, and love. If these musings continue for long, or if they lead to a break with reality, they will not be transient phases of adolescence but will be due to schizophrenia.'

'Early non-specific signs that may disquiet the relatives include day-dreaming, seclusiveness, undisciplined attitudes, violent unfeeling criticism, lack of energy, and lack of interest in work and play. The patient himself may complain of these and also of self-consciousness, general uneasiness, apprehension, puzzlement, hopelessness, depression, moodiness, poor concentration, and of physical symptoms such as constipation, dyspepsia, poor appetite, abdominal pains, headaches, and poor vision.'

'Although the schizophrenic tends to lose insight early, some patients will for long realise that they are mentally unwell and will complain that they have changed.'

This, thus shows that certain disharmonies of thought, perception, affect, and of interest and habit may have existed for long time in the given individual. Therefore, a thorough scrutiny of the premorbid aspects of the case be done with patience to avoid future hazards. Because, if we miss the diagnosis of schizophrenia of a patient for a day, perhaps, we miss the case/patient for a month at least in initiating proper treatment.

Again, obsessional and/or compulsive colouring may be present in some patients with schizophrenia. But one has to be careful in diagnosis and treatment when obsessional thoughts lead to schizophrenia. A number of cases are found in our culture, particularly amongst adolescents and young adults, where a shift from obsessive neurosis to schizophrenia is evident.

Such persons even in the early stage of their life, frequently report mental sickness for a considerable period of time prior to their diagnosis of schizophrenia. Such sickness might not have got proper attention of his family members. Thus, there may be a 'transitional pre-schizophrenic' (Kolb, 1973) phase of one or two years prior to the manifestation of full blown symptoms of schizophrenia. Obviously, onset in such cases, follow a gradual evolutionary process (except the catatonic type, Kolb, 1973). However, differentiation be made in such cases, based on psychoanalytic orientation, *i.e.*, whether the patient fails to differentiate between the self and the non-self (Mayer-Gross *et al.*, 1974).

Hypochondriasis

Hypochondria is occasionally met with among the disturbances of affect in schizophrenia. Such a prooccupation with ones own bodily functions provides a meaningful purpose. Social isolation may be the root cause of such bodily preoccupation. As the patient has ingrained a strong negative idea about surrounding people, he perhaps, expresses towards his own body the same attitude he has held toward others, and thus uses the same ego defenses. Similar view has been advocated by Kolb (1973). Excessive sexual drive, which remains oppressed so far because of Indian cultural training, gives a feeling of guilt in the person. Such guilt is then centred on his genitals and leads to preoccupations (Kolb, 1973) with defects in genital functioning. The individual may express these preoccupations in bizarre terms, such as "electric current in the genitals", a "sense of shrinking of the body" (Kolb, 1973), and more recently fear of acquiring AIDS etc. is evident mostly in our youngsters (see Chapter IV); some complain of fear of other terminal diseases, like cancer. The concept of body image boundary (Kolb, 1973) seems to have some relevance here, particularly in the early stages of schizophrenic reaction. Kolb (1973) advocated that "in some instances, other body parts come to represent the genital areas through the process of displacement". Such a process of displacement, what Kolb (1973) opined bears a strong relevance to our patients who developed hypochondriasis in the beginning, which later turns out to be schizophrenia, if remains untreated (for detail, see Chapter III & IV). Such guilt anxiety, in some cases becomes severe so much so that the patient is led to self-mutilation 'in those occasional fantastic acts of personal dismemberment' (Kolb, 1973).

With the advent of the modern physical methods of treatment and management facilities, it is realised that earlier the recognition of the illness, the better the services the patient could be rendered to. Gillis, (1949), (cited by Mayer-Gross *et al.*, 1974) mentioned that 'when treatment was restricted to institutional care and occupational therapy, early diagnosis was scarcely important, but with the coming of the modern physical treatments, and the realisation that the best results are obtained in early cases, it has become of the first importance to recognise the illness at its beginnings. When the onset is sudden and results in a catatonic stupor or frenzy, or in a florid outburst of delusions, then diagnosis will be easy, but doubt will arise when the disease has begun insidiously and has been present for months or years before the patient is taken to a doctor. Although the primary symptoms are almost pathogonomonic, in their mild form they are difficult to detect and they may be masked by the patient's reaction to them.'

Some of the major symptoms of schizophrenia will now be mentioned briefly.

Symptomatic Diagnosis

The presence of thought disorder, (Bleuler's loosening of association), is a first rank diagnostic sign, if found in a state of clear consciousness. Conversation with such patients may be found to be interfered with by 'vorbeireden' (see Chapter-II), blocking of the stream of thought, narrowing of concepts, drifting into irrelevant side-lines, vagueness of thought and all such other peculiarities of thought disorder described earlier (see Chapter-II). In some cases, thought–blocking may sometimes assume the appearance of a Petitmal (Mayer-Gross *et al.*, 1974). However, absence of other clinical pictures in favour of Petitmal helps ruling out such a confusion. Attempts have been made to investigate schizophrenic thought disorder both qualitatively and quantitatively (for detail the reader is referred to Hamilton, 1976). Psychological tests have been constructed to assess disorders of 'conceptual thinking'. Vigosky suggested a sorting–test of coloured wooden blocks which he claimed could reveal the nature of loss of the patient's ability to think in abstract concepts and a regression to 'thinking in complexes' (Hanfmann and Kasanin, 1942). Hanfmann-Kasanin test of thought disorder also consists of blocks which could be sorted by colour, size or shape. They reported that schizophrenics had difficulty in abstracting a quality which could be used for sorting. Also, once having found one such quality for thought sorting such patients could not get away from it to discover another. Similar findings have also been reported by Goldstein, (1939) who applying a test battery (similar to the one he used for his research in organic brain lesions) confirmed Hanfmann-Kasanin's findings of an impairment of abstract attitude in schizophrenics. However, the diagnostic value of all these tests are limited as because these are applicable only to a minority of patients, *i.e.*, patients with pronounced and permanent thought disorder. Secondly, it reveals only a part of the total and complex abnormality of function. Thirdly, these results are affected by mental age, and fourthly, these cannot be quantified. Furthermore, because of non-availability of parallel tests, findings obtained on such tests cannot be verified. Lastly, for clinical purposes these tests do not seem to have any advantage over the simple method of using stories and proverbs. In case of the latter the patient is asked to explain proverbs given to him, or to make a mental effort like making a story, or repeating the gist of a fable. In doing so, patient shows poor ability to think in terms of abstract concepts and also indications of over inclusion in his thought process.

Results obtained applying the Rorschach-ink-blot test may be diagnostically useful. This is a test of thought processes and is also markedly influenced by affective factors. This is based on the mechanisms of projection. Some of the Rorschach signs considered to be pathogenomonic of schizophrenia are extreme variation in the form quality of responses, 'contaminated' responses, and 'confabulation' in answers. All these response characteristics are definitely closely connected with thought disorder. 'Position' answers are found in Rorschach protocols of a schizophrenic, but this is less certain. The reaction to the coloured blots is also rather characteristic. Likewise, variety of movement responses and bizarre responses are also significant.

In practice however, there are certain main difficulties in the way of the diagnostic application of this test. These are very often, such patient's fail to understand instructions properly; often patients are found to reject quite a number of cards. Of course, rejection of cards itself is significant clinically, provided rejection does not become the rule, rather remains as exception in a Rorschach administration session. In case of total rejection the clinician is handicapped since he has not got any information in hand for interpretation. Such rejection is quite likely in case of other psychiatric cases, *viz*., depression. Likewise, 'confabulatory' responses are found in other patients, *viz*., Mania, and 'position' responses are noted in 'Organic' patients as well. Therefore, one more limitation of this test is that, there is no single and definite Rorschach protocol which is typical of schizophrenia as a whole. After all, the expert clinician will have to associate the obtained findings with his own observation and insight about the patient in hand. However, some authors claim (Skalweit, 1934; Klopfer, 1946) that in early and doubtful cases, the Rorschach test findings with other clinical signs, have a diagnostic significance.

Based on communication patterns between family members of schizophrenics, Wynne and Singer (1963) have proposed scheme to examine thought disorder. In this, schizophrenic thought disorder was classified into amorphous or fragmented forms. For detail the reader is referred to Wynne (1968).

Diagnostic value of thought disorder may sometimes be questioned when a disorder of thinking of a similar type to schizophrenic may be seen in many conditions of clouded consciousness, in the epileptic and the hysterical twilight state, the sub-acute delirious state and in manic confusion. In these conditions the primary disturbance of consciousness sometime is not easily recognised and may be overlooked. Even then, the history of the illness and the total clinical picture help in deciding the issue without ambiguity. For example, absentmindedness and a tendency to loss the thread of thought may be seen even in normal individuals in conditions of excessive fatigue as well as in neurotic patients and both may at times provide a suggestion of the schizophrenic. Needless to mention that such persons can always supply an account of their inner experience at the time the phenomenon occurs and this clearly distinguishes it from the corresponding schizophrenic change (which is different in its origin and mechanism) (Mayer-Gross *et al.*, 1974).

Next, in diagnostic value of symptoms mention should be made of disturbance of volition and the self (Mayer-Gross *et al.*, 1974). Passivity feelings such as feelings of an influence, that of thoughts from outside are being put into his mind etc. are obviously pathognomonic. If the patient complaints of weakness, lack of energy, failing will power etc. these symptoms may be mistaken for those of exhaustion syndrome or mild depression. If the patient makes no complaint but simply remains inactive so much so that appears lazy but without showing any strange/uncommon conduct, then the possibility of schizophrenia is very high. Passivity phenomenon may very closely resemble with some of the complaints of depersonalised or derailised patients (Mayer-Gross *et al.*, 1974). However, depersonalisation may be the prodormal symptom of a schizophrenic illness.

Excessive activity and hyperkinesis in schizophrenia are likely to be mistaken for manic excitement. However, a closer and continued examination will show the existence of elements irreconcilable with a manic state. Underlying thought disorder will show itself in the stream of talk, even reducing it to incoherence. This overactivity will appear to be accompanied not by elevated but by incongruous or inadequate affect (Mayer-Gross *et al.*, 1974). The movements themselves may turn into stiffness, monotony or a stereotyped repetitiveness. If however, manic excitement leads to clouding of consciousness, which may also accompany schizophrenic excitement, diagnosis on the basis of the present status may be difficult. The same is true of the hyperkinesis of epileptic twilight states (Mayer-Gross *et al.*, 1974). However, the differentiation of schizophrenic akinness and hyperkinesis from similar phenomena will be discussed later in the chapter on differential diagnosis (Chapter VII).

Presence of primary delusions in patients, though is pathognomonic, it is very difficult to be sure of their presence. Such a problem of identification is more so when delusional ideas expressed by the patient seem to be closely associated with environmental/psychological situation around him. If however, the patient is highly intelligent and sufficiently clear in his mind, he may be able to describe the sudden appearance of such delusional ideas; but fails to explain rationally as to how it is derived from his surrounding environment. Thus, his perception seems to be illuminated by his own circumscribed thought process. Sometimes similar phenomena are to be met with in epileptic and other schizophrenic – like psychoses (Mayer-Gross *et al.*, 1974). Also, distinction from paranoid and hysterical reactions may then be difficult. However, auditory hallucinations are often found to be present from an early stage and this acts as an aid to the diagnosis.

Diagnostically another significant factor to be mentioned is emotional disturbances. The commonest emotional disturbance is impoverishment of affect. Also, delayed affective response, or incongruous affect are characteristic features. When it appears as the numbing of feelings of sympathy and regards for other people (Mayer-Gross *et al.*, 1974) it becomes most significant diagnostically. These feelings may die off in other organic mental diseases too, but in that, there is always a parallel deterioration of intellectual ability and judgement, whereas in schizophrenia the latter remains unimpaired. Conversely, in epilepsy in early cerebral arteriosclerosis, or in G.P.I., the emotional responses may remain well preserved even when signs of dementia are already manifest. Ecstasy and excessive emotions in acute paranoid states are difficult to distinguish from similar experiences seen in epileptic psychoses. However, it indicates schizophrenia only when the patient himself gives a description of his unexpected and certain appearance, "in a clear sky unexplained by circumstances, and unconnected with his preoccupation and interest" (p.319) (Mayer-Gross *et al.*, 1974). Mention should be made here that such an experience of the patient, at this point, may also be distinguished from the passionate outbursts of hysteria.

At the time of Kraepelin, catatonic symptoms though received much significance diagnostically, recently these have lost diagnostic value considerably since such symptoms have been observed in lots of organic diseases (Mayer-Gross *et al.*, 1974). However, these symptoms are still considered rather typical, only when symptoms like, stereotypes, mannerisms, word salad are found to be present in the clinical picture in long-lasting cases. Stupor and other akinetic symptoms may be found in depressions and in hysterical psychoses, and are then hard to differentiate. Incidentally mention may be made here that eleven out of thirteen patients diagnosed as 'Benign stupor' by Hoch were found to be schizophrenics when followed up by Rachlin (1935). However, the psychological attitude of the schizophrenic towards his motor behaviour (Mayer-Gross *et al.*, 1974), *i.e.*, his peculiar indifference, dissociation between thought and conduct and the profound symbolism expressed in catatonic movements are of some diagnostic significance.

As diagnostic aid mention should be made of hallucinations. Hallucination, like hearing one's thoughts repeated is of much clinical significance, otherwise hallucinations probably are the least characteristic signs of schizophrenia. Of course, the predominance of auditory and especially tactile hallucinations suggest the diagnosis of schizophrenia (Mayer-Gross *et al.*, 1974). According to Kurt Schneider (1957) first rank in diagnostic importance were the hallucinatory voices that conduct a commentary on the patient's actions; hearing thoughts spoken aloud "echo de pensée", broadcasting of thoughts, bodily feelings of influence, thought withdrawal, passivity feelings in relation to affect, instinct, and volition.

Finally, the phenomenon of 'Splitting' (explained in detail in Chapter-IV and V) remains an important diagnostic sign. Splitting gets expressed through dissociation of emotions from ideas of expression from emotions, of conduct from intentions, of some parts of mental life from the rest. Such dissociation differs from dissociations noted in hysteria. In the latter, the dissociation is, as a rule, transparent in nature and thematic in its content. Also hysterical dissociation makes use of dynamic mechanisms (Mayer-Gross *et al.*, 1974). Furthermore, dissociation in hysteria is more massive, while that in the schizophrenic is trivial (see Chapter-VII, differential diagnosis). For detail of symptomatic classification the interested reader may consult DSM-IV-TR (APA, 2005).

Summing up: Less definite and more vague the neurotic picture, the more these may be considered as precursors of schizophrenia. To establish the diagnosis of schizophrenia the examiner must attend particularly to the quality of interpersonal contact, to the perceptual organisation, and cognitive functions of the patient. The patient may have to be seen on several occasions or one has to obtain descriptions of his behaviour in different settings (at school, work place, family), before ruling out the presence of schizophrenia.

5 CHAPTER

Theories of Schizophrenia

In 1904 Stransky opined that psychic life had got two major elements, *viz.*, emotional or thymopsyche, and the intellectual or noöpsyche, and in normal individuals these two elements maintain a close relation between them. Stransky held that in some psychological illnesses these two elements of the mind not only loss their early functional connection but also new ones are formed. Usually this loss is partial and takes place slowly. But in dementia praecox a complete change in the relationship between these two components of the psychic life occurs so much, so that the normal interaction becomes unstable, and some new fixed connections are formed. This conditions is called 'intrapsychic ataxia' or 'intrapsychic incoordination' (Stransky, 1914). Stransky was of the opinion that in dementia praecox, especially in its early stage, the striking feature was not so much of poverty of affect/affective expression, or simple emotional devastation, but incoordination between these two elements of the mind.

This theory goes contrary to that of Bleuler's (1911) which emphasized that 'affective changes' are one of the primary symptoms seen in schizophrenia. This will be explained later in this chapter.

Weygandt (1907) believed that dementia praecox is a volitional psychosis. To explain this disorder, he used Wundt's concept of 'apperception' and stated that a weakening of apperception would lead to a thorough going disturbance of psychic life as that noted in schizophrenia.

Bleuler (1911) explained schizophrenic symptomatology by means of association psychology. He believed that this was due to brain disease. But in some cases there was no pathological brain process and these he attributed to a mild quantitative deviation of the brain function from the normal. Accordingly, he described primary symptoms and secondary symptoms; the former he attributed to the direct expressions of the disease of the brain, and latter to those which could only be derived from them. The primary symptoms were—(a) disturbance of association in terms of impairment of both quality and number of connections of associations, (b) clouded states, (c) affective changes, (d) possibly the tendency to stereotype, (e) possible hallucinations (Bleuler considered that everyone has a general predisposition to hallucination which might get released through schizophrenia), (f) physical changes like vasomotor disorders, papillary changes and so on.

Again, Bleuler divided schizophrenic symptoms into fundamental and accessory. A fundamental symptom is that which occurs in schizophrenia and in schizophrenia only, whilst an accessory symptom occurs in other diseases as well. The fundamental symptoms he described were – (a) disorder of association, (b) disorder of affect, and (c) ambivalence.

All the symptoms of schizophrenia could be traced back to the primary symptoms which produced secondary symptoms as a result of their interaction with healthy functions. Thus, *e.g.*, the loosening of association leads to the train of thought taking an unusual path. When it is very severe leads to the fragmentation of thought. Illogical thinking and incoherence occur, since the normal mechanisms of displacement, condensation, and generalisation take place readily. Because of weakness of thinking complexes of thought becomes independent, and at the same time, the affective loading of these independent complexes leads to their taking over the decision of thinking. This means that psychic activity is sometimes being dominated by this complex and sometimes again by another complex, and thus there is a splitting of personality. This splitting of personality has an obvious affect onto total sympatomatology of schizophrenia. Because of weakness of thinking autistic thinking dominates psychic activity. Excessive autistic thinking and the disorder of association work together to produce delusions out of the fears and wishes, which often are disguished symbolically and loaded with split-off unconscious affects.

Though Bleuler demonstrated psychological connections between the fundamental and accessory symptoms, unfortunately many important schizophrenic symptoms, *viz.*, the apophanous experiences, thought withdrawal, experiences of control and so on were left out of consideration. Secondly he believed that schizophrenia is a disease of the brain. Also mentioned that in those cases where there was no pathological brain process, there was a mild deviation of the brain function. At the same time, while explaining the genesis of delusions he had mentioned about the role of unconscious affect. If however, brain is the locus of such illness, what is the role of unconscious affect in that. One obvious question would be what would be the seat for unconscious? If Bleuler accepted both brain and unconscious affect together to explain schizophrenic symptomatology, then it appears that he joined up the known, the seen with that of unknown and the unseen. Nevertheless, his attempt to interpret psychologically schizophrenic symptoms may be taken as a model of its kind.

Berze and Gruhle (1929) attempted to keep a complete psychological explanation of schizophrenia and postulated that this disorder was a primary insufficiency of psychic activity or hypotonia of consciousness. Hypotonia of consciousness leads to poor intellectual activity and this in turn changes affectivity. Both quality of association as well as its formation are affected. Weakness of perception gives rise to perceptual incompleteness and hallucinations. The loss of feeling of possession of activity in perception gives rise to a disorder of feeling. This also gives rise to a feeling of alienations. Some of the most common complaints of schizophrenics, such as weakness and emptiness in the head, thought withdrawal, disorders of volition were used by Berze and Gruhle to support the theory of weakness of psychic activity. Blueler conceived of such disorders as originating from a weakness of logical thinking, whilst these authors attributed these disorders to a change in the overall state of psychic activity. However, this theory is too general, and appears to be vague, and thereby its contribution as well to our knowledge of this illness is not a significant one.

Based on the concepts of constitution Kretschmer (1952) regarded Schizophrenia as the extreme end of a continuum, the other end of which is represented by normals. Since Kretschemer's (1952) contention that schizophrenics tend to be slender, considerable effort has been given in determining the importance of physique in the etiology of this disorder. Later, Sheldon (1954) also added a further support to Kretschmer and reported that about two-thirds of schizophrenics have a slender build. But such a relationship between physique and schizophrenia is difficult to evaluate. According to Kretschmer, schizoid personality and schizophrenic have the same body type. Therefore, schizoid personality virtually be regarded as a mild variety of schizophrenia. Secondly, if we restrict schizophrenia to such a condition as quiet hebephrenias and catatonias with a few active symptoms, then only it could be considered to be an exaggeration of a schizoid personality. In practice, however, it is not possible to understand most schizophrenias in this way. Thirdly, schizophrenia generally occurs among a younger age group than is characteristics of other functional psychoses; the younger age group is generally more slender than the older age groups. Fourthly, schizophrenics often pass through a stage of gradual withdrawal and introversion which may not be conducive to muscular development. However, Davidson, McInnes, and Parnell (1957) opined that slender boys with below average muscular development tend to display more anxiety and "showing off" behaviour than boys with more fatty tissue or a stocky physique. Sensitivity and anxiety together may lead to the avoidance of normal social interaction as well as to the development of conditioned fear responses which in turn, impair normal socialisation. In some cases, under certain stressful conditions, the net effect may be a predisposition to the development of schizophrenia. However, even now it requires sufficient scientific evidences to justify that most slender children suffer from inadequate socialisation, or that most slender individuals become schizophrenic. Unless that is done, the specific importance of physique as a key to etiological significance seems doubtful since etiology of schizophrenia could largely be taken as an interaction of factors whose specific importance is not very clear and also that these probably vary in different contexts.

Of course, this idea that schizophrenia is grossly exaggerated behaviour of abnormal personalities has also been put forwarded by Adolf Meyer as early as 1910 (Meyer, 1951).

Meyer (1910) looked upon mental illness as a reaction to stress; a reaction which is a "faulty response or substitution of an insufficient, or protective, or evasive or mutilated attempt at adjustment". His view has been conceived by others as vague and woolly and some of his pupils have called his approach, though proudly, as the 'Common sense' approach.

Dementia praecox was regarded by Meyer as mainly a disorder of the young. He opined that it is a direct result of the prepsychotic personality in that the individual develops faulty habits of behaviour due to heredity, poor family background, and bad social environment. The individual is unable to express his thoughts adequately. He thus, acquires faulty habit of thinking and theorizing in an abstract way. He develops very poorly integrated social relations, becomes excessively self-centered, and sensitive to others comments, appears to be excessively shy especially about sexual matters. Such a faulty thinking and lack of social relationships leads to indulgence in fantasies which can not be fulfilled. He develops dependency and cannot stand normal stresses of maturing and adult life. The world becomes extremely stressful to him and reacts to such stress with all those faulty habits he has developed over the years, and thereby manifests disorganisation of personality. The patient retreats into personal fantasy (a means of getting relief from environmental stress) which gives rise to delusions and hallucinations.

Summing up: Dementia praecox, according to Meyer, may be considered as the faulty habits of a life-time carried to an extreme.

It might appear difficult, however, to understand the genesis of the strange acute schizophrenic delusional phenomena and many other symptoms in this simple way of explanation. Nevertheless, his contribution to enrich our knowledge about this illness is worth mentioning since his insistence on the importance of the individual and his environment, as a genesis of schizophrenia, can surely be taken as a "useful corrective for the organically minded psychiatrists who can not lift their eyes from the cerebral cortex" (Hamilton, 1976). Moreover, Meyer's view is much in line with the recent theories of abnormal behaviour which are based on the principles of learning. Such theories claim that such a behaviour has been wrongly learned by the patient from the environment where he has been brought up. In other words, manifestation of abnormal behaviour is a manifestation of one's faulty learning experiences and such behaviour can be modified, if the patient is helped to re-learn the wrong habits he has acquired.

With a view to distinguish between the paranoid personality and the paranoid state due to psychological illness, Jasper (1910) introduced the concept of psychic process. He opined that even in the absence of coarse brain diseases, a definite irreversible, 'non-understandable' change of personality is caused by the psychic process. This process is analogous to the physical psychotic process caused due to an organic brain disease. The latter also produces an irreversible change in the personality if the change in a person was understandable as a development of the previous personality; Jasper called this as 'development' of the personality and contrasted this with 'process' in paranoid states. However, it must be mentioned here that though Jasper did not say that the psychic process was synonymous with schizophrenia, in a later work he did mention that in a large number of 'process' cases the psychological changes of schizophrenia were present.

According to Conrad (1958a,b) schizophrenia is a disorder of the brain. He has applied Gestalt theory to explain the psychopathology of this disorder. He divided acute schizophrenia into three phases, *viz.*, the trema, the apophanous phase and the apocalyptic phase (for detail see Hamilton, 1976). In the trema, the patient experiences a loss of freedom. He feels he is being surrounded by barriers, and unable to communicate with others. He feels that his environment is changed and occasionally he behaves in a senseless way. Severe anxiety may occur or marked depression with suicidal ideas and severe feelings of guilt. A general feeling of suspicion may pervade all social contacts, the patient may feel that there is something behind all his social experiences and finally, a delusional mood may occur. The trema may last for several months or may be a very brief prelude to the apophanous phase.

In sum, in trema, the coherence of the patient's inner and outer world is found to be loosening.

The word 'apophany' is used (Conrad, 1958a,b) to designate the delusional and other paranoid experiences of the acute schizophrenic shift. Apophany can affect both the outer space (the objects which he encounters) and the inner space (the things which he thinks about) of the patient. Delusional perceptions, *e.g.,* are the most obvious example of external apophony. Of course, the patient's experiences of false acquaintance and false alienation of people and object are also of this kind. In the latter, the patient misidentifies persons in his environment and either gives them the identity of someone else or denies their identity even though the individual is known to him previously. All these external apophanous experiences give rise to an impression in the patient that he is surrounded by a set of properties manipulated by some almighty.

In apophany of internal space, the represented material becomes manifest. It seems as if there is a barrier which presents the process spreading from the sensory aspects to that of the representational aspects of psychic life. When apophany affects freely rising memory images, some of them come into prominence as delusional inspirations as because they are experienced as thoughts, inspired from without, so much so that an ordinary 'brain wave' (Hamilton, 1976) becomes a delusional inspiration. Thought broadcasting may be conceived of as the reverse of delusional perception. Instead of perception becoming manifest to the patient, his thoughts become manifest to his surrounding people. Finally, when all personal identification is lost, the thoughts turned out to be hallucinatory voices.

Since in delusional perception the perceptual coherence is loosened, one would expect that in severe schizophrenic process this coherence would break up completely. In such a case of fragmentation of psychic life takes place which Conrad (1958a,b) called the apocalyptic phase (Hamilton, 1976). Such an apocalyptic phase corresponds very well to a catatonic illness. In this phase there is a destruction of the sense continuity, so much so that only fragments of the total experience during such a phase can be subsequently recalled. If this phase continues, it is likely to pass into the terminal phase of acute deadly catatonia.

To explain the residual or defect states Conrad (1958a,b) (also see Hamilton, 1976) had used the concept of energy potential. Energy potential refers to each individual's own particular ability to apply and direct his energies. In residual states, according to Conrad, there is reduction of the energy potential. Conrad's (1958a,b) use of the term 'energy potentials' is more from a psychological viewpoint. During recent years this concept has been applied by different authors to explain emotional status of individuals, both normal and pathological. Emotional excitement or drowsiness either, as manifested by different categories of psychiatric patients has been explained by these authors keeping in view the physiological basis of energy potential. This will be explained in detail later in this book. However, a similar viewpoint as that of Conrad has been given by Petrilowtisch (1958) and Pauleikhoff (1957) to explain schizophrenic psychopathology. They regarded psychic events and states, called the sphere of experience, in the individual as figures. Figures occur on a ground, which is called 'structure' or 'personal structure'. According to Petrilowtisch (1958) manic – depressive illness produces and increases or decrease in the sphere of experience only, having no effect on the personal structure, whereas, in schizophrenia there is a blockade between the 'structure' and the 'sphere of experience' (Hamilton, 1976). This leads to the psychic phenomena becoming more independent. Independent in the sense that there is an emotional experience of a diffuse kind, *i.e.*, delusional mood. This gives rise to an intense feeling of personal concern with few symptoms. New experiences of an 'as if' character (Hamilton, 1976) are present with an insight into illness. As the illness progresses, delusions appear which leads to new experiences having the character of reality. There is very little personal concern; a wealth of symptoms with a defective insight into the illness become apparent both in acute and chronic schizophrenias though such changes have been far from specific as yet. Nevertheless application of the Gestalt theories in schizophrenic behaviour is interesting.

Psychoanalytical Approach

Explanation of psychological illness, according to this approach, is based upon Freud's ideas about the development and structure of the mind. Before discussing Freudian-view of schizophrenia, let us give a succinct view of his concept of development and structure of mind. He believed that adult sexuality is achieved by a process of libidinal development. In this process, the child gets pleasure from different parts of the body and bodily functions. The first state is called the 'early oral stage' in which the source of enjoyment to the infant is sucking. The infant, in this stage, has no concept of an object and thereby cannot differentiate between the ego and the world. He shows neither love nor ambivalence towards objects but stays in a state of primary narcissism. The 'late oral sadistic' phase ('cannibalistic stage') is the next stage in which the infant derives sexual satisfaction from biting and swallowing. The only way by which an object can be dealt with at this phase is total incorporation. The next stage is 'early anal sadistic stage' in which the infant gets pleasure from controlling his bowels more particularly in the elimination and pinching off of the feces. Now he is capable of object love with incorporation. In the next stage, the 'late anal sadistic stage', the infant gets satisfaction from retaining his feces. This is followed by the early genital phase in which the infant obtains sexual gratification from the genitals. The child now is capable of love for an object; but this object love is limited by the fear of castration. When this fear is overcome and sexual gratification is connected with the genitals, the child can be said to have achieved the 'final genital stage'. Now, the child is capable of love without ambivalence.

Along with this libidinal development side by side there is the development of a structure of the mind. A fully developed mind consists of the ego, the superego, and the Id. The ego consists of the conscious self, and those contents which can readily be made available to consciousness. It is the reality-bound part of the mind. The superego is the conscience (ego-ideal), which is partly conscious and partly unconscious. It consists of all the punitive and critical thoughts and attitudes which can be said to have been taken in or introjected from parental models. The Id consists of all the instinctive materials which has never been allowed to become conscious or which has been repressed from consciousness. Thus, Id is entirely unconscious. It wants to gratify the instinctive drives by means of primary process, which ignores time, place, reality, and logical connections. During the course of libidinal development, a stage may not be properly passed through, so that a 'fixation' point occurs at this level. Fixation may be due to excessive, or inadequate gratification at the libidinal stage concerned. Due to some disappointment in life and loss of a loved object psychological illness occurs. The libido which is attached to the object floods the mind of the individual and a regression occurs which leads back to the fixation point.

Having such a background of the Freudian concept of the development and structure of the mind, let us examine Freudian explanations concerning development of schizophrenia. In schizophrenia regression extends back to the early narcissistic level. As because, at this stage the child does not distinguish between self and environment, in the schizophrenic there is a loss of object relations. The inner perception of the loss of object relations gets itself expressed in the form of the classical schizophrenic delusion or fear that the world is coming to an end. Also bodily hallucinations, depersonalisation, feelings of grandeur peculiar of schizophrenic thinking, hebephrenic-symptoms and some of the catatonic symptoms such as, passivity feelings, negativism, and automatic obedience are all considered to be regressive since they all demonstrate the loss of ego boundaries which is in keeping with primary narcissism. Some of the other catatonia motor activities are considered as revivals of archaic types of motor behaviour.

According to Freudian view, two kinds of symptoms are found in schizophrenia (see also Hamilton, 1976), *viz.,* those due to regression, and those due to an attempt to restore the lost object relations. Thus *e.g.,* world reconstruction fantasies, and some catatonic symptoms, such as stereotypes are regarded as efforts to regain object relations. Hallucinations can be regarded as substitutes for perceptions in that objective reality is lost either partly or entirely, while some ideas obtain a perceptual quality, giving rise to a substitute reality. Sometimes hallucinations are wish-fulfilling, but since auditory hallucinations are mostly unpleasant, this can only apply to a small group of hallucinations. Freud was of the opinion that anxiety connected with hallucinations are produced by the reappearance of a part of the reality which has been repudiated (Freud, 1924).

Paranoid delusions are conceived of deriving from a formerly repressed form of object relationship, *viz.,* homosexuality. Since the desire for homosexual relationship is still present in the individual, this group of thinkers therefore, consider this as a form of object relations (Freud, 1924). Based on the Autobiographical accounts of Justice Paul Schreber which has been published later (Schreber, 1955), Freud elaborated his theories of the psychopathology of delusions. According to Freud the patient can deny his basic desire of a homosexual relationship in four different ways and accordingly paranoid delusions can have four different contents. The initial homosexual thought of the patient is, 'I love him', but the patient denies this and his thought becomes, 'I do not love him'. This may later develop into 'I hate him', and then into 'He hates me', so that a delusion of persecution occurs. Again the thought 'I do not love him' may develop into 'she loves him 'and not me' and thus delusion of jealousy occurs. If however, the thought 'I do not love him', develops into 'I love her, she loves me', then it may be said that an amorous delusion or erotomania has developed. Finally, the thought 'I do not love him', can develop into 'I love no one', which is followed by 'I only love myself', so that a delusion of grandeur develops. Paranoid delusions can also be regarded as projections of elements of the patient's body or personality. Thus, *e.g.*, the persecutor may be the homosexual object, which is regarded as a narcissistically hypercathected organ such as feces or the buttocks. This objects is projected which also represents the projected superego.

Jung (1909) along with Bleuler employed psychoanalytic ideas to interpret the delusions and behaviour of schizophrenia. He originally opined that this illness was psychogenic, but that toxic factors might play a secondary role. But later he argued that the immediate cause for this illness is a severe affective disturbance which finally leads to a weakening or disturbance of the ego. Though on the whole, Jung's view on the psychology of schizophrenia appears to be less complex than Freud's, ultimately it appears that he agreed with traditional psychoanalytic views that schizophrenic symptoms could be traced to a weakening of the ego. However, his use of the word association test in schizophrenia may be regarded as one of the important milestones (Hamilton, 1976) in the development of experimental psychopathology.

The above mentioned classical theories of schizophrenia advocated by Freud have been revised by some psycho-analysts later. These analysts also have modified Freud's theories of the structure of the mind. Thus *e.g.*, Federn (1952) has put forward a new concept of the ego. According to him, ego experiences itself as both subject and object. Ego feeling (feeling of 'selfness') permits the individual to distinguish between himself as the subject and the external as the object, as well as to distinguish between himself as an object and the representations of objects. The ego acquires its energy from the libido, the destructive drives, and the life processes. In schizophrenia, the energy supply of the ego is set to be weakened, as a result the ego boundary breaks up, giving rise to an inability to distinguish the self from the environment. Since the objective can not be distinguished from the subjective, the patient's conception of reality is falsified. The ego state of the patient resembles to those of the ego states normally occur in infancy. Therefore, for Federn, schizophrenia begins with the development of a false reality, whereas for Freud the false reality is a reconstruction following the initial regression to primary narcissism. However, Federn's concept that ego experiences itself as both subject and object is very much in line with the views on ego given by Sartre (1957). Also, Freeman, Cameron, and McGhie (1958) on the basis of their research findings reported that Federn's views are very useful in understanding chronic schizophrenia.

Again, Freud's theories of libidinal development have also been modified. For a detailed account of it, the reader is referred to Klein (1952) and Fairbairn (1952). Klein's view of mental structure, *e.g.*, is necessarily considerably different from that of Freud. She believed that the ego is present from birth and the infant mainly uses the mechanisms of introjection and projection. However, Klein has pushed back the development of object relations and ego functions into a period of infancy which is so early that her ideas are beyond proof. Of course, similar criticisms do hold good about many of the Freudian concepts he has made use of while explaining the development and structure of mind (Hamilton, 1976). Thus, *e.g.*, one basic objection to all Freudian theory is that aspects of mental functioning, such as unconscious cerebration or self-awareness are turned into fixed entities with some inner sources of perceptual motion. Secondly, like most other psychological theories of schizophrenia, psycho-analytic theories also mostly gloss over many of the outstanding acute symptoms only but do not take into account the great diversity noted in chronic clinical pictures. Thirdly, psycho-analytic theories claim that all schizophrenic symptoms could be traced to a loss of ego boundaries. Such a formulation appears to be vague and suffers from the limitations of over generalisation (Hamilton, 1976). It appears, as though it can account for everything and nothing at the same time, since all the paranoid phenomena are by definition disturbances of the relation between the self and the environment. There are many other psychoanalytic theories of schizophrenia, a complete critical review of the same is beyond the scope of this write-up. However, the main thrust of this view and some major criticisms have just been mentioned above.

Existentialism

Coming to existentialist approach to schizophrenia, as a brief account of existentialism it may be stated that existentialism as a philosophical movement began in 1927 with the publication of Heidegger's (1953) book Sein Und Zeit ("Being and Time") (see Hamilton, 1976). This philosopher developed many of Kierkegaasd's (1813-1855) ideas but in order to express those it seems to me that he rather invented a very complicated jargon. He should have expressed the basic ideas in lucid form, more so in context to its application in explaining psychological illness like schizophrenia.

There are two basic propositions in philosophy, *viz.*, realism and idealism. The realist (materialist) believes that mind is a product of matter and the sensations are produced by matter. To the idealists, mind is primary, and the matter is secondary so that sensations are not entirely produced by a material world which is said to be independent of mind. An extreme variety of idealism is called 'Solipsism', in which the individual is source of his own existence and considers his sensations to be present in his imagination. Kant, a great philosopher in his explanation of idealism suggested that we perceive things as phenomena, but we do not perceive things as they really are, *viz.*, things-in-themselves. To know a thing as it really is one has to make a transcendental leap from the thing for us to the thing in itself.

Therefore, human experience consists of the elaboration of perception, so that the mind orders the perception of object in time and space. From the above, it follows that there are two types of psychology, *viz.,* (a) that which deals with mental phenomena; and (b) that which deals with transcendental mind. If so, then mind in the latter sense can not be investigated. It has to be analysed only by means of the apriori concepts which are present in the mind. Obviously, the necessity to appeal to empirical facts is nil if one follows this kind of philosophy. Heidegger believed that by means of self discovery one is able to detach oneself from the everyday aspects of things (*i.e.,* from the Kantian phenomena). This detachment he opined, creates a distance from things which allows of their proper appreciation. This self detachment is expressed as 'the insetting of a nothing'. Thus, the understanding of the things – in themselves can not be said to have achieved. But the limitation of this whole system is that there is a lack of an adequate method of testing the results. How one can be sure that he really has discovered his trueself? (Hamilton, 1976).

Now, leaving aside psychiatric criticisms of the philosophy, let us consider its application to the problem of schizophrenia. Existentialists are of the opinion that the most striking feature of this philosophy is its morbid subjectivity, and they claim that this type of subjectivity (who I am? etc.) is sometimes found in the shut-in, shy adolescent who finds it difficult to make proper interpersonal relationships. Therefore, it may not be surprising to state that ideas resembling existentialist thinking may be found in disturbed adolescents and young intelligent schizophrenics.

Biswanger gave a detailed account of existential studies of a 5 schizophrenics during 1944-53 which he published later (1958) in a book, entitled schizophrenia (also see Hamilton, 1976). He claimed that the basic concept in the understanding of the development of schizophrenia is break in the coherence and sequence of experiences which otherwise normally proceeds as a natural sequence of connections. In other word, it appears that Biswanger also accepted the view to loosening of association as a basic reason for schizophrenic behaviour. If so, then question arises that have we learnt anything new about schizophrenia out of existentialists views? In other words, the philosopher's view of schizophrenia has been presented to us in a disguise by Biswanger. Otherwise, nothing significant can be said to have come out which could be helpful in understanding and explaining schizophrenia.

Zutt (1952) had introduced the concept of the physiognomic aesthetic sphere of life. By this he designated those aspects of experience which are not dependent on intellect or emotions. Individual has a specific position in the world and that is to be physically manifest. The human being can only become manifest in a given position provided there is a distance between him and others. In other words, Zutt meant that boundaries must be maintained (Hamilton, 1976). Later on, Zutt and Kuhlenkampf (1958) viewed the existence of the paranoid patient as a breakdown of such boundaries and as a result the individual loses his separate identity: private and public gets merged. Friends and foes can no longer be differentiated with certainty. Uncertainty leads to feeling of insecurity. Fear and suspiciousness develop (Hamilton, 1976). However, it is apparent that both the existentialists and psychoanalysts have emphasized the necessity to maintain a 'boundary' so as to lead a normal life, though the former has interpreted it from the point of view of physiognomy and the latter from unconscious psychic viewpoint. According to the former, due to break down of such boundaries the human existence is no longer able to cope with the 'crowding in of the physiognomic' (Zutt and Kuhlenkampf, 1958); having lost its position it is said to be physiognomically over powered. According to the Freudian view the break down of ego boundaries leads to manifestation of symptoms which is overpowered by unconscious states of the mind. However, it appears from the above that there is a commonness in views in both these schools of thought regarding schizophrenia, in spite of diversity. Accordingly, it may be justified mentioning here that in existentialist formulation of schizophrenia there is repetition of known facts propounded by other schools of thought. It appears, as though, Freudian formulations of schizophrenia have been described (Hamilton, 1976) to support existentialist view in a very indistinct and bizarre manner. For a detail account of the above mentioned theories the interested reader is refer to Hamilton (1976).

Social Determinants

Based on a social approach, Laing (1960) and his colleagues (Laing and Esterson, 1970) have proposed a theory of schizophrenia. They were of the opinion that social tensions, exploitations, and estrangement of a divided and oppressive society may be responsible for this. There is a saying that sick societies can produce sick people. Now question arises what are the aspects of the sick society which are responsible for producing sick people? Buss (1966) has given a succinct view about such aspects of the sick society, which may be described as follows :

(a) Social Disorganisation. Basic assumption here is that chaos created by social changes or social disruption causes psychopathology, and accordingly one could assume that unstable communities foster more schizophrenic children than stable ones. Using high crime rate, poverty level, cultural confusion, and absence of religious values as indices of social disintegration, Leighton (1959), Leighton, Harding, MacKlin, MacMillan, and Leighton (1963) reported a considerably higher percentage of abnormal individuals in socially more disorganised regions. Likewise, Clausen (1966), Clausen and Kohn (1959), Jaco (1954, 1960) have also found a higher incidents of schizophrenia in disorganised communities.

One basic limitation of these theories is that this could not separate the causalities distinctly. Thus, *e.g.,* it still remains a speculation as to whether social disorganisation leads to psychopathology or it is the other way around? Secondly, some authors (Roman and Rice, 1967) are of the opinion that social disorganisation does not cause psychopathology directly. Disorganisation effects family's outlook which in turn influences personality devevlopment. However, the role of family in causing schizophrenia has been discussed in detail in chapter on etiology in this book.

(b) Social Isolation. As early as 1934, the famous sociologist Faris suggested social isolation as a cause of schizophrenia. He opined that being rejected or otherwise restricted from contacts with persons outside the individual's family leads to the 'Shut-in" personality pattern of the schizophrenic (Faris, 1969) social isolation like, a long period of enforced solitude as that experienced by prisoners may lead to the development of schizophrenic behaviour. For example, long-term prisoners show little joy when their sentences expire. Likewise enforced social isolation like that of induced sensory deprivation, *i.e.,* doing nothing and just being cut off from all contacts with society is likely to land to schizophrenic breakdown. Of course, schizophrenics, are for the most part neither prisoners, nor subjects of experimentally induced sensory deprivations. Social isolation, here means lack of intimate social contacts. This may also cause the same type of seclusiveness as that noted in isolated prisoners.

Research evidences in support of this hypothesis have been far from consensus. Thus, *e.g.,* Kohn and Clausen (1955) reported that schizophrenic behaviour was noted in the childhood of many patients even before social isolation took place. Thus, they believed that social isolation, rather than a cause of schizophrenia, could be a symptom indicating that an individual's interpersonal difficulties have become so great that he can no longer relate to others. It however, appears that Kohn and Clausen (1955) while considering social isolation as a symptom rather than a cause of schizophrenia have emphasized the concept of one's 'predisposition' to schizophrenia. If it is so that well before starting social isolation schizophrenic behaviour is apparent in an individual, then obviously he had a predisposition to this illness (see chapter on Etiology). The very spirit of Faris's (1969) view was not that social isolation is the cause of it. If however, an individual is otherwise free from any predisposition to such an illness, social isolation may be a sufficient reason to start Schizophrenic behaviour in him. Such isolation should also include isolation even within one's family set-up, no matter whether or not he has a good social contact with people outside his family environment.

(c) Social Class. Hollingshed and Redlich (1958) based on their epidemiological studies reported a substantially greater number of psychotics in the lower than in the upper socio-economic classes. Similar findings were obtained by Sorle, Langner, Michael, Opler, and Rennie (1962). Likewise, Dohrenwand and Dohrenwand (1969) reported that the incidence in lower socio-economic groups are equivocal. Some have pointed out that child rearing practices may predispose lower class children to more intense stress, while others believe that the devastating effect of poverty causes its victims to withdraw from the harsh realities of facing it. Still others opine that schizophrenic types have greater tendencies to drift towards lower socio-economic class (Myerson, 1941) because of their social ineptness. In recent years, however, quite a few patients with schizophrenia come from higher socio-economic strata.

The social drift hypothesis of Myerson was corroborated by the findings of Gerard and Houston (1953). However, in an almost identical study some other investigators (Lapouse, Monk, Terris, 1956; Clausen, 1966; and Clausen and Kohn, 1959) failed to find any evidence of drift. An alternate explanation may be that class differences so far noted may be attributed to economic reasons only, not in the sense of poverty causing schizophrenia but in the sense that very rarely one can find schizophrenics of upper classes who report to the OPD or rural health centres, and thus, they are less likely to become subjects in epidemiological studies. Such an explanation does hold good in Indian set up also, where very rarely schizophrenics who come from upper socio-economic strata report to the OPD or rural health centres for their treatment. Mostly they prefer psychiatric consultation privately and attend private clinic/chambers (known as Surgery in London) of the physician and/or private nursing home as and when advised by the physician / psychiatrist. Thus epidemiological studies reported so far based on the patients attending OPD and/or rural health centers fail to give a complete picture of it. These give us a partial view of the total picture.

Cross-cultural Determinants

Culture is socially transmitted from one generation to the next and thus it may be described as a society's total way of life. Culture prescribes a blueprint for living for its members. Its tradition helps shaping its members beliefs, attitudes and thinking and as a whole governs interpersonal affairs of the members. Therefore, it would be of no wonder if one finds that a society's abnormalities closely parallel the culture it reflects.

In psychoses numerous culture bound and unique syndromes have been described by researchers. One example of such a unique behaviour pathology is Koro, also known Suo-Yang (Kleinmuntz, 1974). This is attributed to sexual overindulgence like, excessive masturbation, and is believed to be avoided by abstention from sex (Wittkower and Dubreuil, 1968).

In many respects 'Koro' of the inhabitants of the Malay-Archipelago (South-East Asia) and that among Southern Chinese who migrated to Malay, and 'Jhinjhinia' of the inhabitants of West Bengal, India, resemble Freud's concept of 'Castration Anxiety'.

Even delusional contents of schizophrenics is significantly different in varying cultures and such differences can be attributed to the belief system prevalent in the culture (Kiev, 1972). Thus, *e.g.*, delusions of patients in some South African societies are in the form of becoming Chief or Witch doctors, or being poisoned. Also schizophrenic symptoms in South African societies contain mythological content. Delusions of patients in Western countries, by contrast, include influences operating from a distance, through electricity, X-rays, hypnotism, and outer-space vehicles. Delusions of patients in India mostly include influences by some supernatural power (in some cases, the patient specifies the Supernatural power, like Goddess Kali etc.), and being poisoned by people around. In some patients, mostly in the young ones, an underlying guilt and/or wrong ideas about sexual functions in him/her are found to colour his/her beliefs.

Though people of different castes and creed live in India, India has a distinct culture of its own. But there is a paucity of Indian literature pertaining to pathoplastic effect of socio-cultural norms upon manifestation of psychiatric symptoms in general, and schizophrenic symptomatology in particular. Chauhan, Jain and Kumar (1983) conducted a study on 100 male general psychiatric patients of Agra (North India) mental hospital to see the role of delusions in various functional psychiatric disorders. Applying the Present State Examination (PSE) scale based on the guidelines of WHO (1968) they found that proneness to incidence of delusions in the Schizophrenic category was noted in 'acute reaction' 'disorganised', 'chronic', and 'paranoid' varieties. Delusions of persecution, suspicion, and reference were found to play prominent role in the schizophrenic patients, though delusions of control, and guilt, as well as religious and sexual delusions were found to be present in some patients. Percentage of various types of delusions found in their study in different groups of schizophrenic patients have been detailed by Chauhan *et al.* (1983).

But the number of subjects investigated in this study was 100 only and the number became further reduced when schizophrenics were separated from amongst the 100. Moreover, the patients were taken from one particular hospital and the socio-economic status of the patients was not mentioned in the article, hence, it is not possible to infer whether these findings would be applicable to schizophrenic patients irrespective of their education and socio-economic status. However, in India, mostly in adolescents and young patients an underlying guilt and/or a wrong idea about sexual competency colour the false, firm belief of the patient. Also fear of punishment from some supernatural power is found to be present in a good number of Schizophrenics in India. Some support for this idea may be gleaned from some of the Indian research reports, such as that of Sharma and Agnihotri (1986).

Like delusions, the commonest hallucinatory theme noted in the Indian schizophrenic patients is magic and religion followed by murder and assault, and sex and body organs. Presence of sexual theme in these patients reflected a conflict between the rigid traditional sexual morality and sexual liberalism (Sharma and Agnihotri, 1986). In Indian cultural sexual attitudes and actions are equated with ethical values. This culture encourages more of suppression of sexual impulses rather its overt expression. The latter is considered as a taboo. Delusions and hallucinations being considered as manifest wishes in disguise (Henderson and Gillespie, 1950), the present findings of Sharma and Agnihotri once again support the contention that delusions and hallucinations are well understood in terms of the social milieu of the patient.

Despite scientific and technological advancement religion seems to form an important part of life of Indian people, especially the large rural population. Superstitions and misconceptions like, 'Jadu-tone', Witchcraft and evil spirits are much prevalent amongst less sophisticated section of Indian society. Accordingly, preponderance of the hallucinatory themes of magic and religion is noted amongst females, and less educated persons coming from rural areas and belonging to lower socio-economic strata (Sharma and Agnihotri, 1986).

Mostly less educated, unmarried males manifest the theme of murder and assault in their hallucinations. They represent about one-third of the total number of schizophrenics investigated in Sharma and Agnihotri's (1986) study. In some parts of India people structure their environment, define their identity, interaction, and achievement in terms of fear and violence (Kala and Wig, 1978). Besides, amongst the illiterate, masculinity is equated with aggression (Sharma and Agnihotri, 1986) and unmarried males are free to act out their aggression in the way they like because of less social and family restrains on him compared to married individuals. Thus environmental structuring seems to be significant in producing certain themes of hallucinations in psychiatric patients.

Sharma and Agnihotri's study is subject to criticisms as because the number of patients investigated was 100 only and they hailed from a particular province of India known as Varanasi (Uttar Pradesh), and thus generalisation of the findings is not possible. Secondly, hallucinations were categorised by one of the investigators instead of an independent observer. However, these findings do point out that psychiatric patients symptoms can be more meaningfully understood only when we consider the social milieu the patients come from, a contention which has been supported by both Indian (*e.g.* Bhaskaran, 1963) and Western (*e.g.* Lambo, 1955) researchers.

Mention should be made here that not only across culture, even within culture variations in delusional contents have been reported by researchers. For example, among the "Bush" people in the North of Ghana the delusions were found to be dealt with the ramifications of the fetish system, whereas in the South of Ghana, the delusions are mainly about control of electricity and the wireless (Tooth, 1950). Such a difference in the content of delusions may be attributed to the fact that Western influences are more apparent in the South of Ghana than that of the North. Likewise, variations in the content of delusions are also found within Indian culture, *e.g.,* between the South Indian and the North Indian patients. The content of delusions of the South Indian patients is primarily guilt induced punishment whereas that for the North Indian patients is primarily aggressions and challenge. However, even in our own culture contents of delusions have shown a change, over the last 30 years or so, from ideas of persecution by God, devils to that of nonspiritual forces. Possession, *e.g.,* is viewed differently by patients having different cultural contact. In the West, possession was considered as a sign of distress (Wijestinghe *et al.*, 1976) whereas for the patients in India possession was found to be distress relieving (Carstairs and Kapur, 1976). Vagreecha and Asthana (1987) studying possession by ancestral spirits in rural Rajasthan reported that it is a culture bound reaction to stress situation in the beginning and it proceeds to work as a community therapy, finally resolving the initial stress after a few years of practicing such behaviour. The well accepted feeling of being persecuted by spirits or witches noted among the Kwakiutl Indians of Chnada has often been mistakenly described as paranoid by Western specialists (Carstairs and Kapur, 1976).

Symptom differences have been noted among schizophrenics of different ethnic background (Opler, 1956, 1959). Thus, *e.g.,* Irish-American schizophrenics were reported to be less hostile, more subdued, and less bizarre than their Italian – American counterparts. These symptom differences appeared to be related to varying family patterns (Kleinmuntz, 1974) among these groups. Similar ethnic diversity in symptoms was found between Japanese schizophrenics raised in Japan and those of Japanese descent in Hawaii. The former were described as physically assaultive, while the latter were found to be suspicious and brooding. The importance of such group differences in symptom manifestation is that it dissipates the idea that these differences are due to genetic factors. Such symptom differences are attributed to social factors also. Phillips (1966) in this context has pointed out that "persons of the same racial stock carrying the same diagnosis, develop different kinds of symptoms depending upon the society in which they live" (p.478).

Of course, similarities in the symptoms of behaviour pathology among diverse cultures are also noted. Anthropologists, *viz.,* Leighton (1969), Levine (1963) compared abnormalities among Nigerian (Yoruba tribes) and rural North American cultures and reported that the prevalence and varieties of mental illness were found to be similar in those widely diverse cultures. Some of these similarities in symptoms include hearing voices, talking to oneself, seeing imaginary people, suspiciousness of poisoning and thereby refusal of food, inappropriate affect, overconcerned about religious rituals, and memory loss etc. These abnormalities have their neurotic and psychotic counterparts in Western societies, although their explanations may not necessarily be always same in these two cultures. Thus, for instance, the Yoruba believe that mental illness is due to superhuman attacks from God. This is due to breaking of taboos and failure to observe ceremonial duties. The Yoruba, thus, believe in Witchcraft or the practice of magic (which is called 'juju' throughout West Africa). They also believe, on the other hand, that mental illness is contagious and usually through direct contact with fluids (*e.g.,* foam at the mouth) gets transmitted from one sick person to the next. At the same time it is interesting to note that in the "Yoruba Western Symptomatology, *viz.,* phobia, obsessive – compulsive symptoms and depression are virtually unknown (Kleinmuntz, 1974). Likewise, in spite of having a wide variation between the Western and the Indian culture, we find that (reported earlier in this chapter), there is a similarity in symptom manifestation (originating from sex guilt) in the young boys and girls of both these cultures, though symptoms have been explained and named differently in these cultures.

However, reported literature on cross-cultural contents of delusions and hallucinations is insufficient and findings are not free from controversies. Further research employing well-controlled design is necessary. Till date, available cross-cultural data report that content of psychotic delusions and hallucinations is influenced by the culture in which the person belongs to.

Stimulus-Response Approach

This approach advocates that schizophrenics failed to respond appropriately to incoming stimuli. Normals, though have many associations to incoming stimuli, can select the single most appropriate response at a given time, whereas, schizophrenics failed to make such choice. Some support of stimulus-response approach may be gleaned from the research reports of several authors. However, for a detailed review in this regard the reader is referred to Broen (1968).

Faulty information processing may be the cause of schizophrenic's distortion of reality. (Bernheim and Lewine, 1979). Language deficiencies in schizophrenic patients may result from a deficit in one or more basic cognitive processes, such as, attention, perception, or memory (McGhie and Chapman, 1961; Shakow, 1979; Silverman, 1964; Kleinmuntz, 1974). In their descriptions of schizophrenia Kraepelin and Bleuler, both observed an impairment in attention which has been later supported by many other researchers. Thus, *e.g.*, Shakow (1963) in a series of studies with institutionalised schizophrenics compared the performance of schizophrenic patients to that of non-schizophrenic subjects in a reaction time (RT) paradigm. The subject was required to press a button when he heard a bell and to release it when he saw light. The interval between the bell and the light, the preparatory interval was independent variable and the speed with which the subject released the button after presentation of the light was the dependent variable. Shakow reported that the schizophrenics were slower than non-schizophrenic subjects in most of the reaction-time tasks. Also, variation in the length of preparatory interval and in the pattern of preparatory intervals within a series of trials did show differential effects in which schizophrenics were found to show poorer performance throughout compared to the normal controls. Furthermore, it was noted that schizophrenic patients performed relatively better in those tasks which required less autonomy, whereas the normals performed better in the more autonomous tasks. Based on these findings Shakow (1979) formulated his theory on 'Segmental Set', the basic tenets of which are–(a) the segmental set of schizophrenics produces slowness or lack of readiness to respond to external stimuli; and (b) such lack of readiness is due to their inability to filter out irrelevant and distracting stimuli. Since filtering mechanism does not work adequately, each and every stimulus gets equal significance to the schizophrenic patients and he attempts to respond to idiosyncratic way to each of these stimuli, no matter what the nature of the stimulus is. In other words, because of lack of proper filtering of irrelevant stimuli the schizophrenic seems to have overload of information and his behaviour appears to be overloaded by irrelevancies.

In our laboratory in a reaction time paradigm applying four different experimental conditions, namely auditory simple, auditory discrimination, visual simple, and visual discrimination tasks, we (Chatterjee, Chattopadhyay, Biswas, Bhattacharyya, and Roy, 1979) found that schizophrenics had slower reaction times throughout compared to normals irrespective of experimental conditions. In our personal research we examined the nature of time estimation in task-oriented time in schizophrenics and compared the same with a matched group of neurotic patients, and also with a normal control group. The tasks selected were cancellation, tapping, and drawing a person. Three stimulus times, *viz.,* 10, 20 and 30 sec were used. We found (Chattopadhyay, Biswas and Mitra, 1982) that schizophrenics overestimated all the stimulus times irrespective of the task assigned to them. Neurotics also overestimated, but the magnitude of overestimation was significantly greater in patients with schizophrenia. Similar was the findings in our previous study (Chatterjee, Chattopadhyay, and Biswas, 1980). Not only in task-oriented time, even in non-task-oriented time, schizophrenic patients showed poor perception with a tendency to overestimate (Broota, Kaur and Batra, 1988). Broot *et al.* investigated 30 patients in the age range of 23-30 years and employed three standard times, *viz.,* 10, 20 and 30 sec like that of ours previous study (Chattopadhyay *et al.*, 1982); findings were consistent in the sense that schizophrenics overestimate longer time, no matter whether the stimulus presented is task-oriented.

Another interesting finding of our study was that the trend of overestimation was not found in the patients with schizophrenia when very short time interval (0.5, 1.0 and 1.5 sec) was used as stimulus time. In latter cases a consistent trend of underestimation on the contrary, was observed in the patients with schizophrenia in comparison to patients with neurotic disorders and normals (Chattopadhyay, Biswas and Basu, 1980). Neurotics however, in our study overestimated all the stimulus times (irrespective short or long time) consistently. Schizophrenic patient's autistic separation from external event is likely to prevent them from their full utilisation of sensory and motor cues. Irrelevant thoughts cause distraction in them. This causes inability in them to hold a 'set' (Shakow, 1962) for that long a time necessary to respond to environmental stimuli, which make them extremely slow (Chatterjea, Chattopadhyay and Biswas *et al.,* 1979). Thus, time estimation and reaction time have long been considered as important aspect of schizophrenic pathology (Shakow, 1962; Zubin, 1970). Studies on time estimation and reaction time experiments show similar result in the East (*e.g.,* Broota *et al.,* 1988) and the West (Zubin, 1970).

Not only in RT and time estimation tasks, in two-flash threshold (TFT) task also, in our study (Chatterjea, Chatterjee, Roy, Bhattacharyya, and Biswas, 1980) schizophrenics showed poorer discrimination capacity than the matched normals. All our findings were very much in line with the previous research reports (*e.g.,* Shakow, 1963) supporting once again the contention that schizophrenics show lack of readiness to respond to external stimuli.

In a study, Chapman and McGhie (1962) asked their subjects to repeat sets of six numbers or letters with different series presented visually or auditorily. When visual and auditory presentations were concurrent and the subjects were required to respond selectively to one or the other, schizophrenics did show worst performance compared to that noted in non-schizophrenic psychiatric patients, and in normals. In another experiment (Chapman and McGhie, 1962) these subjects were instructed to turn a wheel at a constant rate that was comfortable for them. Then they were asked to repeat the task while listening to a variable auditory rhythm. While comparing the variability in turning rates between the two conditions, the schizophrenics were found to be significantly more distractible than the non-schizophrenic hospital patients, and also the normal controls. In connection with stimulus-response approach in a series of experiments Garmezy (1966) demonstrated that schizophrenics exhibit a persistent withdrawal from psychologically noxious events and so significantly lessened responsiveness to social rewards. Garmezy advocated two learning formulations in explaining the avoidance behaviour of schizophrenics. First, he proposed that such patient is brought up in "An environment in which the ratio of rewards to punishment was so heavily weighted in favour of the latter that there would be little likelihood that approval or praise would develop strong secondary reinforcing properties" (Garmezy, 1966, pp.170-171). Secondly, Garmezy offered that schizophrenic shows strong resistance to extinction. This is because many of his prepsychotic responses have been both rewarded and punished simultaneously (learning theory approach will be discussed further later in this chapter). Garmezy's view is very much akin to those of Bateson's (1972) double-blind hypothesis and Laing's (1970) checkmate formulation which they have offered in explaining the origins of schizophrenic's avoidance behaviour. These hypotheses stipulate that there are communication problems between the child and his parents, especially between mother and her son. The communication problem is such that the son, who is dependent upon his mother for love and affection, is punished for both showing outward signs of love toward her and for not displaying such affection. These observations however, seem to lack credence because there is considerable disagreement in the literature about what constitutes a double-blind situation (Broen, 1968; Schuham, 1967). Be it, whatever it may, in the presentday society, especially in Indian set up it is evident that parents and more particularly mother because of their high expectations from their children (irrespective of basic potentiality the children's possess) create an atmosphere in the family which is similar to that of Bateson's double-blind situation. Such a situation makes child confused as to whether he is any more loveable to his mother. This in turn, makes the child feel embarrassed and afraid. Such feeling, no doubt, has deleterious effect onto the growth of positive mental health of the child. However, further research is necessary to (a) demonstrate whether families that foster schizophrenic children are in anyway unique in developing double-blind situation; and (b) to see whether mothers who place their children in such a family situation themselves possess schizophrenic trend ("Schizophrenogenic" mother, a primary initial concept given by Fromm-Reichman, 1948). If the answer to the latter question is in the affirmative, then question comes whether these mothers also transmit genetically schizophrenic predispositions to their children along with the behaviour they display.

Genetic Approach

Genetic research to find evidence for the inheritability of schizophrenia began as early as 1916. A review of earlier studies is available (Gottesman and Shields, 1982). Thereafter, in the 1920s studies on twin subjects began to establish compelling evidence for a genetic component in schizophrenia. These later studies compared the degree of concordance in monozygotic (MZ) twins (in which at least one of the twins affective) with the rate in dizygotic (DZ) twins and found a higher rate of concordance in the former (*i.e.* MZ) group of subjects. Since the concordance rates were less than 100% even in identical twins, it became clear that inheritance was not necessarily the only, single significant factor for schizophrenia. Further research on twin subjects confounded the heredity-environment issue which claims that not only the identical twins share the same genetic material, but their environment may also be more similar than that of the non-twins.

To resolve the heredity-environment issue, in the 1960s adoption studies (in which persons with similar genetic material are reared in different environments) began (Gottesman and Shields, 1982). In one such approach, adopted children of schizophrenics mothers were compared with children who remained with their schizophrenic mothers and results showed a similar rate of schizophrenia in both groups. This shows that environment itself may not be considered as single, significant factor in causing schizophrenia. Still later, family studies have been taken up (Gottesman and Shields, 1982) with the assumption that if genetic plays an important part in causing schizophrenia, then siblings should have higher rates of schizophrenia than is found in first cousins (varying degrees of similarity in genetic material). Results support the importance of a genetic component in the etiology of schizophrenia. However, mode of transmission could not be determined (Farone and Tsuang, 1985) from these studies.

For the transmission of schizophrenia, it is postulated that, a specific pair of genes is necessary. This approach is also known as the single-major-locus (Farone and Tsuang, 1985) model. However, to fit into the standard Mandellian pattern, this model requires restructuring (Farone and Tsuang, 1985). In contrast to this approach, there is multifactorial polygenic-threshold theory (Gottesman and Shields, 1982) which supports the family prevalence data in schizophrenia without considering the concept of single-locus for the critical gene pair. The latter approach hypothesizes that the genes at many different loci combine to produce a liability for schizophrenia (Gottesman, McGuffin, and Farmer, 1987). This model includes environmental factors as partially responsible for the development of schizophrenia. This view seems to run parallel with many other modern genetic theories which subscribe to a general "diathesis-stress" model (McCartney, 1989) in which the diathesis is a constitutional predisposition to the syndrome, and environmental events cause stress. The diathesis alone is not sufficient to produce the syndrome. To produce syndrome, stressful environmental events need to have interaction with the diathesis. This approach, according to some, has improved the heuristic value of genetic model (Strauss and Carpenter, 1981).

It has been evident from our personal research that stressful environmental events can produce psychopathological episodes (Chattopadhyay and Das, 1983). Stressful life events scale (Singh, Kaur and Kaur, 1981) was administered onto 20 drug free psychotics, 20 drug free neurotics, and 20 normal controls, and the findings revealed that significantly highest stress scores were noted in the neurotics compared to both the psychotics and normals. Neurotics had shown significantly higher than normal stress scores. These findings support previous research reports (*e.g.,* Paykel and Ulenhuth, 1972). However, novelty, unlike previous studies, which was revealed through the present study was that nature of stressful events was found to have relations with the nature of psychopathological reactions. Thus, our study revealed that neurotics showed significantly highest scores with regard to both recent and remote events, and that too, mostly concerning undesirable events in their life. Normals showed higher stress scores on desirable events only, whereas for the psychotics no such difference could be found with regard to recent – remote events, or desirable – undesirable events either.

However, the mechanism whereby stressful life events produce illness is presumably physiological (Kobasa, 1979) and hence, physiological measures should be incorporated to verify whether the stress originating from the desirable and undesirable events can cause any change in the organism and its subsequent manifestation of symptoms.

Biochemical Approach

The discoveries that various chemicals, *viz.*, LSD could produce hallucinations, and that hallucinogens bear some relation to brain neurotransmitters (*e.g.*, Osmond and Smythies, 1952) prompted researchers to postulate that neurotransmitters such as, dopamine, serotonin, and epinephrine could be held responsible for various mental disorders. Dopamine hypothesis is considered to be the most influential biochemical hypothesis of schizophrenia today. This hypothesis first appeared in 1983 (Carlson and Lindquist). It predicts that there is some hyperactivity along dopaminergic neuronal pathways in the CNS (Strauss and Carpenter, 1981). This hyperactivity is caused either due to the release of too much dopamine at the synapse (the hypersensitivity of the postsynaptic dopamine receptors), or due to other errors in the use of or inhibition of dopamine within the system (Crider, 1979). Most of the evidences for recent biochemical models are pharmacologic in nature, and dopamine hypothesis is no exception to it. This theory is derived primarily from the pharmacologic research evidences, that psychotic symptoms can be produced by dopamine agonists, and antipsychotic or antischizophrenic drugs can inhibit dopaminergic transmission (Strauss and Carpenter, 1981). Though pharmacologic research evidences have brought dopamine hypothesis to a limelight, from etiological point of view, a number of problems with this hypothesis are noted. First, the exact action of the antipsychotic drugs is not yet fully known. Second, whatever knowledge we have regarding their action that may not be enough to state that their action is as simple as the inhibition of dopaminergic transmission. On the other hand, they may even affect multiple areas of brain-operations (Strauss and Carpenter, 1981). Third, there is no direct evidence of dopaminergic system's hyperactivity (Crider, 1979), and the indirect peripheral measures (*viz.*, measuring chemicals in cerebrospinal fluid, C.S.F.) taken may not be valid (Haracz, 1982); also it is very difficult if not impossible to conduct very definite in vivo experiment with the gadgets till now available to the researchers. Fourth, Strauss and Carpenter (1981) reported that performing autopsies on the brains of schizophrenics is inadequate and as such the abnormalities noted may reflect changes related to schizophrenia but not causes of schizophrenia. Fifth, research evidences to document dopaminergic hypersensitivity have not been consistent (Haracz, 1982) throughout.

Of late, Seeman (1985) has reported evidence for an increased number of post-synaptic dopamine receptor in the brains of schizophrenic patients. Though some controversy has been raised over this issue as to whether such an increase could be an artefact of taking neuroleptic medication (MacKay, Bird, and Spokes, 1980), Seeman however, claims this findings unconfounded with the administration of neuroleptic drugs.

In our personal research on large number of drug free schizophrenic patients and matched normal controls we (Dasgupta, 1984; Dasgupta, Chattopadhyay and Ghosh, 1983) have found that schizophrenics had a significantly higher level of Plasma Cortisol than those of the normals. Normals were subdivided into three groups (*viz.*, low, medium, and high anxious) and patients showed higher level of cortisol compared to all three groups of subjects, and more so when the patients were compared with the low anxious normals. All these patients were outpatients of local medical colleges and hospitals of Kolkata, Eastern India. However, on Prolactin measure, the schizophrenics were found to have a lower score than the normals. Though Prolactin and Cortisol both are stress hormones, a reversed picture in the finding (*i.e.,* lower prolactin in schizophrenics) could probably be because of the fact that there was a balance between stress induced stimulation of serotonine and dopamine induced inhibition of secretion (Meltezer, Sacher, and Frantz, 1974). That is, in spite of presence of higher level of anxiety in the schizophrenic patients, excessive dopaminergic transmission (which is undoubtedly a prolactin inhibitory factor) from the limbic and nigro-striatal systems has probably suppressed the level of prolactin amongst the schizophrenic patients. Similar findings were also obtained by others before (Rotrosen, Angrist, Clark, Gershon, Halpern, and Sacher, 1978; Gruen, Sacher, Altman, Langer, Tabrizi and Halpern, 1978).

Neurophysiological Approach

A good number of research reports are available which claim that schizophrenic subjects are different from control subjects on many of the neurophysiologcial measures, *viz.,* electroencephalogram's (E.E.G.s) evoked potentials, eye-movements, and other related measures of arousal (*e.g.,* James and Barry, 1980). Likewise measures of cardio-vascular activity, namely, heart rate, heart rate responsivity, vasomotor responses and respiratory activity claim differences between schizophrenic children and normal controls. These findings led James and Barry to conclude that psychotic children have a neurophysiological hyperactivity to stimulation compared to normal control subjects. Holtzman (1987) reported that schizophrenic subjects appear to suffer from a generalised deficit on psychophysiological measures (*e.g.,* electrodermal responsiveness) compared to normal subjects. However, considering the impact of these findings in understanding the complexity of the syndrome involved, it appears that the findings are not consistent and far from conclusive. The reasons for such inconsistent findings in the literature could probably be because of lack of adequate control (*e.g.,* failure to employ standardised recording procedure, limited reporting of medication regiments, and failure to include appropriate controls groups) in conducting such experiments.

Information processing theories are closely related to neurophysiological theories. Since these have already been mentioned in stimulus-responses approach, need not be repeated here.

Learning Theory Approach

The basic tenets of the stimulus-response approach have just been mentioned above by noting how the concepts of need and drive, reward and punishment operate in the acquisition of schizophrenic avoidance behaviour. Here let us confine our comments to examine as to whether this approach can act as a rapprochement between the systems of traditional psychoanalysis and recent learning models.

Psychoanalytic theory postulates that schizophrenic person has a weak ego (Bellack, 1970) which mediates the environment and the Id and superego by developing defense mechanisms (Robinson and Robinson, 1965). Some such defenses are denial, repression, isolation, projection, sublimation, and reaction formation. The ego defenses in schizophrenics may be weak. This leads to disturbed ego functions and loss of contact with reality as is manifested through inadequate reality testing, impaired judgement and inaccurate regulation and control of desires, emotions, and so on (Bellack, 1970).

Learning theories postulate that all behavioural expressions, healthy or maladaptive, are learned or represent distortions or deficits in the learning process of the individual. Therefore, such behaviours are subject to modification through processes which extinguish the original learning experiences and lead to the establishment of a more effective behavioural responses (Pavlov, Watson, Thorndike, Hull, Skinner, Bandura, Krashner, Lazarus, Ullman, Wolfe, and Eysenck). In the present context one of the early etiological theories of schizophrenia was formulated by Adolph Meyer (1944) who proposed that schizophrenia is the result of learning increasingly abnormal behaviours. Later, others also have proposed this operation or dysfunction of basic learning mechanisms in the genesis of schizophrenia using the concepts like, failure to develop appropriate secondary reinforcers, direct reinforcement of deviant patterns of behaviour modelled by parents, and so on. Ferster (1961), for example suggested that the lack of parental responsiveness retards the development of the conditioned reinforcers and generalised reinforcers necessary for the development of more complex behaviour pattern. Thus *e.g.*, parent's failure to respond to, or inconsistent responses either is likely to weaken the child's appropriate social behaviour. This is mostly found in such families where parent(s) are ill, depressed, or otherwise preoccupied. If this lack of responsiveness is pervasive enough, no wonder that, the child may show even total extinction of some appropriate behaviour (*e.g.*, social interaction). Thus, much of the bizarre behaviour of the schizophrenic patients is conceptualised as the result of his lack of exposure to these stimuli which normals attend to. As a result the patient responds to such stimuli unexpectedly and his behaviour turns out to be inappropriate. Thus, *e.g.*, apathy, which is often seen in the behaviour of some schizophrenic patients may result from their failure to react to stimuli which others find important (Ullmann and Krasner, 1969a,b). Another basic deficit in the behaviour of schizophrenic patients is their inattentiveness to social stimuli. This is also conceptualised as resulting from their experiences with the environment. Appropriate behaviour is viewed as an operant behaviour and this has been extinguished through the interaction process of the schizophrenic individual with his environment.

The main criticism of Ferster's (1961) approach is that it is descriptive in nature. Of course, in a latter study Ferster and Demyer (1962) demonstrated that autistic children respond to techniques (applied to them for therapy) based on learning principles.

Because of its emphasis on individualized treatment the behavioural approach has been criticized for being "excessively individualistic, low in cost effectiveness, and too narrow in the range of behavioural change that are obtained across situations" (Kanfer, 1985, p. 9).

In reply to the critiques it has been reported that "individualistic" approach is of course important considering the fact that even between schizophrenic and autistic individuals there are highly variable characteristics, which can not be ignored. Secondly, certain other major advantages of the behavioural approach, some of which relate to these criticisms have been put forward, and for a detailed account the reader is referred to Johnson and Koegel (1982).

A major weakness of psychoanalytic theory is its inferential, retrospective method. Moreover, many of the concepts, especially these concerning infants and young children, are difficult to test empirically and therefore, must be considered speculative in nature. Also, many of these concepts are inconsistent with well-established notions concerning early cognitive development (Shapiro, 1981). Again, traditional approach assumes common histories and similar developmental causes for all individuals; it gives some diagnosis regardless of the fact that behavioural manifestations of the disorder for each individual may differ. Thus, it appears that the diagnosis rather than specific behaviours, determine the focus of treatment (Kanfer, 1985; Johnson and Koegel, 1982; Schreibman and Koegel, 1980).

Traditional psychoanalytic model and recent learning theory model have certain points of convergence rather than divergence only. Both these models consider infancy or early childhood as the most crucial period of life, since the disturbance is likely to be formed during this phase. Secondly, learning theories seem to have commonness with psychodynamic and family parenting theories in that they often imply that the most significant factor in the genesis of the disorder is the parent-child interaction. Thirdly, it is common in most psychoanalytically oriented theories that the basis of the disturbance is formed in infancy or early childhood through environmental, especially parental – child interaction. If disturbances are formed through interaction, as the psychoanalysts claim, then such formation of behaviour can be taken as an outcome of environmental learning which facilitates in shaping a particular habit pattern. This is so stated because, psychoanalysts also claim that when stresses occur later in life, *i.e.*, during adolescence and young adulthood in schizophrenia, the individual regresses to the early stage of development. What prompts the individual to regress? The answer is – his past experience of lesser stress (pleasure in that particular phase of the development) where the individual felt relatively more comfort. This very tendency to regress once again proves that the individual retained in his mind the past pleasureful experience and his encounterment with a stressful environment later in life prompts him to regress. Such retention of past experience may be considered as effect of learning, which behavioursits also claim.

An Attempt at Synthesis

From the above discussion, it is clear that there have been numerous trends in the relative influence of biological versus psychological factors in schizophrenia. As a result there have been a massive but diverse literature which is difficult to integrate, and as such attempt to draw conclusions is challenging. However, based on two basic types of factors – the biological (*e.g.*, genetics) and the socio-psycho-environmental (*e.g.*, learning) – two major components of vulnerability / susceptibility may be proposed; inborn and acquired (Zubin and Spring, 1977). The variables that contribute to the former components are – neurophysiological in nature whereas those contribute to the latter components are pre- and perinatal trauma, disease, family experiences etc. The combined contribution of the two factors (*i.e.,* inborn and acquired) determine the degree of vulnerability / susceptibility. Every individual has some degree of vulnerability, and under appropriate conditions he/ she may manifest schizophrenia (Zubin and Spring, 1977). By appropriate conditions is meant occurrence of a crisis event and a given individual's threshold to tolerate the crisis. In other words, schizophrenia is triggered when an event produces a crisis to the individual so much so that the intensity of the crisis exceeds the individual's vulnerability threshold. Thus an individual who has had received enough stimulation from inborn and/or acquired factors is likely to experience an episode of schizophrenia when exposed to critical life events. Such an individual is considered of having low vulnerability threshold. An individual, on the contrary, with fewer contributing in born and/or acquired factors may be considered as individual with high vulnerability, threshold. Almost similar to the "vulnerability" concept of Zubin and Spring (1977), Mednick (1970) proposed a concept of "High-risk" children for schizophrenia.

In Copenhagen, Denmark, Mednick and Schulsinger (1973) in a prospective and longitudinal study intensively examined 207 normally functioning children of chronic and severely schizophrenic mothers. They also examined 104 controls and followed them up for about 20-25 years. They found that a good number of high-risk children had suffered from severe psychiatric breakdown.

In another study, Mednick and Schulsinger (1968a,b) reported that children who later suffer from psychiatric breakdown 70% of them suffered one or more serous pregnancy or birth complications (PBC). The PBCs included anoxia, prematurity, prolonged labour, placental difficulty, umbilical cord complications, mother's illness during pregnancy, multiple births, and breech presentation. Researchers have singled out particular brain structure as being "Selectively vulnerable" to the effects of anoxia. Most prominently these areas include, the hippocampus, the amygdala, and the Purkinje cells of the cerebellum. Of these, however, hippocampus has been singled out as the most vulnerable area (Spector, 1965). Spector evaluated the effects of anoxia by studying "biochemical lesions", *i.e.,* "the initial chemical changes in tissues following the application of harmful agents and preceding anatomical evidence of the damage (p.552)". The chemical changes as a function of anoxia, he noted, have been losses in certain enzymes which precede "histological evidence of cell injury by approximately 10 h (hours). It is noteworthy that chemical changes appeared in the hippocampus immediately after anoxia, whilst the other areas showed earliest loss of enzymes after 1-6 h (p.552)." Friede (1966) also reported a similar research evidence indicating hippocampus as the most selectively vulnerable area.

By applying psychophysiological measures Mednick and Schulsinger and others (1977) noted a marked correspondence between PBCs and the anomalous electrodermal response pattern. This suggests that PBCs trigger some characteristics that may be genetically predisposed. The PBCs seem to damage the modulatory control of the organism's stress – response mechanisms. These are characterised by rapid response onset, poor habituation of the Galvanic skin response (GSR), poor extinction of the conditioned electrodermal response, and very rapid (GSR) recovery. This pattern of poor autonomic nervous system's modulation may be considered as a significant etiological factor in the development of mental illness in general, and schizophrenia in particular.

The theories propounded by Zubin and Spring (1977), Strauss and Carpenter (1981) on the contrary, reflect a shift from that of biological approach to a psychological approach. They opined that an exclusively biological approach does not seem to be totally successful in explaining the genesis of and/or behaviours in schizophrenia. There is strong evidence for the influence of psychological factors as well. Such controversy in the literature has currently stimulated research with a multidimensional approach to the problem. Thus, *e.g.*, Zubin and Spring (1977), and Zubin and Steinhaurt (1981) attempted to establish some vulnerability "markers" in schizophrenia. Markers are defined as trait characteristics of schizophrenic or pre-schizophrenic persons, indicating their degree of vulnerability. The "Markers" would be dopamine levels, from the biochemical sphere, EEG evoked potentials and GSRs from neurophysiological sphere, and acquisition abnormalities from learning theory approach, and so on.

6 CHAPTER

Aetiology

Schizophrenia, under one name or another, has been known to us for several years but as yet, hardly one finds any agreement amongst researchers in formulation on the etiology of the illness. Nevertheless, uncertainty and vaguences in formulation of its etiology can be said to be relatively less today. This is because recent research evidences have made available to us many cues and scientifically sound evidences which lend support to various hints than there was when Kraepelin first drew attention around dementia praecox. Based on the available literature one can formulate its etiology under the broad headings of genetic, biological, psychological, and sociocultural.

Genetic Factors

Kraepelin and Bleuler both believed that a genetic background was a necessary condition to produce schizophrenia. Evidence from numerous twin studies carried out in China, Japan, Scandinavian countries, Great Britain, and the United States provides support to the view that monozygotic (MZ) twins are found to be concordant for schizophrenia about four times as often as dizygotic (DZ) twins.

The most impressive evidence which demonstrates the influence of genetic factor is the statistical data of Kallmann (1946) obtained from the extensive study on twins. Kallmann's observation may be summarised as follows : (a) if both the parents are schizophrenics, their offsprings are likely to develop schizophrenia 68 times more than the offsprings of normal parents. In a later study Kallmann and his associates (Kallmann, Falek, Hurzeler, and Erlenmeyer-Kibling, 1964), however, reported that this figure may range from 40-71 times more instead of 68 times; (b) if one parent is schizophrenic, the risk of the child for developing schizophrenia is over 16 times more than that of a normal union; (c) the closer the blood relationship, the higher is the incidence of schizophrenia in relatives of a schizophrenia. In case of MZ twins this incidence was found to be as high as 86% in Kallmann's report. In sum, Kallmann concluded that there exists a genetic predisposition to schizophrenia. Several other investigators tend to agree (Slater, 1947; Stormgren, 1948; Hurst, 1951; Book,

1953) with Kallmann. On the other hand, genetic studies have been criticized by several authors on statistical and methodological grounds. Thus, *e.g.*, Pastore (1949) raised objections to Kallmann's statistical analysis technique, while Bellak (1948) was of the opinion that the selection of patients for this study was biased. Likewise, an objection to the overall validity of twin studies as well as to the accuracy of diagnostic methods was raised by Jackson (1960). Also, it has been pointed out that twin studies lack information on the early biological and family experiences of the twins (Kolb, 1973). Furthermore, these studies have ignored altogether the role of psychodynamic forces in twin development. Of course in reply to this objection one might say that in their writings both Kraepelin and Bleuler mentioned about psychological factors and their role in producing schizophrenia. But the spirit of their statements show that both of them believed that there is a genetic background which may interact with subsequent psychological factors to produce schizophrenia. In other words, psychological factors may only act as precipitating factors provided there is a genetic predisposition in the individual. But this, however, is not the case throughout.

Eugene Bleuler though rejected the notion that schizophrenia could have psychological origins, did believe that manifest content of schizophrenic thinking could be understood in terms of Freudian theory. He coined the term Autism (Bleuler, 1913) which he conceptualised as a form of schizophrenic thinking characterised by the individual's creating a world of fantasy. Silvano Arieti (Arieti, 1959) carried this notion one step further and proposed that the schizophrenic's "inability to make things unconscious" is one of the important characteristics of this psychosis (p.457). Freud (1896) said that projection played an important part in this disorder and postulated that the schizophrenic withdraws his libido from external objects and redirects his energy into the ego or self (1914).

As opposed to Kraepelin and Bleuler, Sullivan (1953, 1956) opined that schizophrenia is an indirect result of faulty interpersonal relations between the child and the parents. Especially crucial in this interaction is the anxiety which the child picks up from his mother through the process of empathy. This anxiety is distressing and may lead to ineffective behaviour, namely, the schizophrenic's avoiding persons and situations that evoke it. Such avoidance, in turn, prohibits the establishment of interpersonal responses that for most people serve to eliminate anxiety. Consequently, such persons withdraw even further their contact with others in the society and resorts to the personal interpretation of reality. This is what Sullivan called 'Parataxic Distortions'. Such misinterpretations of reality lose consensual validity in the sense that such patients report that others now fail to recognize or understand his language and thought.

Based on case-history studies of schizophrenic families Laing (1970) has given a more recent psychodynamic formulation, which can best be described as humanistic – existential approach. His theory does not consider schizophrenia a biochemical, neuro-physiological or psychological phenomenon (Laing and Esterson, 1970). He, on the contrary raised the question of whether the experience and behaviour that psychiatrists called schizophrenia can best be understood as a socially intelligible phenomenon (Kleinmuntz, 1974). The following is an example of his belief in an interpersonal view of schizophrenia. "If one look at some experience and behaviour without reference to family interaction, they may appear comparatively socially senseless, but that if we look at the same experience and behaviour in their original family context they are liable to make more sense" (Laing and Esterson, 1970, p.12). Thus according to Laing the experience and behaviour that is called "Schizophrenia is a special strategy that a person invents in order to live in an unlivable situation" (Laing, 1967, p.115). He called this the person's 'position of checkmate', a state of affairs that is not likely to be perceived as such by someone in it. Thus, Laing emphasized that the social system within which such persons are brought up must be the object of study if one wants to understand schizophrenia well. In sum, psychodynamic formulations of schizophrenia is an indirect result of faulty interpersonal relations and atypical social situations in which such individuals are brought up.

One could argue that the difference in the occurrence of this illness between MZ and DZ twins could be accounted for by taking in view the fact that certain special environmental factors are found to be related to MZ twins and not to DZs. For example, in the course of psychological development the former may be more liable to confusion of identity and weak ego formation (Hamilton, 1976). But based on the studies of MZ twins reared apart Shields and Slater (1967) failed to support the aforesaid argument in favour of special environmental factors. Sixteen of such pairs have been investigated and the concordance rate in them was found to be 62.5% which, according to these authors was of the same order as that of MZ twins brought up together. In studies, *e.g.,* those of Incuye in Japan (Kolb, 1973), where culture itself dictates that twins be separated and one be reared by someone else than the mother, the frequency of occurrence of schizophrenia was found to be higher in both the MZ twins than in DZ twins reared separately from birth. These findings, therefore, reject the influence of environmental factors and support the influence of genetic factors. Again, studies reporting occurrence of schizophrenia in cases of adoption adds a further support to the view that schizophrenia is genetically determined. Thus *e.g.,* Kety, Rosenthal, Wender, and Schulsinger (1968) looked into the prevalence of mental illness in the biological and adoptive families of adopted schizophrenics. They reported that the adopted children who became schizophrenic, their biological relatives (with whom the children have had even minimum contact) had shown an increased risk of developing schizophrenia as compared with the general population, and not the adoptive relatives. Comparing the extent of mental illness among the parents of schizophrenics with the parents of neurotics, Alanen (1966) found that the former group was significantly worse. Based on these findings it could be argued that if schizophrenia is psychologically and sociologically transmitted, then the adoptive parents of schizophrenia would show a large amount of mental illness, but if it were genetically transmitted they would not. Also, one could argue further that if child-rearing practices are important in the development of schizophrenia then the characteristics of the biological/primary parents of schizophrenics would be found in the adopted parents of schizophrenics. To verify this Wender, Rosenthal, and Kety (1968) and Wender, Rosenthal, Zahn, and Kety (1971) investigated 10 couples whose adopted children had become schizophrenics, 10 couples (biological) whose child had become schizophrenics, and 10 couples whose adopted child was found to be normal. They rated these parents on a graded scale ranging from 1 (normal) to 3 (mild character neurosis), and Grade 6 (Border Line Schizophrenia) to Grade 7 (Schizophrenia). They found that the mean grade for the parents in the first group was 3.3 for the fathers and 3.5 for the mothers, while for the second group it was 4.2 and 4.9 and for the third group 2.6 and 3.0 respectively. This shows that the biological parents of schizophrenics had the largest score for abnormality, the adoptive parents of normals had least, while the adoptive parents of schizophrenics fell in-between. Difference between the biological and adoptive parents of schizophrenics was significant statistically, but not between the adoptive parents of schizophrenics and those of normal children. These findings, no doubt are very important but certain methodological limitations were apparent in these investigations. Thus, the sampling of cases was not systematic, the interviewers knew to which group the parents belonged. Furthermore, the authors themselves pointed out that the parents of schizophrenics were found to be frank and outspoken, while the others were guarded during the interview. Heston (1970) suggested that since 45% of the siblings, children, and parents of schizophrenics are found to be either schizoid or schizophrenic, in genetic research on schizophrenia schizoid (but non-psychotic) persons also must be included. He opined that due to defect in a single autosomal dominant gene, about 4% of the general population will be affected by the schizoid – schizophrenic personality complex. The majority of geneticists have given a support to the view that genetic transmission of predisposition to schizophrenia is polygenic. Chen, Hung, Wei, and Koong (2001) hypothesized that since polymorphic activities of debrisoquine and hydroxylase (cyP2D6) were suggested to be associated with some complex diseases like Parkinson's disease, and schizophrenia being a complex disorder, it may be that cyP2D6 gene is a susceptibility gene for patients with schizophrenia. The study was conducted on 162 Chinese patients with schizophrenia and 94 non-psychotic control subjects from Taiwan. The authors suggested that cyP2D6 gene may not be a susceptibility gene in Chinese patients with schizophrenia. Likewise, Shibata, Joo, Fjujii, Tani, Makino, Hirata, Kikuta *et al.* (2001) in a study on large number of genotyped Japanese samples of schizophrenia (n = 193 – 203) and healthy controls (n = 199 – 215) found that polymorphisms in the GluR5 Kainate receptor gene (GRIKI) did not play a major role in the schizophrenia pathogenesis of the Japanese population. Though the genetic contribution to schizophrenia has been accepted by many authors, the manner in which that contribution is expressed in the biological make-up of the individual remains as yet unknown.

Biological Predisposition

This will be discussed under three main headings: (a) Constitutional, (b) Psycho-physiological, and (c) Neurobiological or neurohormonal factors.

(a) **Constitutional**. Some authors are of the opinion that constitutional weaknesses exist in this illness. This they suggest based on the data which indicate that schizophrenic mothers have a higher incidence of deviant fetal growth in-terms of perinatal mortality and malformation in the newborn when compared to mothers from the general population (Kolb, 1973). A majority of children considered to have childhood schizophrenia show indications of delayed or uneven functioning of their motor, postural, sensoriperceptual and conceptual performances. In this context Bender (1953) mentioned that schizophrenia in childhood results from "a developmental lag of the biological processes from which subsequent behaviour evolves by maturation at an embryological level, leading to anxiety and secondarily to neurotic defense mechanisms". According to her, the fundamental pathological process in it is a diffuse encephalopathy, but no anatomical evidence confirming this has been described (Kolb, 1973). Secondly, whether these physical and psychological impairments mentioned above are due to delayed maturation as a consequence of a defect in genetic endowment or to unrecognised brain damaged in early childhood has yet to be ascertained. Thirdly, there exists doubt as to whether clinicians in general would agree to include all children showing such defects under the heading schizophrenic reactions. Fourthly, it is a matter of controversy whether childhood schizophrenia is the same as adult schizophrenia, or whether it is a reactive pattern in which reaction is particularly to a cold emotional climate in the home which the child experiences during the first two years of life. Bender (1953) opined that childhood schizophrenia is not a separate and distinct clinical entity, rather it is a group of related and overlapping clinical syndromes.

Of late, some Indian researchers, *e.g.,* Tripathi and Jahan (2004) have taken interest to demonstrate that if criminality as a predisposition is present in the schizophrenic patients, whether that would cause any difference in behavioural manifestation of symptoms of patients with schizophrenia in comparison to those patients who do not show any criminal records. In this study, two groups of schizophrenic patients were investigated of which 30 patients were with criminal record and 30 without criminal record. Mean age of both the groups was 34.36 (± 2.84) years and 35.46 (± 2.87) years respectively. Mean duration of stay in the jail for the convicted group of patients was 4.9 (± 2.6) years. Schizophrenics with criminal record were found to be significantly more dissocial, impulsive in comparison to non-offenders, a finding which provides support to previous research reports obtained on both the patients of the Indian culture (Sethi, Gupta, Raj and Nathawat, 1971) as well as on the patients of the West (Eysenck and McGurk, 1980). However, this study goes contrary to many others (*e.g.,* Sethi *et al,* 1971; Rahman, 1992) who reported that schizophrenics, with criminal record have typical personality characteristics of criminals of which extraversion was found to be a character feature of criminals. However, in Tripathi and Jahan's (2004) study, maximum number of patients were paranoid in both Group I (77%) and Group II (57%). Most of the patients without criminal record had insidious onset (88.33%) and deteriorating progress (66.67%) whereas patients with criminal history all had insidious onset and fluctuating (60%) progress. Furthermore no informant was available for detailed information about premorbid personality of the patients with criminal records (as they were accompanied by jail escorts), and sex distribution of the patients in both the groups was not known. Majority of the patients of both the groups were residents of rural area only. Hence, further studies are needed to have an insight into personality characteristics and involvement in criminal activities of the patients with schizophrenia.

(b) Psychophysiological. The earliest psychophysiological studies of schizophrenia were largely devoted to identify reliable differences between non-psychotic patients and schizophrenics in their nervous system activity. In these studies the nervous system in choice was typically the ANS, and activities of the ANS measured were both tonic and phasic. At this stage it was largely an inference drawn by the clinicians from their observations of the pupillary dilatations and vasomotor phenomena of the extremities mostly seen in some catatonics with coldness and cyanosis of limbs (Kolb, 1973). Likewise, Maricq (1969) reported that there is an abnormal subpupillary capillary plexus clearly visible in the nailfolds of schizophrenics. But later on, instead of employing observation as a method of study, researchers have done experiments where several ANS functions (both tonic and phasic) of schizophrenics have been measured employing bioelectrical recording devices. The reader, in this context is referred to Lang and Buss (1965) for a critical and comprehensive review of the literature.

`In 1960s studies of psychophysiology in schizophrenia were predominantly concerned with such constructs as "arousal or activation", and "attention". The former is typically indexed by tonic levels of ANS activity whereas the latter is indexed by phasic response and by behaviour. Some researcher integrated these constructs in models of mechanisms underlying psychopathology. Thus, *e.g.,* Venables (1964) opined that there is a bimodally disturbed input dysfunction in schizophrenia. Chronic non-paranoid schizophrenic patients with poor premorbid personality are thought to be hyperaroused, and acute paranoid schizophrenics with good premorbid personality are thought to be hypoaroused. Hyperarousal is indexed through elevated levels of skin conductance or heart rate, whereas hypoarousal is indexed through abnormally low levels or skin conductance or heart rate. These two abnormal arousal states were considered to be linked to aberrant attentional response. Venables and his associates (Venables and Martin, 1964; Venables and Christie, 1974) have made significant methodological and theoretical contributions to the investigation of physiological mechanisms controlling skin conductance. Most of the studies have used some variants of the orienting response (OR) to elicit the phasic skin conductance (SC) change. Thus, latency, rise time, amplitude, and 50% recovery, and number of responses given by a patient before habituation (cessation of response) occurs are some such separate components which are usually recorded from each response in the orienting series (Chattopadhyay and Biswas, 1983). Also some investigators change the stimulus intensity to observe the reappearance of the CR (called dishabituation). Another approach has been to alter the significance that the stimulus holds for the subject (Bernstein, 1968, 1969, 1970; Bernstein and Taylor, 1978).

Following the pioneering work of Bagshaw, Kimble and Pribram (1965), Bagshaw and Benzies (1968), and Bagshaw and Kimble (1972) who demonstrated that amygdalectomized monkeys were found to produce hyporesponsive electrodermal records, whereas hippocampectomized monkeys showed hyper responsive record. Gruzelier and Venables (1972, 1973) were the first to apply this concept onto human subjects, *viz.,* schizophrenics, and claimed that a good number of adult schizophrenics failed to produce SCORs. Accordingly, the latter authors designated the hyporesponsive schizophrenics as 'nonresponders' and the hyperresponsive as, 'non-habituators'. Gruzelier and Venables (1972, 1973) showed that approximately 50% of the patients population, they studied, produced no responses (non-responses) and the remaining 50% did not habituate (non-habituators) the orienting response. Zahn (1976) on the contrary, failed to demonstrate "bimodality" in his schizophrenic patients so clearly as that displayed by the patients of Gruzelier and Venables. However, they agreed to a point that "non responders" are more frequently seen in adult psychotics (as much as 50%) compared to normal subjects (may be 10% or even less).

Modifying the Limbic hypothesis (amygdala was considered an excitatory body and the hippocampus an inhibitory body and excitation/inhibition balance of behaviour is a function of the reciprocity of the two) advocated by Bagshaw and associates and subsequently followed by Gruzelier and Venables, Fonberg later (1972) suggested that other reciprocities are incidence in the limbic system besides hippocampal/amygdala reciprocity. Again, Douglass (1972) showed that every effect that could be obtained due to hippocampal lesion, the same effect could be obtained by depletion of brain acetylcholine. Douglass also demonstrated that there is no brain structure more cholinergic than the hippocampus.

Mednick and his associates (Mednick and Schulsinger, 1968a,b; Mednick, 1970; Mednick, Schulsinger, Teasdale *et al.*, 1977) from their longitudinal studies on high-risk children in Denmark reported that these children show longer latency and higher ANS reactivity on the SC tracings. Later on Venables (1975a,b) took great interest in SC recovery score (especially, 50% recovery) and reported that it is perhaps the only known measurable event that appears to be helpful in predicting schizophrenia in high-risk prepsychotic children. According to Venables fast SC recovery which characterized high-risk children (*i.e.,* children who were found to breakdown in later life) indicates their exceptional "Openness" to environmental stimulation. This, he hypothesized, perhaps leads to a condition of "sensory flooding", seen in schizophrenic patients. Hare (1972, 1973) by contrast, was of the opinion that exceptionally long 50% recovery time is indicative of a mental status of the subjects which could be described to be "closed off" from environmental stimulation. However, unlike Venables, Mednick *et al.* presented data obtained on psychopaths.

Employing standard methods of recording (Chattopadhyay, Bond, and Lader, 1975; Chattopadhyay, Cooke, Toone, and Lader, 1980) SC tracings we (Chattopadhyay and Biswas, 1983) have measured different characteristics of GSR in psychotic patients in India. Recovery time in our study was considered to be the time from the GSR maximum to the point of 50% recovery (Edelberg, 1970) to the level just prior to the GSR. This variable of GSR was thus computed trigonometrically from the recovery angle and the amplitude of the response. Significantly shorter half-recovery time was noted in the schizophrenics (Biswas, 1983) compared to the matched normal controls. The half-recovery time noted in this study was even shorter than the range of half-recovery time (*i.e.,* 1.00 to 1.50 second) reported by Venables and Christie (1980) in normal individuals. In our study (Biswas, 1983) 30 (17 male) schizophrenics (unclassified and untreated) in the age range of 19 to 32 years (mean age 27 years) and with duration of illness about 6 months were investigated. These findings confirm earlier studies (Ax and Bamford, 1970; Gruzelier, 1973; Gruzelier and Venables, 1972; Mednick and Schulsinger, 1974a,b). Faster recovery time in schizophrenics may be indicative of loss of hippocampal inhibitory functioning (Gruzelier and Venables, 1972). If it indicates loss of hippocampal inhibitory functioning then one would expect shorter recovery time to be associated with shorter latency, steeper rise angle, longer amplitude, and steeper recovery angle, and Biswas's findings were in the expected direction supporting previous research reports (Lockhart and Liberman, 1979). Biswas (1983) again compared these findings with those he obtained on matched group of anxious and depressed patients and found that schizophrenics showed significant difference with both these groups of patients throughout. Not only in SC measure, in Finger Pulse Volume and Pulse Rate also Biswas (1983) obtained a similar trend of results as that noted on the SC. However, Biswas did emphasize about the importance of latency and recovery time as index measures in differentiating objectively schizophrenic patients from normals and from other psychiatric patients.

Regarding SC response habituation in schizophrenic patients controversial findings have been reported in the literature. That is, research reports depicting slower than normal rate of habituation (*e.g.,* Gruzelier and Venables, 1972; Zahn, Rosenthal, and Lawlor, 1968), within the normal range of habituation (*e.g.,* Patterson, 1976a, 1976b; Patterson and Venables, 1978; Thayer and Silber, 1971) and failure to reach a point of habituation (*e.g.,* Ax, Bamford, Beckett, Feitz, and Gottlieb, 1970) have been available to us. Methodological differences and procedural differences noted in these studies may be attributed to account for such diversity in the findings reported. These factors have been explored by different researchers over the past decades. Thus, *e.g.,* modality of stimulus used and duration of interstimulus interval maintained varied largely from one study to the other. Some authors have mixed up both drug and non-drug patients together and in some other studies sub-classification of schizophrenia was largely ignored. However, some of the later studies have obtained a definite trend of response habituation in schizophrenics by dividing them as 'paranoid', and 'non-paranoid' (Horvath and Meares, 1979). While the former habituated normally but the latter failed to habituate. Likewise, Venables (1975a,b), emphasized the necessity of detecting 'responders' and 'non-responders', and 'habituators', and 'non-habituators' (Gruzelier, 1973) in this type of research. Recently in an Indian study Roy (1981) sub-classifying the schizophrenics into simple, catatonia, hebephrenia, and paranoid reported that in GSR response habituation slopes faster response decrement was evident in hebephrenic group, and least in the paranoids, then came simple and next catatonics in hierarchical position. Thus, there is difference in the GSR response habituation trends amongst the schizophrenics of the East and the West.

Researchers agree to the fact that there is a great need to standardise these recording techniques. Also to account for such disparity in findings one has to rule out the possibilities of contamination of the findings due to drug intervention. In this connection as early as 1977 Spohn, Lacoursiers, Thompson and Coyne reported that phenothiazines reduced SC responses in chronic schizophrenics. However, Gruzelier (1978) failed to support Spohn *et al.* (1977), For a detailed review the reader is referred to Claridge (1978). Again, Frith, Stevens, Johnstone, and Crow (1979) claimed that phenothiazines are effective in bringing change in SC response habituation trend. They demonstrated that of the acute schizophrenic patients, habituators show a positive response to drug treatment, while non-habituators did not. By contrast, Spohn *et al.* (1977) presented data which suggest that SC response amplitude had no relation to response to treatment and to drug withdrawal in schizophrenia. However, the main problem in this type of research is to find an adequate control population for schizophrenia on daily doses of drug. To find such a control is rather next to impossible for obvious reasons. To obviate such problem one may go for recording each patient's SC response components at the pre-treatment level (self control) and to compare the same when the patient is on drug. Applying this method of control, we have found that chlorpromazine helped acute Indian schizophrenics to show a quicker SC response habituation compared to their pre-treatment habituation scores (Roy, 1984). This however, does not answer the question of drug effects in chronic schizophrenics. Researchers should take interest to look for possible differential effects of these drugs on schizophrenic patients and to compare the same with other phenothiazine compounds.

Douglass (1972) and Warburton (1972) suggested that SC orientation reaction (OR) habituation could be a function of highly variable neurochemical parameters (*e.g.,* neurotransmitters). One way to investigate such a theory would be to combine SC recording with other electrophysiological recordings for which the neurochemical innervation is fairly known.

Not much work has been done on neurochemical mechanisms of SC. Early research reports (*e.g.,* Venables and Martin, 1964) suggest cholinergic innervation of the eccrine sweat glands in SC. Since the eccrine gland innervation in acetylcholine, and pupil constriction is also controlled by acetylcholine, pupilographic relationship to both SC recovery (Patterson, 1976a) and SC responding/non-responding (Patterson, 1976b) have been worked out. Non-responder schizophrenics showed hyporesponsive pupils in the light/dark reflex. Also fast SC recovery was linked with very slow pupil constriction and vice versa. Gross attentional disturbances in schizophrenia may be attributed to acetylcholine abnormality in them (Sherwood, 1955; Warburton, 1972) as acetylcholine is central to maintenance of attention (Warburton, 1972). Accordingly, recent trend has been to attribute schizophrenic symptomatology to altered states of dopamine and thus haloperidol efficacy as a pharmacological aid in the treatment of schizophrenia. For a detailed account of dopamine / acetylcholine balance in schizophrenia reader may wish to refer Davis (1975). To explore the possible effects of medication on various components of SC response the interested readers are referred to Claridge (1978) and Gruzelier (1978).

With a view to assess cardiovascular activity of schizophrenia a variety of such variables, *viz.,* blood pressure (BP), peripheral blood flow, peripheral vascular resistance, pulse rate, and heart rate (HR) have been employed. In India, Mishra and Sharma (1995) found higher HR and diastolic BP in schizophrenia (n=138) compared to normals and 1st degree relatives of schizophrenia. Also, in the West, Lang and Buss (1965) reported that schizophrenics are hyperaroused. There is strong evidence that HR tonic level in medicated schizophrenics is elevated compared to normal controls (Fenz and Velner, 1970; Spohn, Thetford, and

Cancrow, 1971; Zahn, Rosenthal and Lawlor, 1968; Tarrier, Cooke and Lader, 1978; Gruzelier and Venables, 1975). Such an elevated HR level in schizophrenics may be viewed as an outcome of application of defence on their part against environmental stimulation, a viewpoint opined by Venables while interpreting SC fast recovery in high-risk children. Venables viewed this as a reflection of their susceptibility to "sensory flooding" (Venables, 1975a,b). Accordingly elevated HR in high-risk children may reflect an attentional defense on their part against environmental overflow of information. Gruzelier and Venables (1975a,b) reported that on Cardiovascular variables, *viz.,* PP and HR a significantly greater level of arousal was noted in the SC OR responders than those of the non-responders. However, both these groups were receiving the same type and average daily dosage level of antipsychotic drugs at the time of experimentation. Tarrier *et al.* (1978) reported that HR variability remained unaffected by antipsychotic drugs. Similar was the viewpoint of Spohn *et al.* (1977) with respect to influence of antipsychotic drugs on HR level of schizophrenics. Goldstein, Acker, Crockett and Riddle's (1966) finding was parallel to that of Spohn *et al.* (1977). McCormick and Broekema (1978) found larger magnitude of HR decelerative response than normals. But Houthan (1975) reported a finding contrary to this. Thus, the empirical picture with respect to tonic level of HR appears to be fairly clear from the reported literature. But with respect to phasic HR responses, the reported findings vary so much so that a consistent and coherent interpretation of findings across studies becomes impossibles. Such divergence of findings probably is related to a number of methodological and sampling differences noted in these studies. Some of these authors ignored largely the sub-classification of schizophrenia while selecting patients while some others mixed together both drug and non-drug patients. Some authors (*e.g.,* McCormick and Broekema) failed to apply a proper control in washing out drug effects. These author's (McCormick and Broekema) patients have been drug free for only 2 weeks, which however appear to be too short a period to consider a "wash-out" of effects of medication their patients received. Standardisation of procedures and careful selection and classification of schizophrenic patients are to be considered primary in future research in this field.

Since the last few decades or so amongsts the investigators of schizophrenia there has been a shift in interest away from focus on ANS activity towards Evoked Potential and Electroencephalographic (EEG) recording. EEG in schizophrenics patients has been recorded since 1930s. Typical early EEG findings in schizophrenia suggested a "non-specific diffuse" record (Ellingson, 1954; Greenblatt, 1944; Hill, 1956) with "weak alpha" and high beta (Berger, 1938). But later Lifshitz (1978) and Lifshitz, Susswein and Lee (1979) suggested that high beta activity is seen more prominently in acute than in chronic schizophrenics. These authors also suggested that high beta could be due to muscle tension of such patients. To obviate such confusion, Itil, Saletu and Davis (1972) recorded EEG from schizophrenics and normals during rapid eye movement sleep and claimed that high beta in schizophrenics is not due to muscle tension. It could be an index for a genetic predisposition to schizophrenia (Dumermuth, 1971; Itil, Simeon and Coffin, 1976). For brief history of EEG technique and some basic background information the reader is referred to Itil (1979) and Fink (1973) respectively. Information on EEG methodology is available in an excellent review made by Itil (1979).

During recent years attempts have been made to integrate EEG findings with theory and experimentation from other areas. Thus, *e.g.,* for use in psychology laboratory tests like, two-flash threshold and spiral after effect have been employed to record cortical activation where a link between EEG abnormalities and abnormal two-flash threshold and abnormal spiral after effect score has been suggested (Itil, 1979). Also, Venables and Wing (1972), Gruzelier and Venables (1975a,b), and Claridge (1978) had obtained data which suggest a link between two-flash threshold and SC phenomena in schizophrenia. Of course contradictory evidences have also been reported. However, recent research findings suggest that EEG techniques would be still more powerful if it is used in conjunction with averaged evoked potentials (EPs). For detailed information, the reader is referred to Buchsbaum (1975), Callaway, Tuetting, and Koslow (1978). Also three excellent reviews have been made available to us on early EPs (Shagass, 1977), middle EPs (Buchsbaum, 1977), and late EPs (Roth, 1977). In addition, Venables (1977) has reviewed literature in this area and Shagass later (1978) has reviewed his own work on EPs in relation to etiology of schizophrenia.

The shape of the EP wave changes depending upon the modality of the stimulus used. Shagass (1977) noted that schizophrenics show elevated early somatosensory evoked potential (SEP) component with less variability than normals or acute patients. Ikuta's (1974) data corroborate an elevated early SEP amplitude in schizophrenics relatives compared with non-relative normals. These findings indicate impaired reticular filtering in schizophrenics which results in abnormal amounts of information accumulation in higher brain centres.

Using paired stimuli where the main object of interest was to see the rapidity of recovery to the second stimulus, the amplitude recovery was found to be usually attenuated in schizophrenic patients than the normals (Shagass, 1978). However recovery latency was found to be augmented in schizophrenics (Shagass, Overton, and Strauments, 1974). These results also showed some relation with patient sub-groups and were best observed in chronic schizophrenics.

Auditory EP studies (Saletu, Itil and Saletu, 1971) have produced data which show evidence of short latency P_{50} components in both chronic schizophrenics and those with active thought disorder. Itil, Hsu, Saletu and Mednick (1974) found a similar trend of data with children at high risk for schizophrenia. However, though on eye estimation resemblance was apparent between latency components observed in high risk children and chronic schizophrenics, in terms of high statistical probability of abnormal peaks data were not strong enough to comment on between group comparison. Employing three sensory modalities (15 electrodes placed following international 10-20 system) Shagass, Roemer, Straumanis and Amadeo (1978), and Roemer *et al.* (1978) noted attenuated P-100 ms components and an increase in N-60 components in schizophrenics compared to normals. The N-60 components was found to be abnormally high in central locations in schizophrenics, whereas it was at its height in frontal leads and very small in central and posterior leads in normals. This shows that not only abnormality is found in EP wave but also that wave shape changes from anterior to posterior regions of brain, and also in terms of laterality. This finding is found to corroborate well with the research reports of Franzen and Inguar (1975a,b), who looked at regional cerebral blood flow in the brain and observed considerable difference between schizophrenics and normals especially during the performance of psychological tests.

Drug effects have been reported to have complex interactions with EP phenomena. Of the EP components, particularly vulnerable to the influence of drugs were found to be N-20 and P30, especially in the SEP. Though variations were noted in the effects of medication in schizophrenics, overall impression which one gets from the reported literature is that patients who show SEP changes also show clinical improvement with medication. Future research has to be taken up in this area with a view to demonstrate whether changes in SEP could be taken as an index of degree of improvement which medicine can bring into schizophrenics.

On visual evoked potentials (VEP) as early as 1960 Shagass started his research and reported (1972, 1977, 1978) that schizophrenics showed increased amplitude and reduced latency in early VEP. These findings have been criticized since the author did not exclude pupil movements (electrocculography, EOG) artefacts from such EP components. Ishikawa (1968) demonstrated that delayed VEP recovery, elicited through paired stimuli, was the characteristic feature of schizophrenics with marked hallucinations. This shows that EP data can be used to sub-categorise schizophrenics. Perris (1974) recorded VEP from both right and left occipital regions and reported that greater asymmetry was observed in psychotic depressives (having a marked reduction on the left) than in neurotic depressives or schizophrenics. Drugs however could reverse the asymmetries.

Of the early EPs, results with the VEP have been somewhat variable. In future research EPs should be recorded separately on different sub-group of schizophrenia and there too bilateral recordings from a multiplicity of placements would be of much value in understanding schizophrenia.

The middle EPs also show by far the biggest waveforms, and these centre around a positive peak at about 100 ms (called, P_{100}), a negative peak at about 140 ms (N_{140}) and another positive peak around 200 (P_{200}). The N_{140} component seems to be related to "stimulus selection" processes (Schwent, Snyder, and Hillyard, 1976), while P_{200} reflects strongly processes of habituation in context to novelty. In 1975 Landan, Buchsbaum and others reported that P_{100} and P_{200} waves show more abnormality in schizophrenics than N_{140}, suggesting that the attention deficit in schizophrenics is not likely to be of selective or discriminative type. Roth and Cannon (1972) observed less reduction in P_{200} wave over trials in schizophrenics than normals. This finding corroborates strongly with others who reported impaired response habituation in schizophrenia compared to normals on other electrophysiological systems, *e.g.*, SC (*e.g.*, Patterson and Venables, 1978).

Future research aiming to find integration of SC and EP recordings involving tasks in which attention demands are carefully manipulated would be a fruitful line of inquiry.

The "late component" waves of the EP are usually occurred at about 300 ms or later (called P_{300}). Associated with it are CNV (contingent negative variations) and RP (readiness potential). Some authors (*e.g.,* Teace, 1972; Chattopadhyay, Cooke, Toone and Lader, 1980) have demonstrated a late negative (N) wave as well. Roth (1977) suggested that late positive wave (LPW) is an index of the subject's "failure to resolve" aspects of attention. In general, however, LPWs are reported to be substantially attenuated in schizophrenia (Roth and Cannon, 1972; Shagass *et al.*, 1978). Shagass *et al.* (1978) further demonstrated that a number of middle and late EP components, across sensory modalities, *viz.,* P_{300} auditory, P_{300} visual, and P_{280} somatosensory, as well as N_{130} and P_{180} somatosensory, and N_{100} and P_{200} auditory, were all found to be attenuated in schizophrenia compared to normals. Similar was the findings of schizophrenic patients in Levit, Sutton, and Zubin's (1973) study when they compared schizophrenics with depressives and normal controls. Likewise, Bahramali, Lim, Rennie, Mearces, and Gordon (2001) found reduced N_{100}, N_{200} and N_{300} amplitudes in patients with schizophrenia compared to normals.

From the point of view of known neuroanatomical involvement of the EPs, the early EPs are generally held to represent stimulus – registration processes. Therefore, the abnormalities in this respect indicate biological or physiological alterations to the organism. The late EPs reflect psychological processes, and thus, abnormalities in these components reflect more of a functional disorder. For further detail about such background information on EPs, the interested reader is referred to Teace (1970, 1971, 1972); Shagass (1972); Callaway (1975); and Roth (1977).

In 1976, Flor-Henry (also see 1978) advocated a temporal lobe hypothesis of schizophrenia suggesting that the schizophrenics can be discriminated from other groups of psychiatric patients using spectral analysed EEG. Further arguments suggesting temporal lobe or left hemisphere involvement in schizophrenia have been put forwarded by Gur (1977, 1978), Roemer, Shagaas, Straumanis and Amadeo (1978), and Taylor (1975). Aydin, Dane, Ozturk, Uslu, Gumustekin and Kirpinar (2001) in a study on 26 schizophrenics, 17 depressives, 13 with bipolar affective disorder, 5 with brief psychotic disorder, and 24 controls reported that Schizophrenics may be associated with a left temporal lobe dysfunction as opposed to those of patients with depressive disorder, brief psychotic disorder and controls. A detailed account of hemisopheric asymmetry and neuroleptic compounds is available in Myslobodsky (1976). Gevins, Zeitlin, Doyle, Yingling, Schaffer, Callaway and Yeager (1979) however, suggested that some of these "laterality" arguments advocated by several researchers are subject to criticisms since these are based on artifactual data. However, a detailed account of hemispheric asymmetry in schizophrenia has been given later in this chapter under neuropsychological factors.

A clinical look to the existing research reports gives an impression that the field of schizophrenia and brainwave activity has now a substantial data base. But little attention has so far been paid to sub-classifications of schizophrenia using such measures. Phenomena of EEG and EPs of different behaviourally restricted sub-groups of schizophrenia appear to be robust enough to warrant substantial investigation in the future. Of course there is a great need to standardise methodology (concerning all different psychophysiological measures, *viz.*, SC, EEG, etc.) between laboratories preferably having made available sophisticated computer-controlled facilities.

Heath and Krupp (1968) based on electroencephalographic records demonstrated structural abnormality in the septal region of the brain of such patients. Since, this area is claimed to be concerned with alerting and repetitive activity, such functions are found to be disturbed in schizophrenics during periods of abnormal behaviour. They have obtained spike and slow wave EEG discharge as consistently recurrent in the septal area of some schizophrenics during period of attacks. Such abnormality, however, they reported, tended to disappear as the patients seemed to improve. However, similar EEG activity has also been recorded from the septal area in patients with other conditions. Needless to mention that similar findings are found in brains of various animals as well.

Feinberg, Braum, Koresko and Giottlieb (1969) reported that stage 4 electroencephalographic sleep value as recorded in schizophrenic patients are found to occur in about 50% of actively ill schizophrenics. This finding as well is unspecific, since such sleep abnormality has been reported in severe depression.

In sum: In spite of notable controversies in the reported research literature, psychophysiological measures are found sensitive in detecting schizophrenia pathology. However, studies in schizophrenia in Indian laboratories, applying electrophysiological methods are less frequently reported, though such studies on other patient categories are available. Thus, *e.g.*, AEPs have been measured applying both visual and auditory stimuli to see hemispheric involvement in head trauma patients (Mohanty, Das, Mukundan and Jamuna, 1993a,b). Research has also focussed on readiness potential and intrahemispheric EEG coherence as biological markers in psychiatric patients (Mischael, Mirza, Mukundan and Channavasabanna, 1995). These findings are useful to make a comparative evaluation of patients with schizophrenia. Of all the psychophysiological measures, in Indian laboratories SC has been employed more frequently, and it is found to be by far the best in sensitivity in detecting, and differentiating schizophrenia pathology when compared with normals and other categories of psychiatric patients (Roy, 1981; Biswas, 1983; Roy, 1984). However, application of electrophysiological measures require sophisticated laboratory gazettes and adequate laboratory facilities; non-availability of these might be the reason for less number of reported research documents in this area in India.

Neurohormonal Factors

Elkes (1961) hypothesized that there exists a disturbance of information processing by the brain. He was of the opinion that the defect exists in the integration of the subsystems subserving attention and motivation in the selective organisation of sense data. He also has suggested that the limbic system and the higher brain stem structures are involved. Elkes however, has suggested that such defective subsystem functions must be interpreted in terms of biochemical or pharmacological abnormalities, since this would help better in revealing dysfunctions which exist in the synaptic transmitters.

The sweat of schizophrenic patients oozes out a peculiar odour. The substance which causes the odour has been identified as trans-3-methyl-2-hexomic acid (Kolb, 1973). Srivastava, Barthwal, Dalal, Agarwal, Nag and others (2001) reported that a significant decrease in nitric oxide (NO) synthesis and an increase in malonaldehyde in the polymorphoneuclear Leukocytes (PMN) of patients with schizophrenia, while antioxidant enzyme activities were not altered in the polymorphonuclear leukocytes of schizophrenia patients. These authors suggested that the decrease in PMN NO synthesis by PMN might lead to oxidative stress in patients with schizophrenia.

Research concerned with the intermediate metabolism of cerebral glucose demonstrates that in the schizophrenics, there is metabolic defects (Gottlieb, Frohman, and Beckett, 1969). Gottlieb *et al.* hypothesized that owing to such metabolic defects schizophrenics are deficient in their capacity to utilise available energy in reaction to stress. Also they have reported that there exists an abnormality in schizophrenic plasma which leads to abnormal production of pyruvate. Again, it has been suggested that the presence of a malcontrolled protein in the blood contributes significantly to the illness by selectively altering neuronal transmission. Urinary excretion of abnormal metabolites, like that of a mescaline – like derivative in schizophrenics has been reported by several authors (*e.g.,* Friedhoff and Vanwinkle, 1953).

Regarding dysfunctions in the synaptic transmitters, Heath and Krupp (1968) hypothesized that brain cell antibodies attach themselves to the spetal region and thereby impair synaptic transmission. These authors particularly suggested that an immuno-globulin designated taraxein obtained from serum of acute schizophrenic patients when administered to healthy volunteers induce EEG changes similar to those they noted in the brain of schizophrenics. However, this work as yet needs replication, as because critics are of the opinion that these findings are not specific for schizophrenics only.

According to some others, the abnormal defect rests in an altered metabolism of biogenic amines necessary for synaptic transmission. Thus, *e.g.,* abnormal metabolism of dopa, it has been suggested (Kolb, 1973), leads to formation of 3.4–dimethoxyphenylethylamine (DMPEA) endogenously and this is capable of inducing psychotic disorganisation. The dopaminergic transmitters exist in the basal ganglia including the limbic system. However, a discussion on the possible link between L-Dopa and schizophrenic symptomatology has already been made before in this chapter.

Neuropsychological (NPL) Factors

During recent years, researchers have taken interest to examine etiological factors of psychiatric patients in NPL perspective. Bilateral transfer deficit has been reported to be a trait marker in schizophrenia. Deficits in bilateral (inter hemispheric) transfer in schizophrenia have been examined with both structural and functional measures. Structural approaches involved the postmortem measurement of corpus callosum size (*e.g.,* Bigelow, Nasrallah and Raucher, 1983), while functional approaches included perceptual studies with visual split-field auditory dichotic-listening techniques (reviewed by Walker and McGuire, 1982) and studies of ipsilateral/contralateral latency differences in somatosensory evoked responses (Tress, Caudrey and Mehta, 1983). But these studies have provided little information about the relationship between bilateral transfer deficit and clinical state (*e.g.*, acute *vs* remitted; patients with positive symptoms *vs* negative symptoms) of the patients. As early as 1988 Guenther, Danos, Godet *et al.* found that bilateral brain dysfunction, as indicated by cortical activation during a motor task, may be associated with negative symptomatology, but it was not known whether such deficit would persist even after successful treatment.

In Indian laboratories research attempts have been made to examine whether bilateral transfer deficits would persist in schizophrenia even after successful treatment (Biswas, Haque-Nizamie, Pandey and Mandal, 1996). In this study, 14 schizophrenia patients (meanage 23.5 years) were examined using a perceptual – motor task (mirror-drawing) and were compared with 1st degree relatives (n=14) of schizophrenia patients, and normal subjects (n=14). All the patients were treated with standard doses of antipsychotic medication. Results revealed that schizophrenia patients who had shown improvement over a 6-week treatment period, did not show any improvement on any measure of bilateral transfer skill, though both the control groups showed differences with the patient group in their response accuracy. This finding indicates that bilateral transfer deficit is an enduring functional loss in schizophrenia.

Existence of split-brain symptoms in chronic schizophrenia has been pointed out by others which is akin to a deficit in bilateral transfer of skill. Still it is difficult to attribute this deficit to either a structural (*e.g.*, Width of corpus callosum; Nasrallah, Jacoby, McCalley, Whiters and Kupoman, 1982) or a functional (*e.g.*, lowered inter-hemispheric integration; Gruzelier, 1987) cause. Cognitive theorists, on the other hand, relate such impairment to attentional deficits (Mirsky and Duncan, 1986) but that may be more characteristic of acute (Gruzelier, 1990) than of chronic patients. Other researchers attribute such transfer deficit to an abnormal pattern of brain lateralisation in schizophrenia (for review see Cromwell, 1987). However, it appears, premature at this stage to attribute the relatively permanent functional loss of bilateral transfer skills observed in the patients of Biswas *et al.* (1996) to lobular lateralised, or callosal deficits. Also, the conclusion they have drawn that the improvement in schizophrenic symptomatology is not paralleled by a corresponding improvement in bilateral transfer of skill, cannot be generalised as because the patients were retested only after 6 weeks of treatment. Furthermore, correlational analyses done by Biswas *et al.* (1996) indicated a negative relationship between the pre-treatment and post-treatment conditions for the dependent measures of error. This suggests that error scores reduced somewhat with intervening treatment. Generalisation of this finding, therefore, awaits further studies to examine patients at different intervals over a long course of treatment.

Laterality has been associated with schizophrenic pathology in many Indian research reports (Biswas, Haque-Nizamie, Pandey and Mandal, 1996; Mandal and Singh, 1993; Tiwari and Mandal, 1998; Shukla, Behera and Mandal, 1993). Though research reports on side bias in schizophrenia, namely, foot, eye, and ear are available (Tiwari and Mandal,

1998, most of the research on side (lateral) bias in Schizophrenia has been concentrated primarily upon the issue of handedness. In a study on 60 (43 men; mean age 29.6 years) chronic schizophrenic patients (duration of illness 2 years) who were all on antipsychotic drugs, and a matched normal control group side (lateral) bias in terms of hand, foot, eye and ear were assessed taking performance and preference measures. The findings indicated a right bias for both measures in control and in the patients (Tiwari and Mandal, 1998). It may be that cultural pressure against the use of the left hand, as in Nigeria (Gureje, 1988) and in India (Mandal, Pandey, Singh, and Asthana, 1992) exhibit a bias toward the right hand. However, this explanation does not adequately account for the right biases of other organs, since cultural, pressure in India for the use of a particular foot, eye or ear is negligible (Tiwari and Mandal, 1998). Therefore, question remains why schizophrenics in this study showed right bias toward other body parts? Could it be that handedness in the most pervasive among biases which might affect other organs also? This finding is not in congruence with Green, Satz, Smith *et al.* (1989) who reported that chronic schizophrenic patients with known structural defect have normal patterns of handedness, *i.e.,* right handedness. Increased incidence of left-handedness has been associated with structural defect (Green, Satz, Smith *et al.,* 1989). Since in Tiwari and Mandal's (1998) study patients had no history of unilateral cerebral insult, so they were likely to exhibit right handedness. Although the schizophrenics in Tiwari and Mandal's (1998) study showed a right bias as did the controls, three-way interaction of the right sided responses revealed a discrepancy between performance and preference measures. The schizophrenics displayed a right bias for preference that was a little greater than for performance for eye, whereas the right bias for preference was a little less than for performance for ear (Tiwari and Mandal, 1998). However, existing inconsistencies in the reported literature on the side bias in schizophrenia urge upon further research, especially with respect to handedness; special attention be paid to individual characteristics of pathology.

With the advent of Geschwind and Galaburda's (1985) model that a potential relationship exists between left-handedness and anomalous cerebral dominance that results in various immune function and psychopathological disorders, there has been a trend in schizophrenia researchers to reconsider the issue of handedness in schizophrenia. Satz (1972) reported that unclassified group of schizophrenics exhibit pathological left-handedness, whereas the others do not. But others have observed that pathological left-handedness is largely associated with early (unilateral) cerebral insult (Green, Satz, Smith and Nelson, 1989). An early unilateral injury may cause hypofunction of the contralateral hand, as well as a shift in handedness. Such shifting as the result of left hemispheric injury in genetic right-handers is called pathological left-handedness. Since handedness is associated with the pattern of cerebral lateralisation, the study of such behaviour in schizophrenia may lead to an understanding of the precipitating factors and the state of pathology. Empirical research evidences, during the last few decades, indicate a greater incidence of left-handedness associated with schizophrenic pathology (*e.g.,* Manoach, Maher and Manschreck, 1988). But contrary to this some researchers have documented a prevalence of right handedness (*e.g.,* Taylor, Rosemary and Fleminger, 1980), whilst some others documented increased incidence of mixed handedness (*e.g.,* Manoch, 1994), and still some others have obtained null results (*e.g.,* Merrin, 1984), *i.e.,* no difference from the controls in handedness.

In sum: Research evidences on laterality and schizophrenic psychopathology is as yet controversial.

The above mentioned controversies in the findings may largely be attributed to methodological variations involved in these studies. For example, variations related to sample characteristics (*e.g.*, sub-types of the patients investigated), severity and prognosis of schizophrenia pathology (positve-negative symptoms), onset of disorder (early-late), or course of pathology (acute-chronic), task demand characteristics (preferernce or performance of hand activities), response format used etc. are some such characteristics. Operationalisation of the concept of handedness also induces certain amount of variation as because the concept of handedness has been equated with hand preference, hand usage, hand proficiency, hand performance and so on. Such control of variables is essential because in a study on the patients of the Central Institute of Psychiatry, Ranchi, India, it was found that (Mandal, Jain, Hauqe-Nizamie, Weiss, and Schneider, 1999) schizophrenia patients with negative symptoms exhibited a generalised emotion-recognition deficit, whereas the patients with positive symptoms showed a deficit in their recognition of 'sad' emotion only. May be that the patients with positive symptoms, as these authors viewed, suffer from some kind of interpersonal difficulties in which they tend to see others as 'happy' because of their own style of coping (response rigidity?). This style of functioning renders it possible for them to keep arousal-provoking perceptual cues from entering into subjective awareness. Alternatively, it may be that the nature of happy expression itself, which is experienced more frequently (Ekman, 1982), is easier to understand than other emotions (Mandal, Bryden, Bulman-Fleming, 1996). However, the interpretations provided by these authors appear to be more of speculative in nature. Also, the number of patients investigated in either of the positive symptoms (n=12; of male, Mean age 33.03 years) and negative symptoms (n=12; 8 male, mean age 37.25 years) groups was inadequate to generalise the findings. More studies especially the meta-analysis of earlier findings and a comparison of studies that used differential deficit designs are required to permit definitive conclusions to be drawn.

Of course, control of such sources of variations experimentally or statistically does not seem feasible in a single study as because such an attempt may create other methodological problems. However, based on Indian research reports, Mandal and Singh (1993) opined that lateral performance is less overtly expressed in actual hand performance of schizophrenics. General conclusions, in this regard, therefore await further studies that examine patients at different intervals over the course of treatment.

Neuropsychologists engaged in exploring the relationship between cortical structures and higher mental functions use two methods–experimental and clinical. Though neuropsychologists believe that the experimental method is more powerful in understanding normal brain functions, the recently available technologies are perhaps, inadequate to draw a definite conclusion. Faces with such problems neuropsychologists are found to be more inclined to use clinical methods for examining the performance deficit in brain-damaged patients rather than the performance accuracy in intact brain subjects. However, clinical methods should be used with caution (Sergeant, 1988).

Of late, there has been increased interest in the study of emotional processing and its neural regulation (reviewed in Cacioppo and Gardner, 1999) in schizophrenia. Despite the universal appearance of some basic emotions (Ekman and Friesen, 1986), Russell (1994) opined that culture influences and shapes more complex emotional experience and expression. Thus, *e.g.,* Mandal, Bryden, and Bulman-Fleming (1996) reported that healthy Indian participants judged fearful and angry facial expressions as more unpleasant than did North-Americans, regardless of the ethnic, identity of the facial stimulus. Correspondingly, it has been assumed (Kirmayer, 1989) that culture and environment may contribute to the symptom manifestation of psychiatric disorders by influencing the outcome or degree of distress.

Impaired emotional functioning and expression has been considered fundamental in schizophrenia across culture. In a recent study, Habel, Gur, R.C., Mandal, Salloum, Gur, R.E. and Schneider (2000) reported that although some variations in performance was observed amongst Schizophrenia patients of three different cultures, similarities were more prominent than differences. However, understanding the variant and invariant features of the disorder, according to these authors, is necessary for elucidating its biological and environmental bias. This study assessed performance of American, German, and Indian patients with schizophrenia and healthy controls on standardised emotion discrimination and experience (mood induction) procedures using happy, sad, and neutral facial expressions of Caucasian actors. Participants were 80 Americans (40 patients, 40 controls), 48 Germans (24 patients, 24 controls), and 58 Indians (29 patients, 29 controls). American and German patients were found to be more consistent in their respective emotional ratings during mood induction, where patients demonstrated more negative affect. The Indian patients group, on the contrary, showed less positive affect during happy as well as sad mood. The Indian controls, on the other hand, had the highest positive ratings in comparison with the other control groups.

In another recent study in India Mandal, Bhushan and Mishra (2001) observed cultural specificity with respect to hemifacial asymmetry and valence of emotion expressions where Japanese showed a right hemifacial bias for positive and left hemifacial bias for negative emotions; Indians and North Americans showed left hemifacial bias for all emotions. Negative emotion expressions were least distinctly definable in Japanese faces followed by Indian and North American faces. This divergence in the findings, according to the authors, may be attributed to Indian culture in the sense that in a collective society like India, there prevails a tendency to intensify positive and lessen negative emotional experiences. Individualism is more the exception than the norm. The higher positive ratings of Indian controls may be a product of such societal distinctions (Mandal *et al.,* 1996). A reverse trend was found to exist in the pathology of schizophrenia. In assessing proximal and paralinguistic responses to positive and negative emotional expressions, patients with schizophrenia were reported to be highly sensitive to negative rather than to positive emotions (Mandal *et al.*, 1996; Srivastava and Mandal, 1990). The results thus supported the feasibility of cross-cultural comparisons of the data obtained.

In sum: Face discrimination performance was found impaired across patient groups, but was more impaired in Indian patients. Lower performance was found in Indian controls, relative to their American and German counterparts, indicating cross-cultural variations in face discrimination in schizophrenia.

Not only across culture, even within culture comparisons with anxious patients and non-patient controls show that emotion identification deficit is specific to schizophrenia (Mandal, 1987; Mandal and Raj, 1987; Mandal and Gewali, 1989). More interestingly, schizophrenics showed deficit in identifying emotions from full facial expressions while retaining their ability to identify emotions from part facial expressions (Mandal and Palchowdhury, 1989). Such a finding once again, adds support to schizophrenic pathology. That is, in "free" condition, schizophrenics have been found to pay more attention to some parts of the face rather than the total facial expression. Therefore, it is most likely that selective attention given to the full face generates information overload in these patients, which may be equated with what Hamilton (1979) had stated as anxiety. Anxiety overactivates the left hemisphere, making it dysfunctional (Gur, 1979) and giving rise to a right-hemisphere dominance (Tucker, 1981), in them. Based on NPL studies it has been confirmed that the left-hemisphere plays a key role in the linguistic ability (Kimura, 1961) and lexical processing (Chiarello, 1988), while for visuospatial ability (Bryden, 1982) and processing non-verbal stimuli, particularly facial expression (Warrington and James, 1967) the right hemisphere has been held responsible. Therefore, it appears plausible to believe that the schizophrenic's deficit in identifying emotions from full facial expression is due to impairment in linguistic ability which is caused by an overactivated left hemisphere. Both the Western (Hamilton, 1979) and Indian researchers (Mandal and Palchowdhury, 1989) have suggested that the information overload reduces schizophrenics' performance to process higher level information.

Neurocognitive domains that show deficiency in schizophrenia patients include vigilance (sustained attention), executive functions, language skills, verbal learning and memory, working memory (Bilder, Lipschute-Broth, Reister *et al.*, 1992; Bilder, Goldman, Robinson, *et al.*, 2000; Riley, McGovern, Mockler, *et al.*, 1999; Sharma and Antonova, 2003) of which specific impairment in executive function is frequently reported (*e.g.*, Stern and Prohaska, 1996). Executive functions are linked to the frontal lobe (David, 1990; Weinberger, Aloia, Goldberg, *et al.*, 1994). Schizophrenic patients show associated executive symptoms such as, impaired response set, difficulty in utilising feedback, poor judgement and lack of initiation.

In a study on 15 residual (illness duration is more than 2 years) schizophrenic patients (both sexes) of Chennai, South India, Ravindran and Rangaswami (2004) reported that compared to matched normal controls (n=15), the patients group showed poor social cognition and difficulty in spatial organisation. Also, difficulty in learning and remembering new information, and significant impairment in planning, sequencing, response set shifting, working memory in social judgment were noted. In this respect, Indian patients show similarity (John, Khanna, Mukundan, and Reddy, 2001) with the patients of the Western culture (Vrtunski, Simpson, Weiss and Davis, 1986; Liddle, and Morris, 1991; Stern, and Prohaska, 1996; Mohamed, Paulson, O'Leary, *et al.,* 1999) in their neurocognitive deficits. The tests used for assessing frontal lobe cognitive dysfunction were Trail making test (Part-B), Picture arrangement, Block design and Similarities sub-tests of the WAIS, Sentence repetition test (Stanford-Binet) and Logical memory (WMS-R). On the Trail-making Test, however, the findings obtained on the Indian patients differed from that of the West (Vrtunski, Simpson, Weiss, *et al.,* 1986), where the Western patients had slowed reaction time than the normals, but Ravindran and Rangaswami's patients did not differ from their normal controls. But contrary to Ravindran and Rangaswami (2004) our research reports on Indian patients with schizophrenia go parallel to Vrtunski *et al.,* (1986). This thus, shows a similarity in results in the East and the West (see chapter on theories of schizophrenia). However, in Ravindran and Rangaswami's (2004) study no separate analyses of the results were done on the basis of the variables like sex, occupation (skilled workers, executives, housewives, clerks, and businessmen were included) and age. The age range of the patients investigated (25-55 years) was quite a wide range. The mean age of the control group was 34.11 years (SD 8.40 years) and that for the experimental group was 31.94 years (SD 7.55 years). However, these findings do suggest that patients with schizophrenia have neurocognitive deficits related to frontal lobe.

Applying Wiscon's card-sorting test in Indian laboratory, Mukhopadhyay and Das (2002) found that patients with paranoid schizophrenia (n=10), despite adequate attention and concentration, showed poorer problem-solving skills compared to matched normal controls (24-55 years). The age range of the subjects in this study was quite wide and not known whether obtained findings were contaminated by the subjects of above 50+ years. In another study, applying Bender Visuo-Motor Gestalt Test (BVMGT) Mukhopadhyay, Mukherjee, Chowdhury, Gupta, Basu and Dutta (1999) found that in schizophrenia predominant fronto-temporal-parietal dysfunction was evident, whereas in the patients with obsessive compulsive disorder predominant temporal lobe dysfunction was noted. This study was on 10 patients only and thus require replication on large number of patients and preferably on different sub-types of schizophrenia to generalise the usefulness of NPL findings in the management of such patients. These findings, however, suggest that patients need remedial measures to increase their functional outcome.

NPL test findings have been utilised in psychosocial intervention programme in connection with siblings of autistic children (mean age 14.4 years). This study (Tarafder, Mukhopadhyay and Basu, 2004) was on 10 subjects only, hence requires replication on larger sample. LuriaNebraska NPL Battery has been applied on Indian patients, and findings revealed that (Masroor, Haque-Nizamie, Nizamie and Khalique, 2002) few items of this test require modification to improve its applicability onto Indian population.

In sum: NPL perspective reveals neurocognitive deficits related to lobe functions in schizophrenia. Remedial measures to be taken to increase their functional outcome. Psychophysiological and NPL methods, preferably with an interdisciplinary research orientation, be employed for quick and accurate identification of the etiology of such patients. Experts to render remedial measures must be well trained having clinical background.

Family Transaction

Whatever biological abnormality the future schizophrenic may inherit through the birth, his personality unfolds over the years of infancy through childhood till adolescence as the consequence of the ongoing transactions between his parents and those others who relate with him. Thus, family transaction influences the emotional and cognitive maturation of growing children. Studies of family dynamics have shown that a significant number of schizophrenic patients have spent their childhood in seriously disturbed family groups in which both patients were found to have personality disturbances. In their study Lidz, Fleck, and Cornelison (1965) found that two-thirds of the families contained one parent schizophrenic. Such families were full of conflicts and were described by these authors as unintegrated. In these families the parents were found to oppose each other by derogating and defying the wishes of the spouse. Such parents put efforts to win the children to their side so as to obtain from them emotional support not found in the spouse. Again in some such families one parents is found to have a serious personality deficit as is shown in domineering, brutal, aggressive, or alcoholic behaviour, while the other passively accepts it. Such parents are found to be doubtful of their own sexual roles, so much so that some have been found to have homosexual inclinations, and others show conflicts over control of incestuous desires. Such family situations do not help developing personal security and sound sexual identification. Nor does it help in developing ability to share and to repress hostile and aggressive drives effectively. In such family environment series of events occur that impair the evolution of mature communication and thought. Such events are very important for understanding schizophrenic reaction.

Though Lidz *et al.* investigated their patients very intensively, the number of patients investigated was very small (about 17 young patients), and therefore warrants generalisation. Secondly, these authors have not mentioned anything about those families which could readily be accounted for if the probands were a group of children having severe behaviour disorders, but not actually schizophrenic. These objections, however, are not applicable to the work of Alanen (1958) which was relatively more thorough. He examined personally 100 mothers of young patients and reported that 84 of the mothers of schizophrenics were at least severely neurotic, with salient symptoms of anxiety and aggressiveness. He found only three abnormal mothers in the control series. Most of the mothers had been disturbed emotionally at the time of birth of the schizophrenic child and during his infancy, and thereby fear and aggressiveness characterised the early relationship between mother and child. Alanen (1958) also reported that these abnormalities were more marked in the mothers of the schizophrenics than in the mothers of the schizophreniform patients. However, Alanen's (1958) study was completely based on Langfeldt's concept of schizophrenia and schizophreniform psychoses.

As early as 1956, Bateson, Jackson, Haley and Weak opined that the origin of the schizophrenic defects in communication rests upon a 'Double-bind' transaction between two persons. Mostly in such transactions, *e.g.,* it is found that child (who develops schizophrenia later) is in a fix in an intense emotional relationship with a parent who shows contradiction between his/her verbal remarks and behaviour, as a result, the child fails to discriminate properly or to respond correctly. At the same time the child can not clarify his doubts since his questioning is treated as a threat to the needed relationship by the parent. As a hypothetical example, it may be mentioned that a schizophrenic adolescent who, tied to his mother verbally, is encouraged to use initiative in his art class, yet when he attempts to go to library, is refrained from doing so as the parent needs him, his absence will make him/her ill. Such a 'double-bind' situation restricts and confuses the proper and clear communication. This also limits the son's proper development of socialisation. Bateson *et al.'s* (1956) view has been supported by Wynne and Singer (1965).

Psychoanalytic theory has held that as a consequence of the lack of early consistency in the mothering process the child's capacity to maintain a stable representation with others is impaired. The need for the mother is intensified and at the same time there is a fear of her loss, and thus, the child remains in a state of 'need-fear' (Burnham, Gladstone, and Gibson, 1969) dilemma. The child fails to develop trust and certainty in his own autonomy. Childhood shyness and the latter shunt – in life pattern have their origins perhaps, in the seeking of security in early clinging coupled with fearfulness of loss. Therefore, the later social relations of such child with others are fermented by intense ambivalence (Kolb, 1973), with his inability to integrate such a perception of 'need-fear' with the consequent 'love-affect' affects.

If the early mothering is so critical then one must seek an explanation for the occurrence of schizophrenia in one or two children mothered by the same women while rest of her children develop with little evidence of psychopathology? In reply to this it has been stated (Stabenau and Pollin, 1968) that in such families there was evidence of intense family crises at the time of birth itself or in the ensuing months which affected the mother and her relation with the child. As possible sources for the development of such crises these authors identified (a) depression in the mother with feelings of guilt owing to her hostility towards the newborn, (b) the birth of another sibling within two years, (c) dislike of the child's appearance, and so on.

Again, researchers do not agree that disturbances in the early mothering alone can be held responsible for the development of full range of schizophrenic psycho-pathology. Thus, *e.g.,* failure to develop and maintain a proper sense of identity, and to discriminate fantasy from reality etc. are more likely to rest on later deficiencies or distortions in the process of the personality development (Kolb, 1973).

However, these above mentioned findings can not be replicated and compared by others in a strict scientific manner, since these are largely based on subjective impressions of the examiners. One must have to rule out the examiners/therapist's pre-commitment to a theory when he/she starts interviewing parents and justify the obtained data. Thus, *e.g.*, Sechehaye (1954) reported that a girl suffering from severe deteriorative hebephrenic psychosis responded to psychotherapy and made a remarkable recovery. Psychological stress precipitated the onset of this illnesses in this girl. Kind (1966), in this context, commented that the scanty success of psychotherapy cannot be taken as a proof that the illness was due to psychological stress; one wonders what could be the weightage of such a finding statistically since it is not possible to dismiss the objection altogether that such recovery could be the results of a spontaneous remission. Secondly Ernst (1956) has mentioned that factors like, duration of breast feeding, time at which toilet training was established etc. have been found to show non-significant difference between schizophrenic and control groups. Subjective data vary a great deal from one investigator to the next. Also one has to rule out the possibilities of contamination of the obtained data which could be due to halo effect of an emotional attitude on the part of the investigator (Ernst, 1956). Recent data obtained employing objective measures, however, claim significant difference between schizophrenic and control groups which has already been mentioned in this chapter while discussing about high-risk children.

In sum, totality of environmental factors play a large part in the etiology of schizophrenia. The experiences of the child may affect his development in such a way that these would make him more or less susceptible to schizophrenic illness. However, some of the evidences regarding psychogenesis of schizophrenia have been mentioned while discussing symptomatic schizophrenia. For a detailed review of literature the reader is referred to Kind (1966).

Family Transaction in Schizophrenia: Indian Scenario

Of the many factors inherent in schizophrenia which determine the outcome poor social support, particularly poor family support system has been associated with poor outcome especially for the patients in India. Furthermore, Indian research reports claim (Sathyavathi, 1977) that interfamilial interpersonal relationships show significant difference between male and female schizophrenics. In her study on 20 male and 20 female schizophrenics (mean age 23.6 years; SD 3.24 years) and a comparative group of 20 male and 20 female (mean age 22.18 years; SD 2.74 years) neurotics Sathyavathi (1977) found that female schizophrenic patients perceived their mothers as resentful (poor mother-daughter relationship in the family), whereas male schizophrenic patients perceived their mothers as co-operative, considerate, warm, friendly. But both the male and female schizophrenics were found to perceive their fathers as more or less equally loving. Neurotics did not show any difference in their perception of father and mother. Several views may be offered for such variation in perception of parents by schizophrenics. Parental conflicts, discrepancies about sexual identity and parental functions, parents presenting negative images of their spouse to children, pathological symbiotic relationships between parents and their children etc. could be held responsible for such perception of Indian schizophrenic patients. This shows that male and female schizophrenics be considered as two distinct groups (instead of bracketing them together as schizophrenics) while formulating psychosocial intervention programmes for such patients. Since number of subjects was small, generalisation of the present findings require further probe into the matter in question, in future research in India on schizophrenia. However, what is evident from the above is that parental personalities and their ways of relating to their offspring is crucial in understanding pathology of our patients.

Interpersonal Interaction and Interpersonal Communication

Childhood interpersonal interactions play a significant role in the development of 'Identity'. In the families of schizophrenia, in our culture, children mostly experience abandonment or rejection, which leads to absence of identity and the person does not find his own existence in reality. Schizophrenic patients have two basic needs which remain unfulfilled through their early life interaction. These two needs are – (i) inclusion need, and (ii) need for expressed control. In a study on 30 male schizophrenic patients (mean age 28.0 years; SD 4.3 years) it was found that (Sathyavathi, 1974) compared to matched normals the schizophrenic patients had significantly greater need to established and maintain satisfactory relationship with people (need for belongingness). But lack of adequate sense of identity compelled them to think that "I'm not liked by, wanted by others". "No one is interested in me", etc. Because of such inner feeling, he prefers not to take risk of being ignored (apprehension of being rejected by others if I want to be with them). He then decides to be away from people. Therefore, he prefers to 'get along with myself', instead of 'get along with others' (initial inner desire remains unfulfilled). Likewise, there is a constant striving among schizophrenic patients to exercise their control over others (with whom they interact), to the extent of influencing others, command over others. So their overt behaviour may show that they are aggressive, commanding but such overt expression is a compensation of their inner feeling that "I will be rejected by others", "I will be neglected by others". This shows that each behavioural symptom of a patient be explained in terms of his inner needs and desires, which mostly in our patients gets expressed in an opposite direction That is, aggressive, overactive behavioural expression (symptom) is to compensate the apprehension of rejection and negligence (inner needs); withdrawal behaviour (symptom) is to compensate apprehension of failure to belong to others (inner needs). Such social bankruptsy of needs to be rectified and taken care of, in psychosocial intervention, to help such patients reestablishing a healthy social identity. Thus, delusions and hallucinations which Indian patients report, are to be dealt with taking into account their social bankruptsy (which of course is culture bound), in terms of fulfilling their inner needs, desires, drives, and feelings. This will be discussed in detail later in this book.

In sum: Disturbed interpersonal interaction and interpersonal communication in the families of schizophrenia are crucial in understanding and in management of the patients with schizophrenia.

Socio-cultural Influences

A person's first exposure to the influences of culture occurs in the family, and forces that operate within that family unit have already been discussed above. Several other factors in the society which may produce sick people include – social disorganisation, social isolation, and social class.

Social disruption leads to personality disorder. Using poverty level, cultural confusion, absence of religious values, and high crime rate as indices of social disorganisation, Leighton (1959) and Leighton, Harding, MacKlin, MacMillan, and Leighton (1963) reported a higher percentage of abnormal individual in socially more disorganised regions. Likewise, Clausen (1966), Clausen and Kohn (1959), Jaco (1954, 1960) also reported a higher incidence of schizophrenia in disorganised communities. But in these studies, it is even now difficult to separate cause and effect. Thus, social isolation rather than a cause of schizophrenia could be a symptom which indicates that a person's interpersonal difficulties have become so great that he can no longer relate to others in the society.

In context to social class and its relation with incidence of schizophrenia, Myerson (1941) first formulated the social drift hypothesis. Corroborating the drift hypothesis, Gerard and Houston (1953) reported that the highest rates of schizophrenia occurred in the areas with the poorest living conditions. However in an almost identical study Lapouse, Monk, and Terris (1956) failed to find any evidence of drift. In some other latter studies (Clausen, 1966; Clausen and Kohn, 1959) authors once again have expressed serious doubt on the idea that schizophrenics drift down towards lower social strata.

That social class is correlated with evidence of schizophrenia has been well documented in the epidemiological studies done by Hollingshed and Redlich (1958). These authors reported a substantially greater number of psychotics in the lower socio-economic classes when compared to those of the upper classes. In many of such other and similar epidemiological studies (*e.g.*, Dohrenwand and Dohrenwand, 1969; Sorle, Langer, Michael, Opler, and Rennie, 1962) findings are the same.

Explanations put forward by different investigators regarding the greater incidence of mental disorders amongst different socio-economic classes are equivocal. Some are of the opinion that class differences in child rearing practice as such may predispose lower-class children to more intense stress; devastating effect of poverty causes its victims to withdraw from the harsh realities of facing it. Still some others believe that schizophrenic types have greater tendencies to drift toward lower social communities because of their social ineptness.

Mention should be made here that there are three types of problems (Dohrenwand and Dohrenwand, 1969) with these epidemiological studies, and therefore, the findings reported so far should be used with caution. The problems are (a) the validity of the measures used to determine psychological disorder is questionable and thus it is difficult to know what are the true rates of disorders in contrasting class and ethnic groups; (b) the appearance of symptoms may not necessarily be an indication of presence of disorder because symptoms might be transient responses to life stress; and (c) these appear to have a secondary gain (*e.g.*, sympathy drawing, unemployment benefits) from symptomatology and such gain tends to be greater in lower than in higher-class groups. Likewise within classes, gain is greater amongst members of disadvantaged as opposed to advantaged ethnic groups and therefore, this may serve in perpetuating abnormalities.

In sum: Epidemiological studies reveal that social disorganiation, social isolation, and social class may serve in perpetuating schizophrenia like symptoms.

Cross-cultural Factors

Not only that culture-bound unique syndromes are found in schizophrenics, also the delusional content in schizophrenics has been reported to be significantly different in varying cultures. Examination of these delusional systems has revealed their close adherence to the belief system prevalent in the culture (Kiev, 1972). One example of a unique behaviour pathology is Koro, also known as Suo-Yang (Kleinmuntz, 1974). This abnormality occurs only in South East Asia, especially among the inhabitants of the Malay Archipelago and among Southern Chinese who migrated to this region. In this the individual is afraid that his penis will withdraw into his abdomen resulting in his death. To prevent the withdrawal the afflicted individual holds his penis in a vise-like grip, preferably with the assistance of his wife, friends, and relatives (Wittkower and Dubreuil, 1968). This has a sudden and acute onset. The condition may last for several days, or even weeks or months. This is attributed to sexual overindulgence, especially to excessive masturbation, sexual intercourse. It is believed to be avoided by abstention from sex. In fact, this is an anxiety state and in many respects resembles what psychoanalysts call "Castration Anxiety", commonly seen in the West. But to anthropologists (Rin, 1963) such symptoms have their roots in fundamental Chinese concepts of sexuality. The Chinese believe that Koro is due to an excess of what they call **Yin**, the "Female Factor", and must be treated with **Yang**, the male factor (Kleinmuntz, 1974).

Recently the present writers have witnessed identical symptoms amongst young boys and girls in some villages (namely, Ramnagore, Aishtala) of Ranaghat and Santipur, Nadia District, West Bengal, India. 'Jhinjhinia' is the term used by the villagers to describe this episode where the victims express a peculiar, sudden onset of numbness over the penis or breasts (as the case may be) so much so that the respective organ gets shrinked into the patients' abdomen. The afflicted individual starts shouting and crying with a fear of impending death (though no death has yet been reported), and seeks assistance from their relatives and friends to hold the afflicted part of the body and others start pouring cold water onto the head of the afflicted individual. Sexual overindulgence leading to guilt appears to be the underlying cause of such acute anxiety attack. Treatment consists of rubbing oil/sacred water, different plants as suggested by village temple incharge/mosque incharge (popularly known as Priest and/or Imam respectively). Similar symptoms (called Jhinjhini) were found to occur in a village of Midnapore about a decade ago (Nandi, Banerjee, Saha, Sen, and Bhattacharyya, 1992). Here too, sex related guilt appeared to be the cause.

'Jhinjhinia' of the Bengalees resembles very well with the 'Koro' of the Chinese (referred by them as 'Sukwang'). Koro occurs most often in immature and anxious adolescents and young adults who had been troubled by anxiety, guilt, and panic about their virility (Sarbadhikary, 1999).

In rural population of India, preponderance of hallucinatory themes of magic and religion ('Jadu-tona', 'Witchcraft', 'Evil Spirit') are noted, particularly in less educated females (Sharma and Agnihotri, 1986). In rural population of Rajasthan, India possession syndrome is reported (Kapur, 1987) to be a culture bound reaction to stress in the beginning and it proceeds to work as a community therapy.

Apart from hysteria in some parts of the country, 'Dhat' (seminal loss) syndrome (Singh, 1985) is commonly reported amongst Indian adolescents and young adults. The 'Dhat' Syndrome first used by Wig (1960) in India got recognized by the WHO (1992) for classification of mental disorders under 'other specific Neurotic Disorders' (Bandyopadhyay, 1999). Researchers prefer to classify patients with Dhat as 'Undifferentiate Somatoform Disorders' (DSM-IV, APA, 1994). In a study (Bandyopadhyay, 1999) on 63 male patients with Dhat Syndrome (taken from the institute of psychiatry, Calcutta) different cognitive aspects were examined and were compared with normal controls and also with psychotic (n=15) and neurotic (n=15) patients. Questionnaire based data revealed high level of anxiety and preoccupation of having a disease (which though does not really exist) in the patients with Dhat Syndrome, but not in other control groups. Therefore, loss of Dhat ('Dhatu' / Semen) in an anxious prone individual makes him hypochondriacal (Bandyopadhyay, 1999). The number of neurotics and psychotics examined in this study was small. Moreover, their age, marital status, education and employment status were not known. This requires replication on large number of subjects matched in the variables mentioned above.

Dhat syndrome is accepted as a 'culture related' / 'culture-specific' / 'culture-bound' psychiatric problem, particularly in India (Bhatia and Malik, 1991) and her subcontinent (Akhtar, 1988), but still there is ongoing debate regarding the possibilities of cultural expression of known psychiatric disorders in such syndrome. However, these require further study to stop speculation on its etiology (Kapur, 2001).

Co-existence of other psychiatric morbidity with Dhat Discharge needs special mentioning. Depression, both like that of neurotic or psychotic is seen to be commonly associated with this problem along with anxiety and hypochondriasis. Such patients usually respond well with anti-depressants (Bandyopadhyay, 1999). Eclectic approach is required for its management (Kapur, 1987), relatively less number of studies on such phenomenon has been reported in the recent years.

There exists attitudinal differences amongst different culture with regard to mental illness/ behavioural problems, namely, homosexuality, and use of mind altering drugs, *e.g,* Ganja. Also cultural differences exist in how quickly and what kind of symptoms are recognized. Among the Yourba, Phobia and OCD are very infrequently noticed, whereas in our culture these are very frequently reported particularly amongst adolescents and young adults. Some of the culturally determined abnormal behaviour (*e.g.,* Amok, Latah, and Kora) prevalent in the South-East-Asia, mainly in Malaya, Indonesia, Singapore, Borneo and the Philippines have been discussed, citing case reports, by Sarbadhikary (1999).

Culture plays a strong role in the course of schizophrenia. Patients with schizophrenia in developing countries like India, Colombia, and Nigeria are less likely to remain incapacitated by the disorder for long term than those who have schizophrenia in developed countries such as the United States, Great Britain. It may be partially due to variations in the genes for schizophrenia across cultural groups; also differences in how cultures treat their patients probably play a strong role in this regard. In developing countries patients with schizophrenia, for example, are more likely to be cared for at home by a broad network of family members who share responsibility for the individual. In contrast, in developed countries, it is less likely that the person with schizophrenia lives with family or that his/her immediate family has other family members nearby who share in the care (Jablensky, 1989). Caring for a family member with schizophrenia is a huge burden. When this burden is shouldered by only a few persons, there can be tremendous conflicts in the family which may exacerbate the symptoms of the patients with schizophrenia.

Another unique disorder is Susto, also known as "Magic Fright" (Kleinmuntz, 1974). This has been reported to occur among Central and South American Indian tribes and non-Indian inhabitants of the Andean Highlands of Peru, Bolivia, and Colombia. Mostly it afflicts infants and young children (occasionally adolescents and exceptionally adults may also suffer). **Susto** is attributed to contacts with supernatural beings, breathing "bad air" in dangerous places, such as cemeteries. In this disorder symptoms are varied and can be divided into somatic (emaciation, loss of strength, rapid heart beat, gastrointestinal disorders), and psychological (intense anxiety, hyperexcitability, generalised phobias, depression) (Kleinmuntz, 1974). Treatment consists of invoking the absent soul and cleaning the body by rubbing it with various plants or animals; especially palliative is the guinea pig (Wittkower and Dubreuil, 1968).

Likewise, **amok**, which occurs among the Malayans and in some parts of Africa (Kleinmuntz, 1974) has culture-specific features. It is characterised by a withdrawn, quiet, passive and gentle behaviour (gradually leading to a greater withdrawal, and meditation) followed by an excited rage (called **amok**) during which the afflicted individual suddenly jumps up, some times with a terrifying yell, grabs daggers or other weapons, and attacks anyone or anything he encounters. He may even commit homicide or mutilate himself; often he is killed by frightened neighbours. The disorders has similarities, especially to catatonic schizophrenia seen in the West. Amok's cultural components have been described by Wittkower and Dubreuil, 1968; Yap, 1966).

Coming to variations in delusional symptoms it is noted that schizophrenic symptoms among some African societies contain mythological content and also delusions in which individuals become chiefs or witch doctors or are being poisoned or bewitched. By contrast, delusions of such individuals in Western societies include influences operating from a distance, through electricity, X-rays, hypnotism, and outer-space vehicles. Again, within African societies delusional contents have been reported to be different (Tooth, 1950).

Thus, *e.g.,* among the "bush" people in the north of Ghana, the delusion dealt with remification of the fetish system, whereas, in the south of Ghana the delusions are about the control of electricity and the wireless. Such a within society variation is due to varying degrees of Westernization, *e.g.,* in the south of Ghana, where Western influences are more compared to the north of Ghana.

Symptom differences have been noted among schizophrenics of different ethnic backgrounds (Opler, 1956, 1959). Irish-American schizophrenics, *e.g.,* were reported to be less hostile, more subdued, and less bizarre than their Italian-American counterparts. Similar ethnic diversity in symptoms was reported between Japanese schizophrenics raised in Japan and those of Japanese descent in Hawaii.

In sum: Differences in symptom manifestation have been evident among schizophrenics of different culture.

Indian Culture Context and Hallucinations and Delusions in Patients with Schizophrenia

With regard to Indian culture it may be stated that though people of different caste and creed live in India, India has a distinct culture of its own. Research findings pertaining to the pathoplastic effects of socio-cultural norms upon manifestation of psychiatric symptoms in general, and schizophrenic symptomatology in particular amongst Indian patients do claim that even the nature and content of hallucinations and delusions experienced by them are largely reflections of Indian socio-cultural set-up in disguise. Despite scientific and technological advancement influence of religion still seems to form an important part of Indian life, especially for the large rural population. Superstititious and misconceptions like 'Jadu-tona', witchcraft, and evil spirits are much prevalent today amongst less sophisticated section of Indian society. Accordingly, preponderance of magic and religious themes are noted in the hallucinatory themes of Indian patients, especially those belonging to lower socio-economic strata. Studies conducted in different parts of India show similar results. Thus, *e.g.,* Chakravorty (1966) in her study on 280 schizophrenics in Calcutta, Eastern India and Sharma and Agnihotri (1986) in their study on 100 patients in Varanasi, Uttar Pradesh, India, found that the commonest hallucinatory theme noted in their patients was magic and religion followed by murder, assault, sex, and body organs (Sharma and Agnihotri, 1986). Gods (*e.g.,* Lord Shiva, Krishna, etc.) and Goddess (*e.g.,* Kali, Durga, and Of late, Santoshi Ma, etc.) were the main hallucinatory objects, for the Hindus, whereas for the Muslims (Chakravorty, 1966) these were Hasan, Hosain, or Scenes of Karbala. Interestingly enough, two of the Muslim patients, Chakravorty investigated, had hallucinations of Hindu Gods. Thus, in spite of having geographical and sub-cultural (*e.g.,* food habits, dress, and rituals) differences in general, these patients show a commonness in their expression of disguised wishes.

Some of these patients also saw ghosts, or simple objects like, pitcher, etc. (Chakravorty, 1966). About one-third of the patients in Chakravorty's study had complex hallucinations consisted of bizarre images, *e.g.,* 'Nara Rakshas', Thirty-three crores of Gods moving around them all the time, dead relatives talking to patients, etc. A few of the patients reported simple hallucinations of spots, lights, shadow etc., while scenic ones consisted of images like Lord Shiva and Parvati together going down the main street of Calcutta in a four-wheeled carriage etc. These contents are very much pertinent to the social milieu these patients come from. A detailed discussion regarding influence of socio-cultural milieu in understanding hallucinations and delusions will be made later in this chapter.

Prevalence of sexual themes in the hallucinations of these patients reflect a conflict between the rigid traditional sexual morality and sexual liberalism (Sharma and Agnihotri, 1986). In Indian culture sexual attitudes and actions are equated with ethical values. Moreover, this culture encourages more of suppression of sexual impulses rather than its overt expression. The latter is considered a taboo here.

About one-third of the total number of schizophrenics investigated by Sharma and Agnihotri (1986) manifestated the theme of murder and assault in their hallucinations. Mostly these patients were less educated and unmarried. It should be mentioned here that in some parts of India people structure their environment, define their identity, interaction and achievement in terms of fear and violence (Kala and Wig, 1978). Besides, amongst the illiterate, masculinity is equated with aggression (Sharma and Agnihotri, 1986) and unmarried males are free to act out their aggression in the way they like because of less social and family restrictions imposed on them, compared to married individuals. Such environmental factors seem to be significant in producing certain themes of hallucinations in psychiatric patients.

Not only theme, but also the sensory-modality used in hallucinations by the patients seem to have a cultural influence. In psychiatry there is a common notion that visual hallucinations are rare in schizophrenia (Mayer-Gross, Slater and Roth, 1974; Oswald, 1962), and their presence raises suspicion of an acute irreversible (Noyes and Kolb, 1963) organic brain disorder (Bleuler, 1950). But in contrast to these views Chakravorty (1966) reported that about 50% of her patients had visual hallucinations, while 44% had both auditory and visual hallucinations, and about 52% of the Schizophrenic patients she investigated had hallucinations in some form or other. Presence of visual hallucinations also showed some relationship to sex though no such relationship was noted with the duration of illness these patients suffered from. Women patients mostly reported visual hallucinations and there too, women with lower education complained of significantly more hallucinations especially in its visual form. However, educational level did not make any significant difference in male patients.

According to Huxley (1959) diabetic deficiency may produce visual hallucinations. Thus, one might think of dietary deficiency in illiterate and therefore poor Indian women who had shown more prevalence of visual hallucinations. But this view does not seem to be acceptable, as because educated and better placed men also had visual hallucinations (Chakravorty, 1966).

In Indian mythology vision has always been perceived as a most powerful and significant modality and on the basis of which Gods/Goddesses are discriminated from earthly organisms on the one hand and between ordinary people and those who are believed to possess supernatural power popularly known as Priests / Sadhus / Tantrikas on the other. Priests / Sadhus are conceived to have a wider jurisdiction of their vision through which they mediate between ordinary people and Gods/Goddesses. This perhaps is the reason for perceiving Idols of Gods / Goddesses as having three eyes instead of two. Moreover, there is a general belief that Sadhus through their unique vision can alter a given Individual's fortune depending upon whether the victim has been perceived by the Sadhu as a benign or harmful. Likewise, to portray a powerful God like Shiva, Indians mostly attribute a third eye on the forehead of the Idol to emphasize his power through which he may even destroy the earth if he so desires. On the contrary, a humble worshipper perceives the light emitted from the third eye of the Gods/Goddesses as blessings which is popularly known as 'Jyoti'. Moreover, in Indian culture alcoholic beverages are quite often used in many of our religious rituals and practices (*e.g.*, by the Tantrikas) the underlying meaning may be to induce a hallucinogenic experience in the Priests / Tantrikas which enable them to prove that their vision encompasses of a larger jurisdiction than those of ordinary people. Thus, the use of 'Soma Rasa' as described in the Vedas might have been a hallucinogenic substance instead of alcohol as popularly believed to be (Chakravorty, 1966). Induction of such a substance makes the persons feel self-elated and thus a peculiar change the experiences through visual modality. Such being the cultural background perhaps it is no wonder that Indian patients in this study experienced more visual hallucinations than their European counterpart.

However, Chakravorty took patients from only one hospital outdoor of Calcutta and she has not mentioned any diagnostic sub-classification of her patients but that they were all schizophrenics. Secondly, hallucinations were categorised by one of the observers instead of an independent observer. Likewise, Sharma and Agnihotri also investigated only 100 patients who reported to a particular hospital of Varanasi. Therefore, Generalisation of the present findings may not be possible until further research on large number of patients with different socio-economic strata are done. However, these findings do point out that psychiatric symptoms can be more meaningfully understood when we consider the social milieu of the patient. This provides a further support to the prevailing notion that auditory hallucinations occur more frequently in the Western schizophrenic patients, whereas visual hallucinations are common in the patients outside of the Western culture. Some further support to this idea may be gleaned from some of the following Indian studies done on the theme of delusions noted in schizophrenic patient of these culture.

Bhaskaran and Saxena (1970) in a study on 140 first admission schizophrenics in a hospital in India found that 71.4% of the males and 47.1% of the females had delusions. Sharma and Gupta (1978) also reported a greater occurrence of males in both the deluded and non-deluded groups. Among the different types of delusions, the persecutory ones were the most frequent in both the sexes (Bhaskaran and Saxena, 1970), though delusions of grandeur were much less frequent in women patients (Bhaskaran, 1959). In the latter study

(Bhaskaran, 1959), 138 (89 males) consecutive first admissions of schizophrenics were investigated. Bhaskaran and Saxena reported (1970) that catatonic schizophrenia was found to occur with greater frequency in females than in males. Interestingly enough sex differences were noted with regard to presence of as well as nature of precipitating factors in the Indian schizophrenics (Bhaskaran and Saxena, 1970). Thus, identifiable precipitating factors were evident in 47% of males whereas it was 57% in case of female patients. While failure in examination, failure in love-affairs, and frustration in occupation constituted the most commonest precipitating factors in the males, child birth, marital discord, and financial strain or loss in the family constituted the commonest causes in the females. Not only precipitating factors, persecutors also in the patients with delusion of persecution showed differences in both the sexes (Bhaskaran, 1959). While in the males these were elder brothers, father, wife, superior officers, or community at large, in the females, they were husband, sisters-in-law, brothers-in-law, mother-in-law, and neighbours. Likewise, Sharma and Gupta (1978) reported that definite groups / agencies (*e.g.,* Naxalites, Police, C.I.A., C.B.I. and Political Party etc.) and close associates more often appeared to be present in males as persecutors, whilst in the females, family members especially in-Laws, landlady, tenant, police and thieves etc. were the usual persecutory agents. Also, in females more often the persecutor was not specified by the patients. This study (Sharma and Gupta, 1978) was carried out on 295 cases of schizophrenia at the K.G. Medical Colleges, Lucknow, North India. A detailed analysis of the content of some of the common delusions, *viz.,* expansive, paranoid, sexual and influence and control was done. Contents of expansive delusions were sub-divided into delusions of authority, and power, of wealth, of social status, and a comparison of the same showed that a greater incidence of the delusions of authority and power, and social status was noted in these patients of which males identified with political and the religious figures (*e.g.,* Lord Brahma, Hanumanji, etc.), whereas the females identified themselves with the Goddesses like Santoshi Ma, Durga, Kali, etc.

Analysis of the content of delusions of influence and control revealed that in the poorly educated and those of low status the content was simple, often being centered around the superstitions of witchcraft, magic and evil spirits. Educated patients and those of higher status, on the other hand, elaborated their delusions and were found to be related to magnetism, telepathy, hypnotism, radio, transmitters, etc. Similar was the findings of Kala and Wig (1978).

As regards the content of sexual delusions it was observed by Sharma and Gupta (1978) that the most commonest type of it in both men and women was the delusion of infidelity of spouse, and a false belief of imposed heterosexual activity. From an initial critical and fault-finding attitude there is a slow progression through suspiciousness ultimately to development of frank delusions. Apart from infidelity in some cases delusions are found to be accompanied by pathologic jealousy. Such a delusion is named 'conjugal paranoia' (Revitch, 1954). However, conjugal paranoia is a distinct syndrome, whereas, morbid jealousy, pathologic jealousy or erotic jealousy either is a symptom that can be seen in different illness such as, alcoholism schizophrenia, affective psychoses, organic syndromes, etc. In addition to delusions of suspiciousness, delusions of 'persecution' and 'reference' remain as key symptoms of schizophrenia and these are found to occur most prominently in paranoid. On the other hand, delusion of 'guilt' and 'grandeur' exhibit characteristic occurrence in depression and mania respectively.

Sexual inadequacy delusions are restricted to the patient's own feeling of inadequacy in context to his/her sex role competency. This is because in Indian culture one learns more to inhibit rather than to express one's experience and ideas about sex. A sense of fear works in young boys and girls especially during their adolescence as to whether they will be able to perform their sex role (function) adequately. On the one hand the individual wants to conform to the social norm (that he is completely naïve about sexual experience before marriage, and hence society should consider him/her as 'good' boy/man, and/or girl/women), and on the other, as an instinct, his/her libidinal urges instigate him/her to have an experience of sex to meet up his curiosity. Thus, the individual is in conflict. As already mentioned above, a sense of fear works as a background factor behind such a conflict, if such an individual fails to maintain heterosexual relation in practical life, obviously he/she develops delusion of reference, *i.e.,* he/she is being talked about by others regarding his/her inadequacy. Such an idea that people area talking about him/her (reference) thus acts as an external threat to the individual. Subsequently it proceeds to a false belief that people are planning to harm him/her (suspicion) and finally to the conviction that people have started causing lot of harm against his/her (persecution).

Sex differences in the prevalence of hallucinations and delusions, in their contents and precipitatory factors, as well as in the nature of persecutors in persecutory delusions may be attributed to the socio-cultural factors governing the rearing of boys and girls in Indian culture. Unlike the Western culture the socio-cultural factors influencing the developmental trends in Indian culture differ in the two sexes which in turn, produces differences in the social attitudes, social behaviour, value-orientation and in overall personality make-up between the two sexes. Thus, *e.g.,* in the upbringing of boys, a high premium is given on scholastic performance so much so that mostly they are pressurised to be competitive with a view to select a few prestigeladen careers like, engineering, administrative services and profession of medicine. Thus, selection of career becomes a prestigious issue with scarce consideration given to the boys' aptitudes, interests, and potentialities. Being driven into academic and occupational pursuits purely on a prestige issue boys/men become victims of insecurity, conflicts and frustration with regard to their achievement, both scholastic and occupational.

Compared to the boys, the atmosphere, mostly found in the upbringing process of girls, tends to be more restrictive in nature. In their social interaction a high premium is given onto social reservedness, non-assertiveness, and conservatism in their manner. Cultural forces make the girls learn to restrain emotional expressiveness, particularly negative emotions. Sex is considered to be a taboo especially during adolescence and post-adolescence and parents/guardians remain highly vigilant over a girl's habits and interaction. Likewise, educational achievement in girls is usually considered secondary if not unnecessary in some parts of India. Even if a girl is willing to go for education, parents insist on her getting married first. In some cases girls are found to be apprehensive that parents and/or husbands after marriage will not allow them to complete their educational and occupational pursuits, which causes a lot of frustration in them. Of late, a large number of girls are getting educated and a good number of them is going for higher education and thereupon occupation, even then they are mostly perceived as weaker gender and are also and expected to take primarily the role of a housewife only, no matter how much financial help one renders to her husband. This causes both physiological and psychological strain in the women.

In India to remain unmarried for long is a social stigma for the girls as well as for the family she belongs to. Sometimes, younger sisters cannot get married to unless the eldest/elder is married. This causes extra tension in the eldest with a feeling that as if, she is a hindrance on the way to her younger siblings marriage and settlement in life. For this reason less qualified girls get married with heavy compensation like, dowry etc. which causes an additional strain to the girls in particular and to her family at large. After marriage, the girl (now wife) is expected to be totally non-assertive, and is demanded of a great self-sacrifice in the interest of her husband as well as husband's family. She has no way of to expressing her resentments and other negative feelings but to repress.

If unfortunately the marriage turns up to be an incompatible one, mostly the girl becomes the target of all blames. For example, marital discord due to infertility. In such cases, mostly villagers make the girl first hand victim without giving least thought about the possibilities of infertility from the male partner. Marital disharmony originating from dowry negotiation puts the girls in severe stress, and many a times it leads to even murder of the girl. In case of marital disharmony it is seldom found that they resort to redress through legal divorce though there is provision for the same. This is because going back to father's house is perceived as a social stigma for the girls after marriage. A true wife is supposed to spend her whole life with her husband no matter how irresponsible or unkind he may be. Thus, marriage in Indian culture is considered a sacred alliance indissoluble for all practical purposes. Unresolved psychic conflicts contribute to the precipitation of schizophrenic reaction especially postpartum schizophrenic reaction (Deutsch, 1945). The reasons for less frequent occurrence of delusion of grandeur in the females compared to the males seem to be socio-culturally determined (Bhaskaran, 1963; Bhaskaran and Saxena, 1970). As already mentioned above, average women in this society face a great deal of restrictive socio-cultural forces from early life, with little opportunity left for realising their full individual potentialities, talents and aspirations. These, in other words, remain non-realised forever. Socio-cultural forces seem to have made women feel that they are for self-sacrifice, self-effacement, and not to think high of themselves, and therefore, their fantasies too are probably (Bhaskaran and Saxena, 1970) other than grandiose in nature. Lesser frequency of delusions of grandeur in women may also be due to their lower educational achievement as compared to men. Similar to this view of Bhaskaran and Saxena (1970) rarity of delusion of grandeur among the non-literate (tribes) has been reported by others (Adeoye, 1955; Smartt, 1956) as well.

Carothers (1948) found that in the natives of East Africa (Kenya) paranoid schizophrenia was nearly 4 times more frequent among the educated than among the uneducated. Also, Moffson (1954) reported that catatonic Schizophrenia far outnumbered the other sub types of schizophrenia in the natives of South Africa. However, these findings have been obtained based on the patients who reported to a given hospital for a certain period of time. Thus, *e.g.*, in Bhaskaran and Saxena's (1970) study 1st admissions of Hindu male and female patients admitted to the Hospital for Mental Diseases, Ranchi, Eastern India, during the later part of 1967 were investigated. The patients were predominantly from the middle and uppermiddle class of Northern and Eastern-India. Moffson's patients were from admissions to West Koppies in South Africa, whereas, Adecy's patients were amongst the Yoruba tribes. Therefore, generalisation of these findings may not be possible until other studies on several other subjects of different socio-economic and socio-cultural background are done. This is so stated because in some parts of India, *e.g.*, Calcutta, Eastern India, the hospital admissions are predominantly represented by the lower-middle and poorest class of the society. Therefore, study reports based on hospital population would provide us only with a partial view of the total picture. Upper middle and rich people usually go for private consultation to maintain secrecy with a view to avoid social stigma in this regard. Unless these patients are taken into account one is not sure whether similar incidence of certain specific symptom pattern would be found to prevail in women patients only. Incidentally to be mentioned that Sharma and Gupta (1978) failed to find any significant association between variables like, age, sex, religion, education, family income, parental deprivation, and migration with the patterns of delusions. Moreover, in their study paranoid delusions were found to be significantly more associated with large sized families (7 and above). Expansive and religious delusions were significantly more frequent in medium sized families. On the other hand, delusions of reference, sexual delusions and hypochondriacal delusions were more frequent in small sized and medium sized (up to 6) families. Also, paranoid delusions and expansive delusions were found to be significantly associated with total number of siblings up to 6, whereas, delusions of reference were found to be related to the total number of siblings up to 7-9 years. Secondly, during the present era women are not facing that much of social oppression in actualising their potentialities as it was during 1950s and around. Since more number of girls are coming for higher education, and subsequent employment, it gives them opportunity to compare themselves with their counterpart. Of course, the latter situation is also not totally free from any problem. Women at present, especially in cities, are found to have a conflict between traditionalism and conservatism on the one hand (as so-called heritage of Indian girls) and modernisation (strive to cope with the society's present demand) on the other. Such a situation is likely to cause conflict in them, which however, is noticed in many of the Indian girls, especially these who come from orthodox, traditional family background.

To see the role of delusions in various functional psychiatric disorders in India Chauhan, Jain and Kumar (1983) conducted a study on 100 general psychiatric patients of Agra (North India) mental hospital and found that proneness of incidence of delusions in the schizophrenic category was noted in 'acute reaction', 'disorganised', 'chronic', and 'paranoid' varieties. Delusions of persecution, suspicion, and reference were found to play a prominent role in schizophrenic patients, though delusions of control and guilt as well as religions and sexual delusions were found to be present in some patients only. However, this study was conducted on male patients and therefore, one can not be sure whether the findings would remain same even after inclusion of female patients. Preponderance of hallucinatory themes of magic and religion was noted (Sharma and Agnihotri, 1986) among females especially in less educated patients belonging to lower SES. This finding can further be substantiated from the study of Kala and Wig (1978) who investigating 200 Indian paranoid psychotics (in Chandigarh) and reported that two common delusional themes, *viz.,* religion and magic on the one hand, and that of technology of science on the other were evident in their patients. This shows that two contrasting system of values exists in this society which produces a revolt of interaction between westernisation and the traditional institutions of Indian culture. Kuba (1975) in this context reported that possession syndrome can occur only when the shamanistic and modern culture mingle. Possession syndromes provide a safety valve (Teja, 1970) for the emotionally troubled individuals as these help in making them integrated (Verma, Srivastava, and Sahay, 1970) in the community.

Laubscher (1937) noted mythological content in delusions of African schizophrenics in Queenland while the delusion of Europeans included more of influence operating from a distance through telepathy and electricity etc. Similarly delusional contents of influence and control by electricity and wireless were found among the sophisticated people of South Ghana (Tooth, 1950), though the delusional content of the "bush" people of North Ghana was reported to be (Tooth, 1950) associated with the ramification of the fetish system. Likewise, the delusions of middle class Brazilians were found to get expressed (Stainbrook, 1952) in terms of economic and class conceptions of power along with such interpersonal influences as that of electricity and physical waves, while in the lower class Brazilians it was concerning Catholic deities. Lambo (1955) observed that delusions among non-literate Yorubans related to supernatural concepts and ancestral cults, whereas in the literate Africans, hypochondriacal delusions were found to be prominent.

Transcultural studies also have shown that there is a greater degree of differentiation of emotional states in the developing countries especially China, Nigeria, India and Columbia (Leff, 1974), Lucas and Collins (1962) in this connection proposed that symptoms can be more meaningfully related to the social background of the patient than can a diagnosis. This statement seems to be more applicable in understanding contents of hallucinations and delusions since these are mostly influenced by the social milieu of the patients.

The above discussion once again lends support to the hypothesis formulated by Phillips. To quote "persons of the same racial stock, carrying the same diagnosis, develop different kinds of symptoms depending upon the society in which they live" (Phillips, 1966).

In sum : Indian patients have shown some specificity in symptom manifestation compared to patients of other culture. For example, delusions of bodily control and being poisoned were reported to be more common in Indian patients than those of the Western culture (Kala and Wig, 1982). This shows that symptom can be related with the social background of the patients.

Background Cultural Factors as Determinants of Symptom Contents in Migrated Schizophrenic Patients

There is evidence that people endeavour to keep their culture intact even after migrating to other cultures. It has been emphasized by several investigators both in India and abroad that the contents of a particular illness are provided by the prevailing culture the patients come from (Cooper, 1933; Carothers, 1948; Yap, 1951; Stainbrook, 1952; Lambo, 1955; Bhaskaran, 1963). Thus, *e.g.,* delusions of ghost possession, which is uncommon in Britain but common in South-Asian countries, has been reported in the Asians living in the U.K. (Hall and Pinninti, 1994; Bose, 1997). Likewise, a greater occurrence of melancholis among Chinese in Java (Yap, 1951), Whitigi psychosis of Cree and Ojidway (Cooper, 1933), Amok and Latah in the Malayan (Yap, 1952; Murphy, 1973), and Piblokto of Peary's Eskimos (Brill, 1913; Ackernecht, 1968) have been reported by both Indian and Western researchers long back.

In a recent study Suhail (2000) assessed and compared the phenomenology of delusions and hallucinations in Indian schizophrenic patients living in Britain and their native British counterparts. Out of 400 case notes examined, 110 (60 British-Indian and 50 whites) psychiatric patients admitted in two psychiatric units in Birmingham were studied using the Present State Examination (PSE) categories. There was no significant difference between both groups in age and gender distribution. Both groups were also similar in the diagnosis received; greater frequency of patients from both groups had received the diagnosis of schizophrenia. However, groups differed in marital status, with more Whites having single. Majority of the British-Indians was born in the U.K. (53%) than in India (35%). There were no cases to allow separate comparison of 1st and 2nd generations of the Indian group.

Analysis of the types of delusions and hallucinations revealed a mixed picture where 92% of Indian patients reported different forms of delusions compared to 90% of Whites, but greater number of White patients (94%) reported the experience of hallucinations as compared to British-Indian (75%). Comparison of two groups on different forms of delusions showed that the groups differed only in the frequency of delusion of persecution, with more British-Indians believing that they were being persecuted (Suhail, 2000).

So far as themes of delusions are concerned the two groups showed differences where greater number of British-Indians were deluding that they were being harmed, more white patients, in contrast, believed that they were having communication with God.

The analysis of delusional explanations indicated that the delusions of British-Indians revolved around black magic and family members, while for the White it was more of telepathic communication.

Of frequency analyses of hallucinations, majority in both the groups experienced verbal hallucinations. White patients however, excelled in hearing voices (ordering them to go for homicide or suicide). However, in themes of hallucinations the groups did not show any difference in their experience.

From the above it is evident that delusions of persecution appeared to be the commonest delusion in both groups. This suggests that thought problems and schizophrenic delusions and hallucionations may be relatively universal manifestations of underlying organic dysfunction. In this sense, Suhail's study confirms previous findings, both from India and other countries (Mirowsky, 1985). But further analysis of Suhail's study revealed that although persecutory delusions were common in both the groups, British-Indian patients excelled in the frequency of such delusions and also in connecting persecutory theme of being attacked, poisoned and harmed. This indicates that in spite of having universal organic dysfunction in schizophrenia, mistrust is a thematic ailments of group culture and individual beliefs. Mistrust develops out of social interaction as to how a given individual since his childhood has been used to face threatening social conditions, what sort of meaning he has been conditioned to attribute to it, and how he learned to cope with such situations. Rationality of mistrust does not depend upon education and wealth (Mirowsky, 1985). Rather mistrust as a reasonable orientation toward others develops where exploitation and victimisation are common, resources and opportunities are less and at the same time protection provided by the situation and agencies is weak. The high incidence of persecutory ideas in the Indian context may be due to the influence of this particular culture where childhood is characterised by repression of hostility (Rao, 1966). In this context Indian authors, *viz.,* Kala and Wig (1982) also suggested that cultures which structure their environment in terms of fear and aggression show preponderance of persecutory ideas in their sample. Aggression and persecutory themes in Indian patients and the involvement of family members in these themes, may be explained taking into account the process of socialisation a child passes through. During the process of socialisation a high premium is placed in obedience to elders and aggression receives hardly any encouragement (Rao, 1966). The authority of elder brother or the mother-in-law is supported by moral injections. Rao (1966) is of the opinion that the direct hostility or aggression is repressed to reappear, in some cases, in the form of delusions of persecution. In this sense, preponderance of persecutory delusions in British-Indian patients (67%) of Suhail's (2000) study corresponds very well with those of previous Indian studies (Rao, 1966; Kala and Wig, 1982), where a greater persecutory idea (82%) was evident in actual inhabitants in India. Interestingly, it may be mentioned here that two of the Suhail's patients relapsed after visiting India. May be visit to their original culture as Suhail (2000) thought, make them further confused with regard to the conflicting values and goals connected with sharing of two cultures, the immediate outcome of which was relaps of the problem.

In general, in delusion of persecution, the target object to the patient is his most close relatives initially, and then gradually it spreads over to causal acquaints through close friends, etc. Indian family tie, which is really unique all over the world, makes children mostly totally dependable onto their parents/relatives; this may be the reason that persecutors in Indian schizophrenic patients are mostly family members. In earlier Indian studies (*e.g.* Rao, 1966), it has been reported that the persecutor was elder brother in case of male patient, and sister-in-law, in case females. In Suhail's recent study (2000), the persecutors were the patient's own parents, siblings, and in-laws. Compared to the Whites (16%), the delusions (control, reference, and persecutory) of twice as many British-Indian patients (39%) dissolved around their family members. Thus Suhail's study conforms very well the previous Indian research reports (Rao, 1966; Kala and Wig, 1982).

One might question here about the impact of family type in causing such delusions. Previously, joint family was the most prevalent family type in India, which however rarely prevails now-a-days, though extended nuclear family is still in existence in India. Although the traditional extended family system is generally disappearing in Indian families living in Britain, still then, all the near kith and kin keep strong contact regularly with each other. Such close contacts do provide one with a unique opportunity of sharing on the one hand (Suhail, 2000) but on the other, it might cause extra tension and worries in the individual over family responsibilities, family relationships, disputes, break-up etc. Rao (1966) in this context reported that in about 20.5% of the cases in Indian family tension is found to be the cause of mental illness.

In another dimension of the delusion, *i.e.,* delusional explanations, the British-Indian patients complained of themes of magic whereas the White patients had greater themes of telepathic communication. This reflects Locus of Control (LOC) of both the groups of patients. The White patients have more independent attitude towards themselves with more power of their own mind; they seem to believe in extra-sensory perception (Suhail, 2000), whereas the British-Indian patients with dependent attitude and less power of their own mind seem to perceive power in external sources, *e.g.,* magic. The latter, *i.e.,* preponderance of magical themes in British-Indian patients supports the hypothesis of a lowered threshold of culturally sanctioned experiences (Al-Issa, 1995). The excess of magical theme is a means to help one's self to escape the responsibility of misfortune, and thus to put the responsibility of misfortunes of some culturally accepted external source. This may also refer to the factor of suspiciousness which an Indian inculcates through interpersonal interaction. This is so stated because in Suhail's (2000) study the British-Indian patients who reported magical themes were found to be suspicious that their relatives (female patients believe that their in-laws, male patients believed that their own family members) were using black magic or cult to harm them.

From Suhail's study it is not possible to predict whether prevalence of traditional beliefs would be present across generations, because due to small number of data Suhail did not split the data of British-Indians into 1st and 2nd generations. Bose (1997) in this context mentioned that even though beliefs in Witchcraft and spirit possession are observed in 1st generation of migrants, it can not be assumed that they will not be retained in the following generations who have spent their formative years in Britain. There is evidence that in the societies undergoing rapid social change through Industrialisation indigenous beliefs continue to be hold even amongst those educated in the Western way (Bhattacharyya, 1986).

From the above, it is evident that one's cultural values and expectations affect the way distress is perceived, experienced and expressed in a given society. Also its effect remains intact even if the person migrates to another culture. Yet, Suhail's study emphasized that the impact of shared environmental experiences in different cultural groups, with regard to psychiatric symptom manifestation, can not be overlooked. For example, in the above mentioned study both the British groups did not appear to be different in many forms of delusions and hallucinations. The two groups of patients were similar in the frequency of delusions of control, reference, grandiosity, jealousy, and hypochondriasis. Again, in delusional explanations of physical objects both the groups were similar. Both the groups were deluding that either TV, satellites, X-rays, Radio, or Computers were presenting, controlling or referring to them.

Regarding the modality dimension of hallucinations, reported research findings have not been consistent across culture. Ndetei and Singh (1983) like that of Muesser and Berenbaum (1990) though reported greater visual hallucinations in Asians compared to the white patients who showed preponderance of auditory hallucinations, Suhail's study failed to provide a direct support to these above mentioned findings. Though the groups, in Suhail's study did not show statistically significant differences in modality dimension of hallucinations, the trend however, was of more ($p<0.06$) White (88%) patients hearing voices compared to British-Indians (73%); significantly greater number of White patients (24% vs 8%) reported that voices ordered them to kill themselves or others.

Coming to the theme of delusions – those pertaining to religion and infidelity are found to be predominant in Indian patients in general (Kala and Wig, 1982), a finding which corroborates well with that of recent research reports (Suhail, 2000). Interestingly in Suhail's study it was found that British-Indian patients displayed less religious themes compared to their White counterparts. Could it be possibly an expression of revolt against Indian religious faith, on the part of the Indians living in the Western society? Or it could be that the Indians living in Britain tried to acculturate them with the societal norms they were encountering in everyday life. However, preponderance of religious theme of delusions is an expression of fear of punishment which arise out of guilt feeling, ingrained in our population through social training. Likewise, delusional theme of infidelity, is an expression of deep level fear of being rejected/neglected by the life partner, which as projection, turns out to blame the life partner as unfaithful. Extra marital affairs are looked down with contempt all over the world, but more so in India and in her subcontinent. Although, Indian culture is going through rapid changes due to technological advancements, a great majority of our population still likes to hold traditional values and customs and thus betraying spouse is considered a grave moral misdemeanour. This could be the reason that British-Indians, though relatively less in number compared to Indians (Suhail, 2000), complain of infidelity which is an expression of their inner fears that their females may adopt Western style of life. This has been supported from the interview reports of Suhail's (2000) patients living in Britain, where people of a traditional society are confronted with a new culture, its norms and values. This causes mental derangements. Thus, psychological conflicts originating from traditional Indian sexual morality and sexual liberalism of the Western society seem to play an important etiological role.

Findings regarding gender differences in the delusions of infidelity are still not consistent. In Suhail's (2000) study 4 out of 5 patients were men in contrast to Kala and Wig's (1982) report where preponderance of females was evident. Further, in another recent study on Pakistani patients, Suhail (2000) observed that more female patients complained of infidelity. Though one major weakness of Suhail's study is its retrospective design, the findings do provide information about impact of culture in symptom manifestation in psychiatric patient.

Interim Summary on Culture Context and Hallucinations and Delusions in Migrated Schizophrenic Patients

Studies concerning the prevalence of the various types and content of delusions and hallucinations in psychiatric patients have found both similarities and differences in kinds and theme of hallucinations and delusions in patients of different culture. Research evidences available on the types of hallucinations indicate that though auditory hallucinations are most commonly found in all cultural settings, these occur relatively more frequently in Western schizophrenic patients, whereas visual hallucinations are more common in schizophrenic patients outside than within Western cultures (Ndetei and Singh, 1983; Ndetei and Vadher, 1984).

Themes of direct persecution were more conspicuous among German patients compared to Japanese (Taleyama, Asai, Kamisda, Hashimoto, Bartles and Helmann, 1993) who complained greater themes related to delusions of reference.

There is evidence that people endeavour to keep their culture intact even after migrating to other cultures. But one might also assume that although the background cultural factors will play a significant role in determining the content of delusions and hallucinations, there will be many shared themes due to their similar environmental experiences.

Summary of Etiological Findings

Since last few decades or so attempts have been made to test the hypotheses about the nature of the fundamental psychological disturbances underlying schizophrenic symptoms with the aid of carefully designed investigations. Some of these investigations have brought together the approaches of experimental psychology, psychodynamics, and genetics, and investigations were done on both the schizophrenic subjects as well as on non-schizophrenic patient controls and normal controls. In 1914, Stransky using a metaphor from neurology proposed that 'intrapsychic ataxia' is the basic symptom of dementia praecox. What Stransky described as a lack of co-ordination between emotions ('thymo-psyche') and thinking ('nöö-psyche'), is now generally referred to as incongruity of affect. Bleuler introduced the term 'splitting', which he found exists within the thought process itself. One of the starting points of utilising the results obtained from integrated approach of investigations was the application of Norman Cameron's (Cameron, 1939) concept of 'over-inclusiveness' in thinking as the essential defect of schizophrenia. Over-inclusion of thinking means the patient fails to preserve conceptual boundaries. As a result, the patient is found to incorporate irrelevant ideas which finally leads to vagueness and confusion of thoughts. Over-inclusive thinking is mostly noted in acute schizophrenics. Over-inclusiveness in schizophrenic thinking can be detected through the findings obtained on object – classification test and test of the sorting kind (Lovibond, 1954; McConaghy, 1959) where schizophrenics take long time to classify the objects and mostly fail to do so when compared to the normal controls. In some cases it is also evident that Schizophrenic patients classify objects completely on trial and error basis on the object sorting test which is at variance with that noted in normal controls. Over inclusion is also noted on the Rorschach Inkblot Test and Proverb Test. According to Payne (1962) over-inclusiveness may 'arise from breakdown in a hypothetical filter mechanism which normally screens out those stimuli, both internal and external, which are irrelevant to a task in hand, to allow the most efficient processing of incoming information'. Indian research reports employing time estimation and reaction time tasks in schizophrenic patients (Chatterjee, Chattopadhyay, and Biswas, *et al.*, 1979; Chatterjee, Chattopadhyay, and Biswas, 1980; Chattopadhyay, Biswas, and Mitra, 1982) have shown consistent results throughout. It was evident that schizophrenic patients' autistic separation from external event prevents them from their full utilisation of sensory and motor cues. Interestingly, such experimental findings employing time estimation and reaction time tasks show similar results in the East (*e.g.*, Broota *et al.*, 1988) and the West (Zubin, 1970). Likewise McGhie (1969), Silverman (1967) and Venables (1964) considered schizophrenia as a disorder of attentional processes. They suggested that in the actue phase the schizophrenic is constantly aware of a wide range of stimuli other than those which should strictly be in the forefront of his attention (McGhie and Chapman, 1961). They also pointed out that these patients 'orientation' to those stimuli does not appear to habituate. Such an awareness of a wide range of 'irrelevant' stimuli form an overall impairment by such patients to efficient performance. Based on his concept of 'segmental set' Shakow (1963) has attributed this impairment in efficient performance to 'inability to maintain a set to respond' by such patients. Similar was the view of Callaway, Jones, and Layne (1965). Milstein, Stevens and Sachdev (1969) provided a supporting evidence to this view by demonstrating that the EEG alpha response to photic stimuli had a shorter latency and persisted longer in actue schizophrenics than in chronic patients and normal controls. In chronic patients, however, the latency of alpha blocking was found to be apparently greater than that in controls. However, these findings require replication as because uptil now controvertial confindings have also been reported. Thus, *e.g.*, shorter alpha blocking latency in chronic schizophrenics (Cromwell and Held, 1969) than in normal controls as well as no difference in alpha blocking latency between chronic patients and normals (Hein, Green, and Wilson, 1962) have been reported. However, such controversies could be because of lack of uniformity in selection criteria of patients adhered to such studies. As for example, the chronicity status in Cromwell and Held's (1969) patients was uncertain as they had a mean hospital stay of 19 months only. Similarly findings on SC OR and its habituation in schizophrenics have been far from consistent so far. Both slower than normals (*e.g.*, Dykman, Reese, Galbrecht, Ackerman, and Sunderman, 1968) and faster (*e.g.*, Bernstein, 1969; Zahn *et al.*, 1968) than normals as well as no difference with normals in SC response habituation (*e.g.*, Venables, 1960) have been reported in the research reports. Possible reasons for such contradictions in findings could be because different authors have employed different modality and intensity of stimulus to elicit response habituation. Thus, *e.g.*, in Zahn *et al.'s* (1968) study a 72-db tone and a faint light were used as stimuli whereas Venables (1960) employed 90-db tone and a 900-ft-lambered visual stimulus. Obviously the latter is expected to elicit a defensive response, whereas the former an orienting response. Secondly, in some of these studies sub-diagnostic categories of patients were largely ignored and the patients investigated were broadly labelled as 'Schizophrenics'. But recent research reports do show that diagnostic sub-categorisation is essential in this type of investigations. Thus, *e.g.*, in amongst Zahn *et al.'s* (1968) patients when the performance of sub-diagnostic categories of patients was examined separately, it was found that responsivity was highest in paranoid patients and lower than normal among hebephrenics. More recent research in Indian laboratories, (*e.g.*, Roy, 1981) also supports the necessity to employ symptomatic sub-classification in evaluating their performance on psychophysiological measures. Employing SC OR measure of response habituation Roy (1981) reported faster response decrement in hebephrenics and least in paranoids whereas, simple and catatonics fell in between respectively. Indian research reports on SC OR habituation do not show consistency with those of the West, *e.g.*, Venabels (1967).

Using the concept of 'selective attention' a large amount of work has been undertaken by experimental psychologists, but studies have been conducted by two separate groups of workers. It is very unfortunate that the transmission of ideas between these groups has been limited so much so that there have been very few attempts, of course with some notable exceptions (*e.g.*, Callaway and Stone, 1960; Teichner, 1968), to promote any cross fertilisation. One set of ideas has developed concerning individual differences in the extent to which aspects of external world are perceived. This approach has also been concerned with the underlying physiological state relating to the perceptual selectivity exhibited by the individual. From this set of ideas dichotomies, like, broadness vs narrowness of attention, augmentation vs reduction, repression vs sensitisation, etc. have developed which may collectively be labelled as aspects of 'cognitive style'. Other approach has been more concerned around the notion of the organism as an information processing system. This approach includes concepts like, initial sensory input channels, short-and-long-term storage systems, central serial processing symptoms of limited capacity (Broadbent, 1958; Egeth, 1967; Norman, 1960; Treisman, 1969) etc. Venables (1964) made an attempt to apply some of these later ideas in the field of psychopathology.

A third approach has developed which is concerned with the concept of Orienting Reflex (OR). The "OR is a system of unconditioned, motor, autonomic and central responses elicited by any change in stimulation independent of stimulus quality (Graham and Clifton, 1966, p.306)". At first presentation the stimulus evokes on OR, but on repeated presentation it evokes a characteristic adaptive reaction, with, for example, vasodilation or vasoconstriction of peripheral blood vessels serving an appropriate function in maintaining the equilibrium of the organism. Thus OR may be regarded as a part of a generalised response system that has effects on learning and perceptual processes. At a very superficial level the main difference between orientation and attention would appear to be that the organism orients to those stimuli which are primarily novel, whereas the organism attends to those stimuli which are important or "pertinent" (Norman, 1960). However, a comparison of the works of Sokolov (1960) and Norman (1960) provides some information regarding closeness of the ideas of workers on orientation and on information processing notion of attention.

According to Venables (1967) some factors of dysfunction in schizophrenic performance might be attributed to a partial failure of a homeostatic mechanism through which the level of cortical activity is controlled by inhibitory feedback from the reticular system. Experimental support to this view has been provided by MacKinnon (1969). Sutton, Hakerem, Zubin and Portnoy (1961) and Kristofferson (1967) have provided an additional suggestion stating that a deficit of hippocampal functioning may be involved in schizophrenic's more difficulty than normals in switching attention between modalities. At this stage it may be too bold an attempt to associate hippocampus as the brain structure most closely associated with the appearance of schizophrenia. Certain intriguing possibilities, however, present themselves. These possibilities are – the hippocampus is particularly vulnerable to disturbance (MacLean, 1968). Secondly, it has been demonstrated that hippocampus is easily injured by anoxia (Spector, 1965), to readily retain corticosterone (McEwen, Weiss, and Schwartz, 1968), and therefore, it is capable of being disturbed by stress. Thirdly, it has been shown that high concentrations of serotonin (Paasonen, MacLean, and Giarman, 1957) and non-epinephrine (Fuxe, 1965) are found in the hippocampus, and also that several tranquillising agents appear to act on hippocampal function (Killam, Killam and Shaw, 1957; MacLean, Flanigan, Flynn, Kim, and Stevens, 1955-1956). More interestingly, Flanigan, Gabricli and MacLean (1957) reported that there is a large uptake of methiomine by the hippocampus and based on this findings Pollin, Carton, and Ketty (1961) demonstrated a worsening of symptoms when methionine was given to schizophrenics.

Furthermore, studies reviewed by, for instance, Slater and Beard (1963) and Flor-Henry (1969) have shown an association of temporal lobe epilepsy with psychosis. Interestingly enough it has also been shown that epilepsy in the dominant temporal lobe is associated with schizophrenia, and in the non-dominant lobe with manic-depressive psychosis. If one compares neuronal model of Sokolov to the short-term memory process in which storage may be in a verbal, auditory or articulatory mode, then it would appear that disturbance of the hemisphere responsible for speech would appear to bring about the greatest amount of dysfunction. Clearly though there is not major structural dysfunction of the temporal lobes in schizophrenics, in patients with tumors involving the hippocampus symptoms that produce a disease picture appears undistinguishable from that of schizophrenia (*e.g.,* Malamud, 1967). This thus, may lead to a conclusion (Venables, 1973) that schizophrenia is an epiphenomenal disease, which at least in some patients may be produced as a consequence of disturbance of function of the temporal lobes by a wide variety of causes.

In Indian laboratories studies on neuropsychological perspectives have been reported in both psychiatric (particularly schizophrenia) and neurological patients. On Bender Visuo-Motor Gestalt Test predominant fronto-temporal-parietal dysfunctions were noted in patients with schizophrenia (Mukhopadhyay, Mukherjee, Chowdhury, Gupta, Biswas and Dutta, 1999) compared to the patients with OCD (where predominant temporal lobe dysfunction was evident). Likewise, on arousal modulation capacity, paranoid schizophrenics despite adequate attention showed poorer problem solving scales compared to matched normal controls (Mukhopadhyay and Das, 2003). A detailed review on neuropsychological methods in cognitive assessment of cerebral laterality is available (Chattopadhyay, 1998). In neuropsychological studies laterality has been associated with schizophrenic pathology (Biswas, Haque-Nizamie, Pandey, and Mandal, 1996; Mandal and Singh, 1993; Tiwari and Mandal, 1998; Shukla, Behera, and Mandal, 1993). Interestingly cultural specificity was observed in hemifacial asymmetry amongst such patients (Mandal, Harizuka, Bhusan, and Misra, 2001).

As early as 1958 Lidz, Cornelison, Terry and Fleck have pointed out about the distortions of communication frequently found in families of schizophrenic patients. Such distortions, Lidz *et al.* attributed to the schizoid or paranoid personalities of one or both parents of these patients. These are likely to undermine the patient's ability to test reality as well as his capacity to assess and respond appropriately to the emotional responses of other members of the family. Likewise, McGhie (1961) also found that the mothers of schizophrenics do differ from those of neurotics in characteristic ways. Of late, Mednick and others have mentioned about high risk children in connection with the schizoid personality potentialities of the parents.

What is common in most psychoanalytically oriented theories is that the basis of the disturbance is formed in infancy or early childhood. Childhood interpersonal interaction plays a significant role in the development of 'identity'. In the families of schizophrenia, in Indian culture mostly children experience abandonment or rejection which gives rise a feeling of self non-existence in reality. Two basic needs, *viz.,* inclusion need, and need for expressed control (Sathyavathi, 1974) remain unfulfilled in such patients through their early life interaction. As a result, when the stresses occur later in life the individual regresses to the early faulty stage of development. Accordingly a basic formulation of psychoanalytic theory is that the schizophrenics have weak ego (Bellack, 1970; Basu and Basu, 1996) which mediates between the environment and the other two aspects of the mind, the Id and the supergo by developing defense mechanisms, such as denial, repression, regression, isolation, reaction formation, and projection (Robinson and Robinson, 1965).

From psychodynamic point of view, because of maldevelopment of ego and superego functions there are abnormalities in perception, thoughts, and action. Abnormalities are found in their affect, communication, as well as in their capacity to evaluate, make judgement, solving problems and in overall adaptation to reality. Behaviour is overshadowed by suspicious mistrust, personal doubting, apathetic or indifferent efforts. All these lead to feelings of uncertainty and inadequacy over adult role competency including sexuality. Inhibitions of aggressions, dependency drives and sexual drives are noted in their behaviour. In some schizophrenics such checked arousal of rage and sexual pleasure are discharged time to time impulsively which in turn disrupts widely other functions. Aspirational demands exceed their talent and opportunity, and their consequences (*i.e.*, lack of achievement) give rise to feelings of deep shame and excessive burdens of guilt. Role of familial and extra familial object relations in causing defects in ego growth as well as in causing distortions in ego and superego functions is very significant and thus effective psychotherapeutic milieu probably owes its success in restructuring the abnormal ego function.

Culture plays a significant role in the course of schizophrenia. Disturbed interpersonal interaction and interpersonal communication in the families of schizophrenia are crucial in understanding and in management of patients with schizophrenia. Apart from inherent cultural values, shared cultural values are also important in this regard. Analysis of such cultural contents are essential in the treatment of such patients, an issue which has been detailed in the section on therapy.

7 CHAPTER

Differential Diagnosis

One has to take into account the whole clinical picture, the past history, and all the circumstances and findings of the patient. Though tables of diagnostic symptoms, and of psychological signs have been made by some clinicians, they are of little use in early cases where diagnosis is most difficult. Some of differentials will now be discussed in brief.

A. Affective Disorders

While differentiating the patients with schizophrenia from those suffering from atypical affective disorders, especially mania, it is useful to consider Schneider's symptoms of the first rank, though these are usually absent in doubtful cases. If however, one of these first rank symptoms is clearly present, then quite a number of the others are also be. It is often difficult to be sure whether a patient has a delusional perception, **'Gedankenlautwerden'** (Hamilton, 1976) or experiences of passivity. Thus, in some patients an apparent delusional perception may turn out to be delusional-like experience, or a sudden delusional idea provoked by a perception, while in others the presence of very vivid auditory imagery may easily be mistaken for **'Gedonkenlautwerdan'** (Hamilton, 1976). Being asked by the examiner some patients though initially admit that they have experiences of passivity, on closer questioning it appears that they have had a mere feeling of 'as if' they were being controlled. Some manic patients have a paranoid attitude and they are found to be irritable. They insist that they were never mentally ill but have been wrongly certified. One has to keep in mind that lack of insight is quite common both during and after the manic episode and thus, it is quite wrong to assume that lack of insight during and acute episode is diagnostic of schizophrenia.

Auditory hallucinations may occur in severe depression. These hallucinations are voices which consists of odd, abusive words, or brief phrases which may even suggest suicide, but these are fragmented. Continuous hallucinatory voices do not occur in uncomplicated depressions. If however, these appear in otherwise fairly typical depressive clinical pictures, one should have to think of the possibilities of dehydration, over dosage with drugs (especially hyoscine and bromide). Dietary deficiencies, and other coarse brain disorders, as well as schizophrenia.

At times the depressive mood is not obvious and thus the confusion in diagnosis becomes more apparent. Obviously, in such cases, diagnosis has to be made based on symptoms like, depressive thought content, and the typical sleep disturbance (Hamilton, 1976). At times, no wonder, if clinicians come across depressed patients (especially middle-aged and elderly) who are able to put on a good front; they may smile and even make jokes. An untrained observer may interpret this apparent discrepancy between thought and affective expression as due to schizophrenia, though after a skillful interrogation the clinician would confirm this as a more obvious expression of the depressive affect. Thus, *e.g.*, while differentiating involutional melancholia from late catatonia and paranoid forms of schizophrenia one might get confused sometimes. Hypochondriasis and delusions may be totally decorative, and their content may have little relation to the underlying affect. Nevertheless, such ideas have little diagnostic significance, so long as affective response is still present and that confirms the diagnosis.

Problem of differentiation does arise in cases of confused mania and in certain mixed states of the affective group. Whatever deceptive clinical picture the patient máy present at the moment of observation, the history of a preceding manic or depressive attack, as well as an account of the pathoplastic effects of premorbid personality will help to decide on the diagnosis. Also one should pay attention in the first place to emotional reaction and expression. If they are of one colour, and seem to come from the same mould, be it either hilarious and elated, or cheerful and comfortable, or angry and irritable, or despondent and sad (Hamilton, 1976), the diagnosis of an affective disorder is more probable whatever the accompanying symptoms may be. One should keep in mind that so long the warmth of a personal rapport is preserved this should be taken as a pointer for the diagnosis of affective disorder. Empathy is never totally lost in the manicdepressive patients.

B. Adolescent Crisis

The patients complain of lack of concentration, forgetfulness, irritability, sleep disturbances, poor appetite and sometimes appear to be brooding as well. Overall, they appear to be strange and odd, though no typical schizophrenic symptom as such may be well evident in them. Since schizophrenia is more likely to occur in a predisposed person who is subjected to acute or prolonged psychic trauma, it is possible that the traumatic experience an individual has had during adolescence may provoke a schizophrenic illness. Of course manicdepressive illness may also be provoked some times by an adolescent crisis (Hamilton, 1976). Depression is no doubt, common in adolescents, but it is usually found to be more of a reactive unhappiness rather than a true depressive illness.

Though crisis during adolescence is a universal phenomenon, the genesis for such crisis is not completely free from cultural influences. Thus, *e.g.*, most adolescents in Western cultures experience disturbances at this phase of life due to difficulties in trying to change their relationships (Hamilton, 1976) with their parents from one of dependency and love to independence and love, whereas, in Indian culture mostly this disturbance is due to fear of sex, shame and guilt over masturbation, and heterosexual relations, and absence of avenues for the boys and girls to discuss their emotional problems concerning sex and sex role with others. Thus, there is no way out but to develop a tendency to suppress what all queries the boys and girls have in them to clarify at this stage of life. This is because, unlike the West, our culture directly or indirectly teaches us to suppress information concerning sex and heterosexual relation. Salinger (1951) has given an excellent account of an acute episode in an adolescent crisis, what he called the 'Catcher in the Rye' Syndrome.

C. Obsessional States

These usually begin in early childhood or adolescence. These patients also report a very bizarre content of obsessional thought; such bizarre content alone does not justify the diagnosis schizophrenia (Hamilton, 1976). These patient's abnormal behaviour especially their abnormal sexual behaviour, as is mostly found in Indian adolescents and young adults, may lead them into difficulties which in turn, give rise to psychogenic reactions and depressive illnesses. Due to the pathoplastic effects of the abnormal personality (Hamilton, 1976), these illnesses may show very atypical clinical pictures, but unless clear-cut schizophrenic symptoms of diagnostic significance occur, the diagnosis of schizophrenia should not be made. Hence in a good number of adolescents/young adults, in India, those who later manifest classical symptoms of schizophrenia, a deep level obsession and related depression are revealed which they have been experiencing for quite long time without remedial intervention.

D. Hysteria (Conversion)

Some adolescent and young adult females (rarely males) show episodes of disturbed behaviour which begins abruptly or subsequent to a typical conversion hysteria attack. Following treatment typical symptoms disappear but behaviour disorder starts. They at this stage of their illness are found to be restless, violent, and destructive. They make repeated suicidal attempts and attempts at self-mutilation so much so that the arms and legs, especially the flexor surface of their forearm are slashed with razor blades, pieces of tin, or broken glass. Despite the nursing vigilance, these patients steal and hide materials which will make good weapons and then start mutilating themselves in order to create a scene (Hamilton, 1976). Sometimes they describe visual hallucinations *e.g.,* they are being threatened by men. However, one may be sceptical about such statements given by these patients.

To differentiate it from schizophrenia it is found that rapport can easily be established with such patients. Females usually develop a marked positive transference to male therapist. They act out in the transference situations (Hamilton, 1976). History shows that such patients have been unstable since childhood and often has had psychiatric treatment for a childhood behaviour disorder. They need to continue psychological treatment for long though momentarily the present episode appears to subside within a year or so. Discontinuation of psychological treatment is likely to lead to a recurrent of violent behaviour. Occasionally these patients manage to commit suicide. Rarely the illness turns out to be a clear schizophrenia. Phenothiazine drugs (Hamilton, 1976) and psychotherapeutic help are useful in this condition. But application of punitive measures, such as seclusion or restraint should be avoided, since these patients invite and enjoy punishment.

E. Hysterical Pseudodementia (Ganser States)

In this the patient gives answers to the questions which are though incorrect, indicate that the patient knows the correct answers. That is why, this is also known as the syndrome of 'approximate answers' (Hamilton, 1976). The patient behaves in such a way which would be considered insanity to a man with no knowledge of psychiatry. The patient however is able to look after himself in a better way than that could be expected from his intellectual performance. This disorder usually occurs in psychopathic criminals who want to avoid punishment. This may also occur in mania and early schizophrenia. Pseudodementia in a young person who does not seem to have any reason for having such an illness would suggest an underlying schizophrenia.

F. Psychopathic Personalities

Psychopaths when put into severe environmental difficulties may show short-lived psychotic episodes. Some psychopaths may be able to live a fairly normal life for a year or two, but then begin to behave badly. This is because they get bored with their non-stimulating existence and as a means to come out from this start drinking heavily, get involved into extra-marital liaisons, take amphetamines or similar other drugs and so on. As a result of such irresponsible behaviour, they get into a further great social difficulties, and this may precipitate, a transient psychosis (Hamilton, 1976), following which they may show fairly adequate adjustment again.

Many anti-social psychopaths show little emotion after a very violent behaviour. Likewise many murderers, following arrest, are found to be apparently unmoved by their crime. This is dissociation of affect. This must not be misinterpreted as blunting of affect and held to be diagnostic of schizophrenia (Hamilton, 1976). Distinction from schizophrenia simplex sometimes appears to be rather impossible, especially if no adequate history of the case is at hand. If however, a change of personality is proven even in early adolescence, the possibilities of schizophrenic nature of illness is ruled out. Psychometric test, *viz.*, the Rorschach test at times reveals violent and sexually perverse fantasies in psychopaths, but this not a pointer of schizophrenia. Psychophysiological findings can be used as aids to such diagnosis in differentiating schizophrenia from psychopaths.

G. Coarse Brain Disease

In this schizophrenialike psychoses are much more common than typical schizophrenia. In coarse brain diseases schizophrenic illnesses appear to be indistinguishable from 'endogenous' schizophrenia in symptomatology and course (Hamilton, 1976).

In schizophrenia – like psychoses confusion arises because of the occurrence of organic hallucinosis. This condition is characterised by continuous auditory hallucinations in a state of clear consciousness. Usually the hallucinatory voices are abusive which talk about the patient in the third person (Hamilton, 1976). The general activity of the patient appears to be fairly normal; also no personality change in this noted. Delusions of persecution occur which may be a resultant of the continuous hallucinatory voices, and thus, the illness as such may appear to be a natural reaction to the continuous auditory hallucinations.

Organic hallucinosis can occur in epilepsy. But a clinical picture resembling some varieties of paranoid schizophrenia is more common in this condition. In paranoid – epileptic psychosis though the patient usually appears dull and bewildered, consciousness is clear (Hamilton, 1976). Voices and primary delusions occur. The peculiar sticky, slow, epileptic speech is found to be present in them sometimes. Of course the typical egocentric characteristic of epileptic personality can very rarely be overlooked by an expert in such patients. E.E.G. is often found to be normal during the psychosis.

Differentiation of the nature of disturbances of thinking and speech seen in epileptic twilight states (Mayer-Gross *et al.,* 1974) from the corresponding schizophrenic symptoms, may not be difficult, since there is a definite disturbance of consciousness. This may be described rather as a restriction in the field of consciousness (Hamilton, 1976). Restriction in the sense that the patient's thinking is dominated by a few overvalued ideas, or it may be a dream – like changes of consciousness similar to that found in delirious states of the mind. Visual hallucinations may be reported which are usually concerned with devastating fire and religious topics, such as, the crucification etc. These patients also report frequently that they hear voices of God, Jesus, and the Angels. Though apparently hallucinations, and delusions can be very similar to these noted in schizophrenics, the total picture differs in most cases; there is no emotional coolness, and also the disturbance of thinking in the epileptic with its characteristics of slowness and circumstantiality do not show any thing common with schizophrenic dissociation. Marked restlessness like general overactivity, violent assaults on others, stereotyped activity, and continuous praying may occur. Sometimes there is stupor which resembles that of catatonia. Twilight states usually follow a series of fits (Hamilton, 1976). If however, the pattern of fits is one of minor grandmal, an untrained observer may overlook the epileptic phenomenon in it. All these epileptic states can be distinguished from schizophrenia by adequate history taking (including the history of such attacks in the past, though not always the immediate past) and by the use of electroencephalographic examinations. The EEG mostly shows abnormal rhythms which may be focal or general.

It should be mentioned here that though for shake of clarity, the syndromes of organic hallucinosis, epileptic paranoid psychosis, and epileptic twilight states have been rather sharply outlined, one should keep it in mind that there can be some degree of overlap (Hamilton, 1976) so much so that symptoms belonging to different syndromes may occur at the same time, or in the course of time one syndrome may develop into another.

H. Brain Injury

If a schizophrenic illness, with progressive deterioration, occurs immediately following a brain injury, then the injury must be considered as causal (Elsasser and Grünewald, 1953).

Even if there is an interval between the brain injury and the onset of the psychosis, the injury can be considered causative, if symptoms occur during the interval. The commonest bridging symptom of this kind is usually epilepsy (Elsasser and Grünewald, 1953). Elsasser and Grünewald (1953) were of the opinion that after brain injury, schizophrenic – like illnesses occur more frequently than true schizophrenia. These disorders take the form of organic hallucinosis or paranoid epileptic psychoses.

Schizophrenia can easily be differentiated from a group of psychoses with a cerebral pathology as because neurological, serological, and physical signs are present in organic mental illness. Moreover, in the latter, the psychological changes proceed in the opposite order, *i.e.*, defects of memory and intellect proceed disturbances of emotion. The affective relationship to environment is mostly well preserved at a time when signs of dementia are seen. This is found to occur in cerebral tumour, presenile and senile dementia, arteriosclerosis, and in post-traumatic and syphilitic conditions (Hamilton, 1976). General paresis in juveniles may sometimes be mistaken for hebephrenia. However, it should be possible to find some specific physical signs, even though the serological findings appear to be ambigious.

Frontal-lobe tumours can cause aphasia; physical signs, such as an extensor planter response or papilloedema appear. Confusion arises especially because of the presence of the apathy, moodiness and impulsiveness in patients with prefrontal lesion, as well as by the fact that early hebephrenics complain of headache not infrequently. Feuchtwanger and Mayer-Gross (1938) found that schizophrenia was more frequent after frontal lobe lesions, while Hillbom (1960) reported that schizophrenia-like psychoses are more likely to occur in patients with temporal lobe lesions. It is however, difficult to estimate the site and extent of brain damage purely by clinical and radiological investigations only. Neuropsychological tests help in localisation and assessment of impairment in cognitive functions (see Chapter-V).

I. Morbid Jealousy

In this the patient has wellheld delusions of marital infidelity. Such delusions are supported by a falsification of memory. Based on such falsification the patient claims to have had an experience which strongly suggests that the spouse has committed adultery.

This illness occurs in both sexes and are evident in Indian culture as well. In Britain it appears to be more common in men than in women. This is an abnormal personality development which conforms to Kraepelin's criteria for paranoia. This illness is also known as the 'Jealous Husband Syndrome' (Hamilton, 1976).

Delusions of jealousy may be the present in a paranoid schizophrenia, but other schizophrenic symptoms, though unconnected with morbid jealousy appear later. On the contrary (Hamilton, 1976), in the morbidly jealous patient the delusion varies in intensity for the rest of the patient's life.

J. Toxic Psychoses

Chemical intoxications, such as mescaline, lysergic acid diethylamide and hashish can produce states which are indistinguishable from acute schizophrenia. Also, drugs like cocaine may lead to hallucinatory psychoses but these have little in common with schizophrenic hallucinosis (Kolb, 1973). But differential diagnosis from alcoholic hallucinosis can prove difficult. However, alcoholic hallucinosis differs from paranoid schizophrenia in the preservation of normal affect, and also that personality may be found unimpaired for long periods. The clinical picture is found to be dominated by the auditory hallucinations which are often of a critical (Mayer-Gross *et al.,* 1974), accusatory or commanding character. Determined suicidal attempts are mostly common.

Excessive bromide consumption may lead to a paranoid psychosis. In this, auditory hallucinations are present in the absence of clouding of consciousness. To prevent any diagnostic error the routine estimation of the blood – bromide and a routine investigation of previous medication are necessary (Hamilton, 1976).

In Amphetamine psychosis, ideas of references, delusions of persecution, are present (Kolb, 1973). Also auditory, visual, tactile, and olfactory hallucinations have been found to occur in some patients (Connell, 1958). Depression, and fear are not uncommon. In most cases, symptoms disappear once the drug is withdrawn. In view of this it has been suggested (Connell, 1958) that for differential diagnosis the urine of all acute paranoid psychotics should be tested repeatedly for amphetamine. Immediate withdrawal of drug, and pharmacological intervention is required. Psychotherapeutic interventions following recovery from such a state, are indicated to correct the motivational forces which compel the patient for the drug.

To sum up: On the whole, though typical toxic confusional state or subacute delirious state presents no diagnostic difficulties, some toxic psychosis, *viz.,* bromide and amphetamine psychoses, may be mistaken for paranoid schizophrenia. The incoherence noted in the subacute delirious state differs from the schizophrenic dissociation by being less influenced by complexes, and also being more uniform whenever tested. That is, in schizophrenic thought disorder as a characteristic feature one gets a correct answer one moment and a confused one immediately afterwards, whereas, in delirious state every utterance shows the disturbance, if at all it is present.

Early hebephrenia may sometimes be mistaken for mental deficiency. Actually problem arises only when deficiency occurred before the onset of schizophrenic illness. Imbecile patients are liable to affective storms frequently in which hallucinations, incoherence and catatonic behaviour may be evident. However, such states usually passes off after a few days or week (only rarely months) and leaves the patient exactly as he was before. Unlike this, hebephrenic illness always leaves a mark. If the patient was not originally defective, the school record alone should help in settling the diagnosis.

8
CHAPTER

Treatment

Dementia praecox was once considered disastrous disorder as because it had an early onset and proceeded unabated and unresponsive to treatment for years together. The picture appears to be still grim, although it is known now that schizophrenia can have a later onset, is responsive to treatment, and complete recoveries are not impossible. With the advent of modern treatment methods, schizophrenics have been introduced to a wide variety of treatment methods, which may broadly be divided into three categories: somatic, psychological and environmental.

Whatever be the mode of treatment one has to decide first whether the patient requires hospital visit (inpatient or out-patient either) or should remain at home. Such a decision depends largely upon the condition of the patient as well as his family environment. Needless to mention that acute onset, excited, unmanageable, or thought to be suicidal, and threatening patients require hospitalisation. Of course, undisturbed patient but non-communicable (severe thought disorder) and unable to take care of self may require hospitalisation, if adequate assistance from family side cannot be provided with.

When the symptoms develop slowly, and are characterised by apathy and withdrawal, the patient may be considered suitable to receive treatment as an out-patient, provided the patient is cooperative to his treatment. Family environment of the patient must be suitable to render sympathy, patience and skilled attention the patient requires.

Likewise, discharge from in-patient treatment obviously does not depend on the complete disappearance of symptoms, but on whether the patient can be given the care and attention he needs outside the hospital set up. When a patient shows sufficient improvement which is considered suitable for discharge from hospital, arrangements should be made for him without delay, to receive the continued supervision and help required for him to return to normal life.

Systematic follow-up is necessary to ensure how much the patient has been able to restore, or regain his work efficiency after treatment. This has to be enquired from his family members or boss as the case may be. But in our culture mostly such an attempt proves to be a failure as because neither the patient and his relatives nor the officer incharge and his associates are above social stigma concerning mental illness.

Individual Psychotherapies

Individual psychotherapeutic method is the oldest and most widely practiced. Individual psychotherapy may be divided into two groups, *viz.,* traditional and innovative. The former group is represented by (a) the Freudians who emphasize on rendering unconscious wishes and impulses conscious; (b) the neo-Freudian followers of Erik Erikson with their emphasis on the idea of identity and identity crisis; (c) the Jungians who popularised the idea of mystical analytic psychology; and (d) Adler and Fromm with their emphasis on social psychological theories. Of the innovative psycho-therapists worth mentioning are Rogers, Maslow, Jourard, Peris, and Janov. Innovative psychotherapeutic approach consists of the humanistic existential, *i.e.,* it focuses on the importance of the here and now and stresses more on individual's potential and positive strivings than on his disorders.

Thus, it is evident that there are different individual psychotherapeutic orientation depending upon the strategies involved in it. Amongst the strategies of individual psychotherapy certain major approaches will now be discussed. Each of these approaches is derived from a particular set of beliefs about the problems of people. Each strategy includes certain specific procedures to restore the potentialities of the patient(s). In spite of such strategic differences every therapist perceives psychotherapeutic relationship as a 'Unique' relationship which is based on a 'contract' (Kurl Meninger, 1958). 'Contract' in the sense that both the therapist and the patient mutually agree to employ all possible means to reach the therapeutic goal.

Psychoanalytically Oriented Psychotherapy

In psychoanalysis the therapist introduces techniques that are directed toward the source of the pathology. Therapist relies more on the patient's past as clues to his present behaviour and emphasizes on restructuring personality of the patient.

Although psychoanalysis is employed in the treatment of neuroses, as such this treatment method has not been satisfactory in the treatment of schizophrenia. However, modifications have now been evolved that may successfully maintain schizophrenics at a functioning level of social adjustment.

The establishment of a working relationship with the schizophrenic patient is very essential. Such a relationship between the therapist and the patient is of a different quality from that seen in neuroses. Tremendous patience and tolerance are required on the part of the therapist in breaking through to obtain the trust of the highly suspicious, withdrawn, and sensitive patient. Although Free Association as a method is employed to facilitate recall of repressed material in neuroses, in psychoses, on the contrary, in the early stages of treatment the patient's verbal communication may be incomprehensible totally to the therapist. At this stage, the therapist should not try, as he usually does with the neurotics, to form an association with the verbalisation the patient produces. Rather the therapist must give a patient hearing and try to relate the patient's verbalisation to the feeling – tone of the particular interpersonal relationships (Kolb, 1973) that have been remaining in the patient and precipitant of such distorted communication or those which are observed by the therapist time to time with regard to the patient's relationship with his/her relatives. The therapist must make it possible for the patient to appreciate that the therapist has understood the feeling – tone of the patient and the patient must find in the therapist a sustaining source of security during emergence of anxiety and hostility.

Though in the analytical therapy with the neuroses the analysis of dream is customary, the same is not advised with regard to schizophrenia. Dream analysis may perpetuate the schizophrenic patient's propensity for withdrawal into fantasy living (Kolb, 1973).

The patient must be helped to face emotionally toned events of everyday life and also learn socially adaptive methods of accepting such events. Contrary to the earlier attempts to resolve delusional and hallucinatory experiences through their content analysis (which is now regarded as unsatisfactory therapeutic procedure) (Kolb, 1973), for quite sometimes efforts are being made to understand the interpersonal situations that may precipitate the patient's expression of delusional and hallucinatory experiences. For a detailed account of this the interested reader is referred to Fromm-Reichmann (1954); Abramowtiz, and Coursey, 1989; Rangaswami (2000).

The transference situation is such a useful and important part of psychoanalytic treatment that the technique encourages its development. But with regard to schizophrenics, the therapist must be ever mindful of the consequences of transference distortions. There is every likelihood that such patients will misperceive the therapist in transient roles as recapitulations of the past identification the patient has made with authority figures. Multiple misperceptions (Searles, 1967) of the patient get projected upon the therapist and thus there arises much difficulty in establishing a therapeutic relationship with the patient (Burnham, Gladstone and Gibson, 1969; Deutsch and Munich, 1996).

There are limitations to this type of psychotherapy with schizophrenics. Complete resolution of the schizophrenic process may be obtained very rarely even by the most experienced therapist. Some authors are of the opinion that psychodynamic treatment of schizophrenia has been considered to be unhelpful or even harmful (Klerman, 1984; Drake and Sedener, 1986; Muesser and Berenbaum, 1990). This is because insistence to revolve conflicts on the part of an enthusiastic therapist to the patient beyond the capacity of the patient may be harmful (Kolb, 1973). The therapist must continue a supportive, though distant, therapeutic relationship when such need is indicated by the patient.

In sum : Persons with schizophrenia seem to profit from multiple treatment methods and thus it is necessary to measure complementary treatment modalities as they interact together overtime.

Client-Centred/Person-Centred Therapy

In sharp contrast to both Freud and Adler, Carl Rogers (1951, 1961) used the term 'client' instead of 'patient', 'subject', 'counselee', and 'analysed' to avoid the connotation of sick and/or experimental guinea pig. Secondly, supporters of this therapy disown the view that psychopathology develops because human nature is regressively self-defiance and destructive. According to Rogers behaviour pathology results from a conflict between the individual's two fundamental evaluative processes, *viz.,* self-evaluation, and those based on the values of others. Thirdly, unlike Adler, Rogers did not perceive therapist as an agent mainly responsible for inducing change in the patient's behaviour and personality. Rogers placed this responsibility onto the client while the task of the therapist, according to Rogers, is to create the proper conditions that allow the client to feel such change. Such conditions enable the client to examine those experiences that are inconsistent with his self-concept and those that were perceived by him previously distortedly, or denied. Thus this therapy purports to develop in the client an empathic understanding of the self and unconditional positive regard towards the self. Fourthly, Rogerians are not impressed with the Freudian tactics of interpretation since they believe that this takes the initiative for progress away from the client. This method is not likely to succeed with schizophrenics (Rogers, Gendlin, Klessler, and Turax, 1967) and other psychotics with long-standing illness.

Supportive Psychotherapy

Its aim is to reduce incapacitating tensions and anxiety by supportive techniques. Techniques employed are reassurance, and use of authority, permissive attitudes that relieve guilt, reasoning, encouragement and advice. Also counselling including attempts to alter attitudes of the key persons in the patient's life as well as manipulation of environment are included in it. Little attempt is made to bring about personality change (from dynamic consideration) but attempt is made to help the patient improve his ability to face reality at his best integrative level. The choice of the selection of this therapy has to be determined by many factors, *viz.,* personality characteristics and the level of its integrity present in the patient, the nature of the illness, age, and life situation of the patient. Chronic institutionalised schizophrenics, excited unmanageable schizophrenics are not amenable to this therapy. Schizophrenics those who are on drug treatment and have shown improvement in behavioural symptoms (*i.e.,* not restless and destructive, but communicable) may show improvement with such mode of treatment in relieving guilt, in revolving conflict and in handling reality with his best potentiality. Care must be taken to see that the therapist doesn't encourage dependence and regressive passivity in the patient.

Early studies (*e.g.,* Karno and Vandenbos, 1981; Hogarty, Goldberg, and Schooler, 1984) have failed to demonstrate positive results of such therapy in schizophrenia. However, this studies are subject to criticisms. Because pharmacotherapy was not controlled, therapists were inexperienced and number of confounding variables were present (Cameron *et al.,* 1998), and the length of treatment was not adequate (Wasylenki, 1992). Gunderson, Frank, Katz *et al.* (1984) the Boston Psychotherapy Study Group reported that received standard pharmacological management did show improvement through supportive psychotherapy or exploratory insight oriented therapy, which was evident through role performance of the patients and also through the reduced rate of rehospitalisation.

In sum: Supportive efforts should aim to promote maturity of personality of the patient. However, limited outcome would be expected if there are harsh environmental pressures from which the patient fails to escape.

Also caution be exercised not to assign patients randomly to therapy. Patients to be assessed properly (Gabbard, 1999), and particular therapy modalities be prescribed only when they are felt to be appropriate by the expert clinician therapist.

Interpersonal Therapy

From amongst the traditional psychotherapies, 'Interpersonal Therapy' formulated by Sullivan (1953) has been especially geared for the treatment of schizophrenics. Sullivan's main focus was on the self-system of the patient and the defenses he/she has developed to cope with his/her anxieties. Interpersonal therapy of Sullivan aimed to correct the perceptions of the patient himself/herself and of others so that the patient earns greater 'consensual validation'. He devised ways of building closer and more trusting relationship even with suspicious patients. Sullivan suggested that the couch of the psychoanalyst, with its invitation to free-association is inappropriate for the schizophrenic patients. Connection between the current interpersonal problems and the affective status of the patient (particularly depression) is the main treatment focus (Cameron, Ennis and Deadman, 1998).

In Indian psychotherapeutic system also, recently there is a shift in emphasis from the intraindividual to interindividual approach, particularly with regard to family members of schizophrenic patients. This is necessary because, as already been mentioned before, Indian research reveals differences in perception of parents, sex role identity etc. between male and female schizophrenic patients. Therefore, Indian researchers have recently focussed more on the importance of psychosocial intervention rather than psychiatric intervention – an issue which will be discussed later in this chapter.

Behavioural Therapy

The origins of behaviour therapy can be traced to the pioneering works of Bekhterev (1912), Pavlov (1927), and Thorndike (1898). The origin of such treatment with humans lies in research with autistic (Ferster, 1961) and schizophrenic (Kazdin, 1977) patients. The principles of learning that emerged from these early researchers continue to be modified and elaborated in contemporary laboratories of experimental behavioural science (Ullmann and Krashner, 1969a,b). Behaviour therapy, briefly speaking, is the systematic application of principles of learning to the analysis and treatment of disorders of behaviour. According to this theory, undesirable patterns of behaviour can be 'unlearned', and replaced by new 'learned' appropriate behaviour.

During recent years one of the most promising developments in the treatment of schizophrenia, especially in chronically deteriorated patients, is the use of behavioural techniques. The methods of training used with schizophrenic patients are often based on operant conditioning. This technique emphasises the active response of the patient but at the same time does not require high level of motivation from them initially.

The power of operant – reinforcement procedures in the treatment of psychotic patients in a word setting was first systematically demonstrated by Ayllon and Azrin (1968). Later, these authors introduced tokens as convenient medium for the delivery or withdrawal of positive reinforcement. Token economy technique will be discussed later in this chapter. Now some of the other techniques employed in behaviour therapy will be discussed.

Operant treatment is concerned with behaviours which are also considered harmful to the patient and to others. These behaviours include physical aggression (Hitting, Kicking, etc.), self-injury (Head Ranging, Face Slapping, etc.) and tantrums (*e.g.,* Screaming, Property Destruction).

Planned Ignoring

In this procedure social attention which is contingent upon instances of problem behaviour (Hall and Hall, 1980) is removed. Cox and Klinge (1976), *e.g.,* found that withholding social attention resulted in significant reduction in problem behaviour like, hair pulling, wrist cutting and hand burning. Martin and Foxx (1973), though reported the effectiveness of this type of intervention programme, such procedure has not been always successful (Martin and Lagulli, 1974).

Differential Reinforcement Procedures (DRP)

This involves reinforcing the patient for a period of time in which the problem behaviour has not occurred (Homer and Peterson, 1980). This technique has been widely used on patients with autism and schizophrenia in reducing aggression (*e.g.,* Vukelich and Hake, 1971), tantrums (*e.g.,* Bostow and Bailey, 1969), and self-injury (*e.g.,* Ragain, and Anson, 1976). In contrast, Corte, Wolf, and Locke (1971) had not been successful in using this technique.

DRP also involves reinforcing behaviours that are not physically compatible with the target behaviour. Lovaas, Freitag, Gold and Kassoria (1965) attempted to reduce head banging behaviour of reinforcing hand clapping (incompatible with target behaviour). The frequency of hand clapping increased following reinforcement, and the frequency of head banging decreased. This technique has been employed successfully by many (*e.g.,* Repp and Deits, 1974), although Measel and Alfieri (1976) reported contrary to it. One limitation of this technique is that it does not state what the patient will do during DRP interval. Also, one has to think of individual differences in perceiving stimuli as reinforcers. The reinforcing nature of the stimuli has to be assessed first. For example, access to arm restraints was found to be reinforcing for a 27-years old woman with a history of self-injury (Ravell, McGimsey, and Jones, 1978). Similarly, problem inherent in differential reinforcement of incompatible behaviour is the lack of guidelines for selecting (Voeltz, Evans, Derer and Hamashiro, 1983) alternative behaviour.

Contingent Negative Consequences

This assumes that if a behaviour is followed by punishment (aversive stimulus), the frequency of that undesired behaviour would reduce in future. To reduce problem behaviour exhibited by Schizophrenics a plethora of negative consequences have been tried out. These include time-out from positive reinforcement (Cayner and Kiland, 1974), over correction (Matson and Stephens, 1977; Johnson, Baumeister, Penald and Inwald, 1982), Contingent restraint (Azrin, Besalel and Wisotzek, 1982) and application of electric shock (Corte, Wolf, and Locke, 1971; Tate, and Baroff, 1966). Applying contingent electric shock an immediate reduction of aggressive behaviour was noted (Foxx, McMorrow, Bittle and Bechtel, 1986) and 15-months follow-up showed a satisfactory outcome. Significant reduction of immediate problem behaviour by applying electric shock though has been reported (Carr and Lovaas, 1983), evidence of complete and long-term suppression of problem behaviour are rare (Murphy and Wilson, 1981; Giuess, Helmestetter, Turnbull and Knowlton, 1987). Furthermore, usually application of electric shock has been rated as unacceptable by caregivers (Pickering and Morgan, 1985; Singh, Watson and Winton, 1987) and thus unwillingness on the part of the therapist in its application is also reported (Foxx and Livesay, 1984). Likewise, failure to obtain clinically significant results with overcorrection (*e.g.*, Rapoff, Altman and Christoppherson, 1980) procedure has been reported. Clinical research however, documented that hallucinatory behaviour could be modified with social interference and aversive procedures (Alford and Turner, 1976; Turner, Hersen, and Bellack, 1977).

The successful outcome of any treatment depends, at least partly, on the environment where the intervention is conducted. Some treatment methods are more successful when carried out in institutional settings whereas others are more successful in community settings. The majority of the treatment research conducted till date has been carried out in institutional environments and thus may have little applicability (Giuess, Helmestetter, Turnbull and Knowlton, 1987) for individuals living in community.

Token Economies

Already mentioned earlier in this chapter that operant reinforcement procedures in the treatment of institutionalised psychiatric patients was first systematically demonstrated by Ayllon and Azrin in 1968 and later they introduced tokens as reinforcers. They named their treatment "The token economy" because their patients were provided with metal tokens that the patients could later exchange for "back up reinforcers", including activities, consumables, rentals and about anything else which the patient requested for and the therapist considers ethical and not detrimental to their treatment (O'Brien, Azrin and Herson, 1969).

Now-a-days operant and conditioning procedures have been the preferred method in the treatment of schizophrenic disorders. Operant techniques have also been applied to children with such problems and results reported are promising. Thus *e.g.,* Ferster and Demyer (1962) using coin-operated vending machines to administer rewards were able to widen the children's behaviour and could bring much of their autistic behaviour under control. Token economy programme has been found effective in eliminating delusions (Schaefer, and Martin, 1975). Similarly, Curran, Monti and Corrivean (1982) recommended that token system is effective in treating chronic schizophrenics and it provides motivation to the patients to learn new skills and coping strategies.

Token Economy Programme with Children

The traditional psychotherapy has consistently failed to produce noticeable change in the behaviour of children with schizophrenia or autism earlier. Long-term behavioural outcome studies, though are few, the work of Lovaas, Koegel, Simmons *et al.* (1973), and Nedelman and Sulzbacher (1972) on autistic children and thereafter some other research evidences reported O'Leary and Wilson (1975) on schizophrenic children clearly demonstrate that this children can be aided by behavioural methods of intervention. The prognosis of schizophrenic children not treated with behavioural programmes has been reported to be poor (O'Leary and Wilson, 1975), and so also the children with autism. It seems too early to make any definite statements about the percentage of recovery found in such children to the extent that take an interact well in family and school environment; long-term follow-up studies estimated that behavioural treatment was superior to play therapy (Lovaas, 1973). Token economy programme has also been applied extensively on children with schizophrenia and outcome study reports are (O'Leary and Wilson, 1975) satisfactory.

Prerequisites of Token Economy Programme

Experimental works on the techniques for 'reinforcing' desired behaviour have shown the importance of the rules that reinforcement should be immediate, relevant, should take place in small steps, and should be positive. A close examination of the environmental antecedents and consequences of the behaviour in question has to be made. The next step is the specification of the goals of treatment and the means of obtaining them. Another essential aspect of this approach is the measurement of the specific behaviour before and during treatment. By doing this, the therapist ensures that the effort given is utilised properly. But prior to specification of goals and before establishing a token economy programme, it is obviously imperative that one decides which criterion behaviours and their components are to be reinforced. It is useful to view these criterion behaviour in a hierarchical fashion. Thus, grouping of behaviour may be done in connection with *e.g.,* self care (bathing, shaving, dressing, and feeding), in connection with occupational (promptness, staying on the task, etc.), educational (basic rudiments of reading, writing, and arithmetic), and social (initiating conversation, participating in games) spheres of life. Social learning treatment techniques will be discussed later in this chapter. Under each of these groupings one has to stipulate further an exhaustive list of those behaviours that are to be reinforced. For example, under self-care, appropriate eating and dressing behaviour may be selected as choice (Criterion) behaviour. Also each of these behaviour must then operationalised. For example, in a research project Paul and Lentz (1977) decided to reinforce appropriate appearance and 11 sub-components of appropriate appearance used were – (a) proper use of make-up; (b) clean finger nails; (c) hair combed; (d) teeth brushed; (e) all appropriate clothing on; (f) clothing buttoned, zipped; (g) clothing clean and neat; (h) body clean; (i) no odor; (j) shaven; (k) hair cut appropriately (Paul and Lentz, 1977). Each of these sub-components was further operationalised. As for example, "Teeth Brushed" was defined as no food on teeth; no grit on teeth; breath that allowed one to stand within a few feet (Paul and Lentz, 1977). Such selection and defining criterion behaviour help in preventing inconsistencies among those individuals responsible for dispensing the tokens. Also, it is important that while operationalising these criterion behaviour the capabilities of the patients be given some consideration. For example, if the patient is to receive tokens for engaging in recreational activities, such as, volleyball, some consideration must be given to his athletic talent. Again, having athletic talent present, age is another factor which one should take into account. For example, a 55-years-old chronically institutionalised psychiatric patient may not be expected to play volleyball, even though he had an athletic talent in young age. In such a case, playing volleyball may be defined (Paul and Lentz, 1977) as standing mostly in one's assigned zone, attempting to hit the ball over the net, not kicking the ball but throwing it to another patient etc. However, one should always be vigilant to see that the operationalised definitions of the criterion behaviour are consistent with the goals of the programme.

Clinicians working with schizophrenic patients especially with chronic institutionalised patients know well that some times it may be highly inefficient to wait for a patient to exhibit the total criterion behaviour before reinforcing them. In such cases, various activities must be arranged and teaching devices must be employed in order to elicit and develop criterion behaviour (Bellack, Herson, Kazdin, 1984). For example, activities can be planned in which the patients are expected to interact both with other patients and with treatment staff members. Patients can be taught how to initiate a social interaction, how to terminate a talk, how to make a brief talk etc. Likewise, self-help classes can be arranged to teach the patients how to shave, how to wash their cloth, etc. Thus numerous learning techniques including instruction, modelling, verbal and physical prompts, fading procedures, response chaining and response shaping (Bellack *et al.,* 1984) are in use. A comprehensive recent review in this regard is available (Baker, 1975). Although all of these techniques may be used to teach a skill, some procedures may work best for a particular skill or for a given patient. As for example, in teaching highly regressed patient to shave, Bellack *et al.* (1984) found verbal and physical prompts were helpful.

At this junctures a basic question still remains unanswered, *i.e.,* how to transfer the attained skills to the natural environment? Unless that is done there is no practical utility of such therapeutic programmes. Furthermore, unless the patients are gradually introduced back into the natural environment and extramural support systems are established, it is likely that the skills developed may deteriorate. To avoid such deterioration of the skills earned, as a useful procedure for promoting transfer back into the natural environment what is done is – as the patient progresses through different steps he is 'weaned' (O'Leary and Wilson, 1975) from token system, and more time is spent in the natural environment. In the initial steps, reinforcement is given immediately while on the more advanced stage, the patients may receive the tokens that they have earned only at the end of the week. Subsequently, the patient may be allowed to work, *e.g.,* 8 hours a day in the community, and is asked to come to the hospital just for sleeping at night. Gradually, at a more advanced stage, the patient is allowed to join a pre-release group, which aims to prepare the patient for self-supporting functioning in the community. The leader of the pre-release group/psychiatric social worker can serve as the liaison person for the patient between community and the treatment staff within the residential treatment centre.

Several other methods may be employed to introduce patients to the community. Community trip may be arranged once or several times a week, for those who meet individualised criteria. To give further exposure to community facilities, trips to restaurants etc. may be arranged. Gradually patients would be encouraged in taking of day, night and even week-ends to spend in the community (O'Leary and Wilson, 1975). Another way of giving residents exposure to the community is to bring the community to them through evening programme etc. (Paul and Lentz, 1977). Of course, these volunteers from the community need to be extensively trained in the principles of a token economy. For detail the reader is referred to Bellack *et al.* (1984). In some countries, the impetus of community model of behavioural therapy is found in their societal, legislative and judicial forces (*e.g.,* Matson and LaGrow, 1983).

Some critics are of the opinion that it is difficult to draw a firm conclusion regarding the outcomes of most of the token economy studies, as because the authors of different studies have used different patients and different category of treatment staff. Also differences in the dependent measures, and programme components within the token economies have been reported. However, Kowalski, Daley and Gripp (1976) reported that paranoid schizophrenic patients seem to show better improvement than other types of schizophrenics in a token economy. As early as 1959 Ayllon and Michael, and in 1960 Isaacs, Thomas and Golddiamond demonstrated the effectiveness of token economy programme in connection with schizophrenic patients. Of late, Paul and Lentz (1977), and Magaro, Talbott and Glick (1984) have claimed that token economy programme was found to be more effective than other psychotherapeutic methods in the treatment of schizophrenia.

The management of a token economy programme, however requires a continual monitoring of all aspects of the programme and a knowledgeable dedicated staff.

Methods of Learning Social Skills

Though the characteristic symptoms of schizophrenia are hallucinations, delusions, incongruent or flattened affect, agitation and so on, impairment in social functioning due to fluctuations between exacerbations and remissions are recently considered to be the hallmark of this illness. DSM-III-R (APA, 1987) states that schizophrenic patients need not have any one specific typical symptoms mentioned above, but deterioration is markedly evident in their social relations compared to their pre-illness stage. Furthermore, unsatisfactory social competence in childhood may predate the onset of schizophrenia (Lewine, Watt, Prentky, and Fryer, 1980). Also, important long-term prognostic indices of the outcome of schizophrenia are considered to be (Zigler and Glick, 1986) the attainment of social competency in adolescence and early adulthood (Presley, Grubb and Semple, 1982). Better social adjustment in schizophrenics would mean that they have been able to manage effectively, at least partly, noxious stressors arising from their life events. Therefore, modern treatment methods strive to enhance social skills of such patients with a view to maximize the tenure of community stay, and to avoid re-admission to institutions.

Social skill techniques are largely behavioural although recently professionals have made an integrated approach (Brenner *et al.,* 1992, 1995) incorporating both cognitive and behavioural methods strategies include : assessment of interpersonal competence; to determine the specific deficits; to set the goal; repeated rehearsal of interpersonal interaction – through instructions, prompts, role playing, contingent reinforcement (which acts as feedback) in vivo assignments (Cameron *et al.,* 1998) and problem solving. These patients fail to supply adequate linkage between speech clauses (Harvey, 1983; Rutter, 1985). They have paucity of material to talk about as they are relatively isolated and can not share experiences from school or work or peer situations. Therefore, speech form and content are generally the targets for such training.

Expressive behaviour is also composed of non-verbal responses such as, proxemics, kinesics, eye contact or gaze, and facial expression (Harper, Wiens and Matarazzo, 1978). Proxemics refers to interpersonal distance. Such distance may be related to many aspects of interaction, namely, dominance, intimacy, submission or fear as well as level of formality. Kinesics refers to our postural movements / gestures manifested during social interactions. For example, head nods, hand gestures, nervous or "autistic", movements (Pubbing a part of one's body, biting one's nails etc.). Needless to mention again that schizophrenics manifest postural rigidity and peculiar gestures.

Through eye-contact we can read one's mind. Thus, *e.g.,* gazing indicates dominance, affection, whereas, failure to maintain eye-contact indicates submission, fear, boredom. Schizophrenics often fail to maintain direct eye-contacts. Our emotions are communicated through facial expression. Schizophrenics often show unexpressive facial exposure. Schizophrenics show marked impairment in the ability to identify affect, especially negative affect from facial expressions (Morrison and Bellack, 1967). Therefore, in social skill training programme both these aspects of non-verbal behaviour are targets for change. Very recently Hogarty has given a systematic treatment strategy for regulation of affect in schizophrenics. Steps involved are: patients are taught to recognise internal events; practical skills are taught regarding community re-integration; the patients learn to maintain stability; then they develop insight into their problem. It starts with individual training and gradually the patient learns to communicate with family and social groups (Hogarty *et al.,* 1995).

A modular approach to social-skill training has been developed by Liberman and Corrigan (1993). It aims to help the patient conceptualise the deficits in social skills. Three basic steps are followed (Liberman and Corrigan, 1993) – receiving, processing, and sending. Goals are – management of medication and thereby symptoms; conversation skills and self-care; involvement in recreational activities. Thus, social skill training is a highly structured intervention technique. In this the patients are taught to perform new behaviours as is done in case of programmes for teaching motor skills, *e.g.*, playing a musical instrument or sports. It emphasizes the importance of demonstration and rehearsal rather than discussion. Complex behaviour is perceived into small units and the training programme proceeds in a gradual hierarchical fashion (easy to difficult behaviours) (Morrison, and Bellack, 1967). Needs and limitations of all the participants are taken into account. Emphasis is given on extended practice and over learning so that response can be performed automatically.

There is disagreement amongst therapists over the number of sessions to be taken per week, and duration of each session. Also, lack of concensus is noted with regard to the size of the group. However, Morrison and Bellack in 1967 and later Muesser and Bellack (1989) have given a detailed account of it. According to them patients may be taken in small groups so as to enable the patients to learn from each other. Gradually, training is conducted 3 to 5 times/week each session lasting for 1 to 1½ hours. Precise schedule is determined by pragmatic factors in the clinical setting. The total duration of training depends on the amount of material to be covered as well as the rate of progress noted in participants. Training programme may be concerning assertiveness, conversation skills, detecting negative affects, and so forth.

The therapist must have a structured plan ready with regard to each session and with regard to the whole tenure of the training programme for the patient concerns. The therapist has to identify some of the events that the patient(s) encounter in his everyday life interaction. This helps the therapist to place the patient in a desired role-playing situation during the session. Teaching each of the response elements of a particular skill should be given one at a time only following a hierarchy (less difficult to more difficult). Thus, *e.g.*, in assertive training programme the patient may be taught first to be assertive with a familiar person in a known situation (*e.g.*, hospital ward, hospital reception room, etc.), then with a familiar person outside the hospital set up, and then with an unfamiliar person in a familiar situation, and finally with a stranger in an unknown situation, and so on. According to Muesser and Bellack (1989) there are 5 steps in this training process. These are instructions, modelling, role playing, feedback and positive reinforcement, and homework. Instructions should always be simple, brief and should emphasize what the patient is expected to do rather than what he should not. Instructions are to be repeated as and when necessary.

Modelling should focus specifically on the target behaviour. The patient is to model the therapist's action and modelling display should be brief. It may be repeated when necessary.

After watching the model behaviour the patient is required to implement it and thus the next step is role-playing (Muesser and Bellack, 1989). The patient is prompted to perform the behaviour required of him. Depending upon the quality of the performance, the patient may be requested to repeat the role. He may be asked to repeat the role, at the maximum 4 times and at the minimum twice in a session (Wallace and Liberman, 1985). Frequent repetition may make the patient feel frustrated with a sense that his performance is not satisfactory. Repetition of role has to be interspersed with feedback and reinforcement between trials (Wallace and Liberman, 1985). Individual care, attention and coaching would be necessary depending upon the level of performance of each patient. Feedback should be specfic to the target behaviour and reinforcement may be even a verbal praise, patting etc. for the patients hypersensitive to criticisms negative feedback should be taught about its acceptance with individual coaching (Wallace and Liberman, 1985) and later through group discussion about their performance.

The whole aim of setting such programmes is to enable the patient achieve transfer of training. But such transfer is not possible unless the patient receives opportunities to practice it in vivo between sessions. That is why homework should be assigned to the patient at the end of each session (Wallace and Liberman, 1985). But arrangement should be made in such a way that full co-operation is received from the members interacting with the patient so much so that the patient gets positive feedback from them. Patients who are successful to comply with the instructions are rewarded and those who fail are taught again with individual care but are not criticised.

In Indian set up, a combined approach consisting of social skill training, psychoeducation, stress management and vocational rehabilitation was employed (Rangaswami, 2000). Sessions were taken thrice/week, each session lasting for an hour and continued till 3 months. Follow up sessions were for once a month, for 6 months, after the termination of the treatment. Both the groups of patients were assessed in a pre-post design using Quality of life check-list, and Brief psychiatric rating scale. The sample consisted of 6 male (mean age 25.66 years) neuroleptic stabilised schizophrenics. The control group was also consisted of equal number of neuroleptic stabilised schizophrenics (mean age 24.79 years). In addition to age, the groups were matched for education, onset, and duration (6-6.2 months) of illness. All the cases were of 1st attack, early onset and diagnosed following ICD-10 criteria and remitted with pharmacotherapy and were maintained on low dose neuroleptics. The patients were not on any additional psychosocial management except that they were on routine monthly follow-up for psychotherapy.

The social skill training employed in this study involved role playing by the patient, modelling, prompting, feedback and social reinforcement.

Psychoeducational family intervention technique was employed with a view to increasing understanding of the illness by the family members and thereby to decrease anger, guilt, and to improve communication pattern.

Stress management package consisted of relaxation training, graded exposure to anxiety arousing situations and assertive training.

Vocational rehabilitation part was concerned with their returning back into the community, where necessary to place in job, to enhance quality of life.

Initially social skill training was started for the experimental group, simultaneously the family was taken for psychodrama. Information giving, clarification and discussion were the methods used for the families.

Social skill training was carried out individually throughout the treatment period. They were exposed to 5 individualised relaxation training sessions and thereafter adviced to carry out the same at home once a day with the help of parents, in a gradual manner, vocational rehabilitation/placement (to job or educational institution) programme was carried out. Skills for sustaining in the job/studies, and job maintenance activities were carried out.

A scrutiny of the results revealed that in the therapy group all were placed back to their respective job/education. In the control group 2 resumed to work, one remained unemployed, and 3 were students. In the control group, 2 had exacerbations of symptoms, but no such problem was noted with regard to the therapy group. Thus, it was evident that the quality of life of the therapeutic group (better household activities, communication, education, relationships, independence, physical care, leisure activities, employment and religious activities and overall mental health an psychiatric care) improved remarkably.

Limitation of this study is that only 6 patients were taken. Secondly, differential effects, of these methods employed, were not assessed. Thirdly, it requires long term follow up (preferably for 2-3 years) to be sure that such a combined approach help to prevent progression and relapse. However, the study deserves credit in the sense that in Indian set up, with significant difficulties of resources required to conduct this type of programme, and with strong resistance the relatives show to participate in such programmes, this no doubt has been a hard task on the part of the author to conduct such a study completely and successfully.

One limitation of social skills training programme may be that the clinicians teach the skills which they feel necessary for the patient. Attempt should be made to see that clinicians can teach the skills which the patient desires to learn. Secondly, there is a general notion amongst clinicians that behaviour therapy brings relatively rapid improvement, but with regard to schizophrenics one should not be in a hurry to prove the effectiveness of the programme.

In sum : Research reports of outcome studies on social-skills training (SST) in schizophrenia have not been consistent. Several studies though have concluded that this training is effective in reducing symptoms and increasing social adjustment, many have documented its ineffectiveness in decreasing relapse rate (Hogarty *et al.,* 1986, 1991; Marder *et al.,* 1996). Contrary to this, Bellack *et al.* (1984) claimed that SST is effective in reducing frequency of relapse. Again, a positive impact of SST on re-hospitalisation was demonstrated by Bradshaw (1993) just after one year, whereas, Hogarty *et al.* (1991) found no impact on re-hospitalisation even after 2 years. Thirdly, many studies suggest a time-limited effect on social-functioning; a weak reduction in symptoms (Benton and Schroeder, 1990), as well as a large effect, based on meta-analysis, have been (Corrigan, 1991) documented in the literature. Fourthly, many studies suggested a time-limited effect of SST on social functioning (*e.g.*, Cameron *et al.*, 1998) and expressed doubts about its long-lasting generalised effects; Wallace and Liberman (1985), on the contrary, reported that training skills are maintained well.

To overcome such inconsistencies in the research reports future research should look into the following, prior to the implementation of SST;

(a) to identify the specific factors responsible for social-skill development;
(b) to be sure that one can attend to and can translate/interpret the cues;
(c) to determine the optimal training, frequency, and duration of SST (Cameron *et al.*, 1998);
(d) to ensure that training is imparted for persons with early onset of illness (Cameron *et al.*, 1998). This would help better learning before the deficit gets firmly established (Marder *et al.*, 1996);
(e) the training be imparted by those professionals who have expertised to understand the relationship between theory (cognitive aspect) and practical (behavioural) underlying these programmes, so as to apply complementary treatment methods.

Cognitive Therapy

Cognitions cause emotional states and various types of psychopathology. Beck, Rush, Shaw, and Emery (1979) used the term 'schema' to refer to the typical tendencies of the patients to depression to view the self and the world negatively. Such a systematic errors in thinking, which Beck *et al.* (1979) designated 'cognitive-model' has been used to explain other types of psychopathology as well. Cameron *et al.* (1998) opined that to maximize the effects of cognitive therapy, the effects of cognitive deficits in the personality development of the patients require clear understanding.

In a recent review of the cognitive therapy in schizophrenia, Alford and Correia (1994) have given the following therapeutic principles :

(*i*) *Therapeutic relationship*. This though, is common in all sorts of psychotherapy, no matter whether analytical, cognitive, or behavioural, here its main focus is to deal with the sensitivity to the negative self-concept of the patient.
(*ii*) *To decide upon intervention* – based on observations to identify problems and to decide about the perspective to be taken.
(*iii*) *To focus both content (e.g., delusional content), and process (e.g., arbitrary inference, specific distortions etc.) of symptoms.*

To identify the symptoms / behaviour and also to develop appropriate coping, Tarrier, Harwood, Yusopoff *et al.*, (1990) employed cognitive strategies, they called 'coping and strategy enhancement technique'. The outcome was positive.

A meta-cognitive approach has been advocated by Perris and Skagerlind (1994). This focuses on the interaction between the biological and psychological factors to address how illness may influence the view of self of the patient. This view is largely based on the Beck's principles of cognitive therapy. However, this approach has not been applied in well controlled design, hence, require verification of the results.

In sum: To maximize the effects of cognitive therapy – social difficulties due to residual cognitive difficulties of the patient with schizophrenia be identified; effects of cognitive deficits in the personality development of such patient be understood clearly; residual cognitive difficulties and their relation to symptoms of schizophrenia require proper identification.

Cognitive Behavioural Therapy

Cognitive and behavioural therapists differ from one another in a variety of ways. Cognitive therapists believe that particular schema of thoughts and interpretations (cognitions) of a person cause emotional states (Beck, Rush, Shaw, and Emery, 1979) and various types of psychopathology. In contrast, traditional behaviour therapists believe that problem behaviour (psychopathology) stems from learning experiences, which is largely based on the patterns of environmental reinforcement and punishment the person has had received throughout. Despite differences, there appears to be a kinship between the two. Recently, therapists believe that behaviour is determined by a broad range of factors (Cameron *et al.*, 1998), *viz.,* biological (*e.g.,* genetics and neurotransmitter), cognitive (beliefs, predictions and attributes), and learning (conditioning). Therefore, the most comprehensive and integrated psychological treatment includes a variety of cognitive and behavioural interventions, called cognitive behavioural therapy ('CBT') (Brenner *et al.,* 1992, 1995).

Approaches so far taken by professionals in CBT as viewed by Brenner (1994) may be grouped under three heads: direct, indirect, and combined. In the direct approach, the target is specific attentional and conceptual skills. Patients are required to perform exercises repetitively. Recently computerised training programmes have also been employed. In indirect approach the aim is behaviour modification. This brings cognitive changes only indirectly. For example, reframing of delusional thoughts. As the name implies, combined approaches incorporate both direct and indirect techniques. In this specific deficits are targeted in context of actual functional difficulties. For example, integrated psychological therapy. The integrated approach is again based on 5 sub-groups (Brenner *et al.,* 1995). The sub-groups are : cognitive functions (simple to complex, *viz.,* attentional functions to discriminative tasks), social perception, verbal communication, social skills and interpersonal problem-solving. It is evident from the grouping that this approach addressed problem in a behavioural fashion.

Positive and negative reinforcement techniques, Token economy, may be applied to alter psychotic symptoms, in impatient set-up. For modification of auditory hallucinations Bentall, Haddock, and Slade (1994) developed a CBT model. This is based on the hypothesis that hallucinations are due to failure to attribute internal mental events to the self. These authors have mentioned three strategies : physical characteristics of the voices; content of the voices; and related thoughts and assumptions about the voice. Likewise, humming as a technique has been employed for the treatment of auditory hallucinations (Green and Kinsbourne, cited by Cameron *et al.,* 1998). This is based on the hypothesis that movement of the laryngeal muscles are causally related to auditory hallucinations. Therefore, it is assumed that interference with these movements would reduce hallucinations.

There prevails a belief that CBT helps to improve social skills, self-care and skills for independent living. CBT though helps to reduce aggressive behaviour in schizophrenia patients, it has little effect on positive symptoms like delusions, and hallucinations (Cameron *et al.,* 1998). But contrary to this Tarrier, Beckett, Harwood, Baker *et al.,* (1993), and Bentall, Haddock, and Slade (1994), reported that CBT is helpful in treating hallucinations, and delusions. The later authors are of the opinion that CBT may help to decrease psychiatric symptoms particularly delusions, but generalisation of such symptoms improvement has not been authenticated. This study was on schizophrenics having drug resistant residual symptoms.

In general, CBT helps to decrease the amount of drug required as well as to increase the interval between relapses. With respect to relapse rate in the 1st year following treatment with four conditions, *viz.,* social-skill training, family psychoeducation, social-skills training and family psychoeducation, and no psychological intervention, Hogarty, Anderson, Reiss *et al.* (1986) found that the one-year relapse rates for the 4 groups were 20, 19, 0 and 41% respectively.

In sum : With a conceptual shift in understanding the causes of symptoms in schizophrenia, there is a shift in application of treatment modalities also. From brief therapies there has been a movement towards long-term and more comprehensive care. This encompasses a number of treatment modalities. Outcome research reports show a favourable trend in modifying behaviour of patients with schizophrenia through application of such combined strategies.

Drug Treatment

The beginnings of modern drug treatment of schizophrenia dates from the introduction of Chloropromazine, the first of the phenothiazines, and reserpine, in the year 1952. The latter is an extract from *Rauwolfia Serpentina Bentham,* indigenous to India, used to be popularly called "insanity herb", by the Indians. In 1931, Sen and Bose published the first report of the use of Rauwolfia Serpentina, in the treatment of mental illness. In 1934, Dr. R.A. Hakim of Ahmedabad, India was awarded gold medal for his success in treating schizophrenia with the major ingredient of which was Rauwolfia (Kolb, 1973). In 1943, a note on the efficacy of this agent in the treatment of schizophrenia, and MDP, and other mental disorders was made in the Indian Medical Gazette, which has later been incorporated in Western literature as well (*e.g.,* Kolb, 1973). It is now almost obsolete for use in psychiatry (Hamilton, 1976). However, an older account of many psychotic compounds is presented by Lewis (1934). For a relatively modern and detailed review of the early experiments in psychopharmacology the reader is referred to Holmostedt (1967), and Ayd and Blackwell (1970).

The prescribing of drugs should be based upon certain general principles, that is why patient must not start medication without consulting a psychiatrist (or physician with equivalent degree). Once the patient has been put on a drug, he/she should continue it at least for a period of 6 weeks (Hamilton, 1976) before considering a change. If however, in some cases change is necessary, that must be up to the discretion of the attending psychiatrist. Though the value of maintenance drug therapy is clear, the limitation of drugs, as well as their side effects, have prompted an examination of careful reduction of dose, or intermittent use of such drugs when possible (Hogarty, Schooler, and Ulrich *et al.,* 1979; Kane, Rifkin, Woerner, and Reardon, 1982; Marder, Wirshing and Miniz *et al.,* 1996). However, targeted intermittent strategies may be feasible in selected cases while in many it may increase the risk of relapse (Scholler, Keith, Sever, and Matthews, 1995).

Hamilton (1976) opined that "It is a useful assumption to make, that any drug which is effective, *i.e.,* has a 'therapeutic' effect is bound to have unwanted side-effects" (p.133). The commonest side effects are extra-pyramidal reactions of pseudo-parkinsonism, akathisia, 'tardive dyskinesia' (an apparently irreversible side-effects of long term dependence on phenothiazine and acute dystonia (uncommon side effects of the more potent neuroleptic, Hamilton, 1976, p.134) etc. Likewise, caution is exercised while administering these drugs under conditions where anticolinergic effects might give rise to difficulties like enlarged prostate, or glaucoma etc. (Hamilton, 1976). However, drugs are to be used, because the benefits the patient receives perhaps outway the disadvantages. Renaissance came in the treatment of schizophrenia with the advent of atypical antipsychotics which can minimize the horrible side effects of typical antipsychotics, even though atypical psychotics have other side effects, as it affects Glucose and Lipid metabolism which leads to weight gain and other complications. Some authors are of the opinion that medication for the treatment of schizophrenia is only effective as part of our overall treatment approach (Cameron, Ennis, and Deadman, 1998). Nevertheless, for acute and unmanageable cases, drug treatment is the method of choice. In this context, Goldstein (1984) pointed out that after care programmes, particularly drug dosages vary according to the length of stay in the hospitals. Goldstein emphasized the involvement of family in particular, community in general, in assessing the primary caretakers role on maintenance of drug therapy. However, more research is needed to examine the interaction of various psychosocial treatment modalities (Awad, 1995) with drug dose maintenance and quality of life.

Other Physical Treatments

Psychosurgery

Schizophrenics have been introduced to a wide variety of treatment methods. Psychosurgery, for example, was greatly applied to schizophrenia for sometimes, and some have claimed even 82% recovery (Freeman, 1953), if treatment is done within 6 months after the onset of the illness. But at the same time it has been reported in the literature that even if surgery is done at its most ideal time, *i.e.,* within 6 months, 18% of the patients are no better off (Suinn, 1975) than they were prior to the surgery. However, this treatment has become more and more reserved for chronic unresponsive patients. Because of the risk involved in it, a serious question still arises, *i.e.,* is it worth the risk? It has been recognised by the physician that the effect of surgery are irreversible, parts of the brain are destroyed. Overall, the treatment is symptomatic, and not curative. If the schizophrenic process has progressed to that extent that gross personality disorganisation marked by persistent emotional dulling, loss of reality contact, widespread delusions, and emotional disintegration, outcome of the surgery is disappointing (Suinn, 1975). However, this form of treatment is used as a last resort.

Electroconvulsive Therapy (ECT)

This has also been used with schizophrenics but with less spectacular results than found with the affective disorders. In a 25 years, follow-up study Bond (1954) claimed that recovery rate improved after ECT when compared to the pre-ECT condition of the patients. It has been suggested that ECT is more effective if the patients are treated within one year after the onset of the illness. Catatonic stupors, hebephrenics, and simple schizophrenics respond poorest to ECT, while catatonic excitement, and acute paranoid schizophrenics respond more favourably. However, there is much controversy now-a-days regarding effectiveness of ECT and regarding recovery rate of the patients receiving this type of treatment (Hamilton, 1976). It is difficult to get convincing figures since in the reported literature factors like, duration of illness etc. have not been controlled and at the same time follow-up has not been done properly. However, ECT is basically considered symptomatic treatment but not a curative one. Patients with risk of suicide are put in this method of treatment (Hamilton, 1976).

Insulin Treatment

Sakel in 1928 administered insulin to excited schizophrenic patients. Sakel believed that the nervous hyperactivity occurs in morphine addicts due to withdrawal of that drug, *i.e.,* because of an excess of epinephrine. This idea was later supported by the symptoms noted in other patients having abstinence syndrome. After a period of experimental work, Sakel published his results in 1933 and opined that excitement is likely to be relieved by large doses of insulin. Though in the beginning Sakel tried to avoid the development of deep hypoglycaemic states, he later found better results if coma is induced. Accordingly he used to administer increased doses with a view to producing insulin shock.

The percentage of recovery following insulin therapy depends largely on the previous duration of the psychosis. The recovery rate is by far the best in patients who have not been ill for more than 6 months. Full recovery in patients who have been ill for more than 2 years is rare (Staudt and Zubin, 1957). However, compared to hebephrenic or simple types of schizophrenia, paranoids show better results (Laqueur, Dussik, LaBurt, and McLaughlin, 1962).

There are certain (Suinn, 1975) contraindications of such treatments. These are – any active infection, chronic or sub-acute infection; serious heart, liver, or kidney disease; diabetes or other endocrine disorder; skeletal pathology; lack of adequate superficial vain; age under 16 or over 45 years; etc. also, presence of some organic pathologic condition in the patient may cause serious complications.

Insulin treatment, however, does not bring any change in the pre-psychotic personality. Researchers (*e.g.*, Stephens and Astrup, 1965) had failed to provide any support for either short or long-term effects of insulin therapy. Recently, insulin therapy has been largely superseded by the phenothiazine drugs. Insulin therapy had its use in Indian hospitals also. The risk factors associated with the use of insulin have been elaborated by Suinn long before (1975).

Crisis Intervention (CI)

To provide services to acutely psychotic patients on an out-patient basis crisis units are designed. Most often such units work closely with hospital emergency room and/or local mental health centres as day clinics with facilities for overnight stay. This arrangement is made to stabilise the patients and to see whether in-patient commitment becomes necessary.

Upon admission most patients are put on some form of pharmacological treatment. When decompensation appears under control dosages are reduced. Efforts are made to return the patient to his pre-crisis setting or to an alternate programme depending upon the merits of the patient. Only when CI appears insufficient so much so that the patient is considered to be a danger to himself/herself or to his/her surroundings, the patient is transferred to a ward to receive long-term indoor treatment facilities.

One form of CI may be provided by a 24-hour walk-in-services, in community mental health centre, where person can receive immediate attention. But not many such centres are available in India according to the need probably because of financial crunch and lack of specialised manpower.

In CI units treatment programmes as well as discharge planning vary considerably across patients. The daily schedule for treatment includes ward rounds with multidisciplinary treatment team, close monitoring in administration of drugs, psychotherapy (individual, group, and family), educational health programmes, and recreational programmes, (Liberman, Kuehnel, Phipps and Cardin, 1984) including activity therapy and art therapy. On an average, such patients remain in such programmes from 1 to 3 weeks and on release are referred to an out-patient mental health centre / and/or community support programme and also to a conference with the patient's family members. Crisis intervention service records (Liberman *et al.*, 1984) claim that 87% of such patients are able to return to their homes without long-term re-hospitalisation. However, such patients require psychotheapeutic intervention and follow-up assessments on long-term basis. Different types of individual psychotherapeutic programmes suitable for schizophrenic patients will now be discussed.

Environmental / Socio-Psychotherapies

This approach refers not only the patient himself, but his family and community also. There are different group methods of treatment. In contrast to individual psychotherapy, group methods, as the name implies deals with more than one person at a time (dyadic transaction). There are many variants of group transactions (socio-therapies) which are directed to the alleviation of conflicts and stresses between him and his social system and thus aids the individual to cope more effectively with the social milieu. Not only the individual pathology of the patient but also those reflected in his transactions within the social system in which he is a member, are most important here to be concerned with. Thus, *e.g.*, the individual may be in need of a clearer perception of the interactions (includes modes of communications, nature of conflicts and defenses employed etc.) existing within his family. The individual may have been deprived of socialising experiences beyond the family, or he may have been projecting his perceptions of the idiosyncratic social relations existing in his family onto those relations beyond the family group. In either case, through the use of one or several of group methods social perceptivity and transactional capacity of the patient is likely to get changed more effectively. Some of the variants of group techniques will now be discussed below.

Family Therapy

Schizophrenic illness is usually accompanied by serious family problems (as already mentioned in the chapter on etiology) so much so that some authors conceive of schizophrenia as an illness not of the patient alone but of the entire family, and thus the family plays an important role in the treatment of the schizophrenic patient. Appropriate and active involvement with the family and other significant members is usually essential, both during the hospital stay of the patient and after his release.

Family therapy educational programme integrated with pharmacotherapy has been found effective in delaying relapse, and in improving social functioning (Goldstein and Miklowitz, 1995). Meta-analysis of family therapy shows that the greater success has been evident in the families of schizophrenic children. Psychoeducation to reduce 'expressed emotion' did show a decrease in probability of relapse (Goldstein *et al.*, 1978) and re-hospitalisation (Leff, Kuipers, Berkowitz *et al.*, 1992).

Of the many factors inherent in Schizophrenia which determine the outcome of treatment, poor social support system, particularly poor family support system has been associated with poor outcome in Indian patients. Rangaswami (2000) in a study demonstrated the impact of psychoeducational family intervention on 1st episode schizophrenics to prevent progression and relapse. The sample consisted of 6 (mean age 25.66 years) neuroleptic stabilised schizophrenia male patients (duration of illness 6 months) under remission referred by psychiatrists for psychosocial management. All the cases had 1st attack, early onset, and remitted with pharmacotherapy and maintained on low dose neuroleptic drugs. Information giving, clarification and discussion were the methods used for the families. Totally 42 sessions were required and thereafter during follow-up they had monthly one session for the remaining 6 months. However, Long-term follow-up (*e.g.* 2-3 years) is needed for such intervention to validate the obtained findings. Rangaswami (2000) also demonstrated that relapse (65-70%) rate following hospital discharge may be reduced to 40% with the use of antipsychotic medication, whereas through psychosocial therapy the relapse rate may further be reduced to around 20% or so. These studies show that schizophrenics having a bio-psychosocial etiology, psychosocial intervention forms an important method of management for them. In the management of such patients, therefore, recently there is a shift in emphasis from the intraindividual to interindividual approach, particularly with regard to families of schizophrenia.

Indian researchers, even decades before have urged upon a shift in emphasis from the intraindividual to interindividual approach in the management, particularly with regard to families of schizophrenia. This is necessary because male and female schizophrenics in Indian studies (Sathyavathi, 1974, 1977) have found to form two distinct groups regarding their perceptions of sex role, differential functions of their parents etc. Sathyavati examined 20 male and female schizophrenics (mean age 23.60 years, S.D. 3.24 years) and compared with 20 male and female neurotics (mean age 22.75 years, S.D. 2.74 years). The male and female schizophrenics tended to perceive their fathers more or less equally loving whereas notably greater number of male schizophrenics perceived their mothers as significantly more loving than their female counterparts. No such difference in the perception of parents by the neurotics was evident. This study however, was on unmarried Hindu patients, and not known whether similar findings will be applicable in respect of married and other religious groups also; further research is necessary in this regard.

The precise intervention has to be determined by the therapist concerns taking in view the special circumstances of the individual case. In general, however, focus may be on the conflict-provoking nature of family relationships, on defective communication techniques employed in the family, on parental attitudes of preventing the patient from exerting autonomy, or on parental withdrawal because of difficulty in identification, and so on. If the patient is married, interaction process employed in relation to his/her wife/ husband and children has also to be taken into account by the therapist. Eventually, the aim of the therapist would be to make the patient aware of that he must deal with his family members as real persons with limitation and assets, rather than acting according to his fantasies. As a word of caution mention may be made here that the therapist should be vary careful not to fall into the trap of accepting the patients fantasies as the whole of reality.

Difficulty may lie in poor communication among family members or in an alliance between family members that excludes others. However, depending upon the situation, the therapist may visit family to observe conflicts and problems of communication in natural setting and advice them accordingly. Sometimes video tape recordings are played back to make family members aware of how they interact. The best way to treat them is to set up family unit in hospital premises itself, as was revealed from the work of Verghese, Bhatia, Raghuram *et al.* (1994) in Indian set up.

In South India, at the hospital set-up of the NIMHANS itself, arrangement is there for rendering family therapy to the patients in a controlled condition. For this purpose they have 'Family Wards', where the patient and the key figures of the family (here 'key' figure means those with whom the patient has got difficulty to adjust when he is released from the hospital) are asked to live together under supervision of a team of specialists consisting of a psychiatrist, a clinical psychologist, a psychiatric social worker and a psychiatric nurse. Patients having family interaction problems are asked to stay with each of their family unit separately in such wards having their separate arrangement for cooking, performing religious acts, etc. Such an arrangement helps the patients and their relatives to get double benefit in the sense that (a) each family unit gets opportunity to exchange their views with the other family unit freely, and (b) with the help of the therapist the patient himself gets opportunity to learn how to adjust in the family when he gets released from the hospital. The patients and the family members during their stay in the family wards are free to move around, but only restriction imposed onto them is to follow the prescriptions of medicine and other interaction processes (amongst the family members) given to them by the physician / therapist, and also that they must return to the hospital wards within a specific time of the day they are asked to. Such an arrangement may not be done at the very beginning when the patient comes for hospital treatment. Initially he is put to a general ward, there he is provided with necessary treatment facilities and is gradually prepared to stay in the family ward. Thus family ward may be considered as a step forward to the patient's getting released for the home. Several times it is found that the patient is completely alright in the hospital set up after receiving treatment but when he goes back home shows relapse. Arrangement in family wards helps much to reduce the incidence of such relapse. After the patient is released from the hospital follow-up is being made separately for the each unit of the family ward.

Long-term family therapy though has a number of approaches, there are some major common components of it. Some such components have been recently reviewed by Lam (1991). These are : (i) a genuine work relationship; (ii) a positive attitude to such a relationship; (iii) to consider family boundaries; (iv) to focus on the problems as evident here and now; (v) cognitive restructuring; (vi) to improve communication; (vii) to apply behavioural approaches in assigning tasks to acquire skills; and (viii) systematic long-term follow-up. Application of behavioural approaches along with cognitive therapy will be discussed later in this chapter.

To maintain liaison with the family members both in the beginning of the therapy as well as during follow-up the psychiatric social worker and psychiatrically trained public health nurse can often play a major and decisive role in this area.

In sum: Family therapy looks at critical issues like patient and family perception and adaptation to illness, patient functioning, family burden and problem solving, and relapse prevention. The therapist must possess an understanding of psychodynamics, communication, and interpersonal theories to avoid medicolegal hazards.

Group Psychotherapy

J. Pratt (1905) (cited by Kolb, 1973) pioneered group psychotherapy through the use of didactic discussion and inspirational group meetings. Pratt initiated this with a view to bring a favourable change in the morale of patients. To start with Pratt arranged for group meetings with physically ill patients (tuberculosis) and later applied the same method onto others with various psychosomatic problems, and finally onto various other diagnostic groups of patients (Kolb, 1973), *viz.*, psychoneurotics, psychotics, behaviour disorders, both children and adults.

There are some specific indications for the use of group therapy (Slavson, 1950). Because of fear, competitiveness, distrust, or antagonism to all authority figures in some individuals, individual psychotherapy is too threatening and such individuals manifest aversion to individual therapist. For such persons group psychotherapy may be successful or even may serve as a means to prepare them for individual psychotherapy. Likewise, persons lacking sibling experiences, having antagonistic sibling attitudes, living alone throughout, experiencing destructive family interaction and so on are considered suitable for group therapy. However, group homogeneity and the number of participants to be recommended for group are still debatable subjects. On the one hand, it is found that too little homogeneity caused scattered interest, and on the other it is also found that extreme heterogeneity, *e.g.*, alcoholic patients getting mingled with patients of psychosis or neurosis may engender mutual trust. The group should be large enough for allowing adequate interaction yet not so large that members remain unattended (considered neglected by the members) (Kleinmuntz, 1974). Homogeneity in terms of age, sex, intelligence, education, socio-economic status, and fairly well balanced in traits are desirable to form such therapeutic groups.

There are different types of groups. These include insight group, supportive, activity, educational and social actions oriented groups (Scheidlinger, 1969).

Early group techniques were mainly in the form of inspirational lectures followed by discussions and didactic presentation of the therapist. Trigant Burrow (1928) applied theoretical principles in group therapy. These principles Burrow derived from the principles of psychoanalysis. Kurt Lewin worked on his field theories and formulated the concept of group dynamics, while J. Moreno developed the procedures of Psychodrama and Sociodrama. Though systems of group therapy differ, probably all groups follow certain common mechanisms. These are – group unification which leads to group identity. This is followed by group interaction based on dynamisms, and finally resolution of dynamisms which produces insights.

In a controlled trial on schizophrenics patients O'Brian and associates (1969) found that after 12 and 24 months, group therapy was significantly better in terms of social effectiveness than individual psychotherapy, though the rates of readmission did not differ significantly. Similar was the view of Nitsun *et al.* (1974) (see Hamilton, 1976) with regard to the effectiveness of group therapy in schizophrenics. However, outcome may not be satisfactory if selection of the group etc. is not adequate; this it claims proper training of the (Hamilton, 1976) therapist.

In sum: Group Therapy may be applied as the sole psychotherapeutic measure or in conjunction with individual psychotherapy. Group psychotherapy has proved useful for many schizophrenic patients especially for those who are inhibited in individual psychotherapy, or who have shown a major problem in group living.

Psychodrama

This form of therapy had its beginning in the work of J.L. Moreno (1959), a young physician who founded the Theatre of Spontaneity in Vienna in 1925. Moreno was inspired in doing this by his unfavourable reaction to Freudian psychoanalysis. The underlying rationale of this method is that role playing is an essential part in everyday life. People change as a result of their spontaneous performance and gain emotional release from such open expression of their problems.

Specially designated and problem-specific stage (Kleinmuntz, 1974) is required for this. The therapist-director gets the psychodrama going by asking the patient to act out a specific scene spontaneously. The patient stages this in front of an audience. The other players in the drama serve as "auxiliary egos" (Moreno, 1959). These players support the ongoing action and help the patient bringing about his conflicts.

In a controlled trial on two groups of schizophrenics Nitsum *et al.* (1974) (see Hamilton, 1976) found that drama therapy showed a significantly greater decrease in restless and aimless movements in the patients and thus helped them for better social behaviour.

This method is found to be particularly helpful to those patients whose ability to verbalise their feelings and experiences (Kleinmuntz, 1974) are limited, *e.g.,* hospitalised psychotics. Psychodrama is also helpful to the patient – audience in working out their own problems.

Industrial Therapy

The whole purpose of this therapeutic milieu is to put the patient on the road to independence. Compared with Occupational Therapy, Industrial Therapy provides a realistic way of assessing the patient's capabilities. It provides the stimulus and activation which is necessary to prevent deterioration (Hamilton, 1976). In a ward this therapy trains him to be disciplined, *i.e.,* punctual and regular in attendance, proper standard of work, and finally providing him with a wage which he has earned (Hamilton, 1976). Aims of this therapy have been clearly described by Bennett and Wing (1963). An excellent general guide to the setting up of industrial therapeutic unit has been provided by Wadsworth, Wells and Scott (1962), and Morgan (1974) has depicted clearly the importance of properly designed equipment and management of the workshops. Running of an industrial therapy unit should be in complete control of one person only. The activities of the therapy unit should be regarded as part of a programme which covers all the patients' needs (Ekdawi, 1972). An adequate system of payments is of the greatest importance here. In this context

Bennett (1970) emphasized the value of payment on a piecework basis. Payments should be accompanied by appropriate facilities for spending money, be it in or out of the hospital. When the patient is ready, he should be prepared for leaving hospital either to a 'half-way house', or hostel, or to return to a home with relatives.

In Indian situation, patients very seldom get opportunities to stay at the 'half-way house', or hostel. So only alternative left to him is to return to home. But home atmosphere at times may be critical. In some families it is noted that relatives find it difficult to tolerate the eccentricities of a patient. A tense atmosphere may easily develop and the patient relapses (Brown, Birley and Wing, 1972). In such circumstances, careful preparation of the family is needed and the family should be followed by continual supervision. Of late some of the NGOs in India are trying to establish such therapeutic milieu but mostly that turns out to be occupational therapy rather than industrial therapy.

Behavioural Family Therapy

Several experimental studies have reported that family is a potentially powerful rehabilitative force in the patient's life (*e.g.*, Evans, Bullard, and Solomon, 1961). As early as 1958-1959 Freeman and Simmons suggested that compared to those schizophrenics living in non-nuclear family arrangements, schizophrenics living in the nuclear family had shown a worse prognosis (also see Freeman *et al.*, 1958). Similarly, in a later study higher rates of relapse for schizophrenic persons living with one's nuclear family (compared to those living with an extended family) has been reported (El-Islam, 1979). Living with siblings of the patient seems to cause lower rehospitalisation rate for schizophrenics than those living with parents and wives (Brown, Monck, Carstairs, and Wing, 1962). High expressed emotion in the family appears to have a deleterious effects on the course of the schizophrenic illness (Brown, Birley, and Wing, 1972; Vaughan and Leff, 1976; Vaughan, Snyder, Jones, Freeman and Falloon, 1984; Karno, Jenkins, Selva De La, Santana, Lopez and Miniz, 1987; Strachan, Leff, Goldstein, Doane, Burtt, 1986). In addition, the residual symptoms of schizophrenia evident in many patients residing with family members can cause distress in the relatives. This in turn, challenges the coping skills of relatives. Moreover, mostly relatives fail to recognise symptoms, like, apathy, blunted affect etc. present in the patients. Relatives frequently interpret these symptoms as indications of lazyness, inferior moral character (Leff and Vaughan, 1985). It thus shows that the family members of the patient are to be concerned in the treatment of schizophrenia as because their interaction helps to modify in a better way the emotional climate which prevails in the family (Leff, Kuipers, Berkowitz, and Sturgeon, 1985; Falloon, Boyd and McGill, 1984). Family members may show resistance to such intervention (Liberman, 1981). This is most likely when the family members have been blamed for causing the patient to become schizophrenic (Appleton, 1974; Terkelson, 1983). However, Therapist has to tackle such resentment adequately.

Certain steps are to be sequentially followed in the behavioural family therapy (Mueser and Bellack, 1989). To start with, family assessment is most important step. Assessment aims to identify the assets and deficits of individual members of the family, including their understanding and perception (Burden) of schizophrenia, as well as the role that specific problem behaviours play in the family interaction. Assessment to be done based on individual interview, and observation (especially when family interacts during therapeutic sessions).

The next stage is to educate the family members of the patient regarding (a) possible causes of schizophrenia, its signs and symptoms, prevalence, course and prognosis; also, it teaches about the role of stress in triggering symptom aggravation; (b) to recognise the prominent indications of relapse; to understand the principles of treatment; (c) the impact and side effects of neuroleptic drugs, and (d) availability and utilisation of community resources including hospital services, psychotherapeutic and vocational programmes and social agencies/advocacy groups. Such an educational session also helps the family members to refute common misconceptions about schizophrenia, *e.g.*, influence of witchcrafts etc. in causing it. This is done in the first three or four sessions, may be extended up to six sessions (Dixon and Lehman, 1995). Methods used in this are – didactic presentation, discussion, hand outs and poster display (Mueser and Bellack, 1989).

The third important stage in this programme is to train communication skills. Such training emphasizes direct verbal communication with other persons of the family either on request or commenting on a behaviour(s) of other person(s). This enables family members to discuss potentially stressful events with minimum of negative affect and thus to create an atmosphere for empathic listening and expression of positive behaviour to one another. The procedures employed here are same as those mentioned before in this chapter in connection with social skills training (Mueser and Bellack, 1989).

The next stage is called problem-solving training. This involves teaching behavioural techniques so as to enable family members resolving their problems. Such an effort to improve family members problem solving skill is likely to lessen the ambient stress in the family. This is also expected to minimize negative emotional undercurrents amongst family members. In the beginning the therapist chairs the session and teaches family members the steps to be followed in defining problem, in finding out alternative solutions, and in its implementation. Everything is recorded systematically. Gradually such responsibility is handed over to family members and the members by rotation chair the session (Mueser and Bellack, 1989). In case of any crisis the therapist is informed and he chairs sessions as a special situation. Thus the main tenet of family therapy is to improve problem solving skills in the family members (through their own weekly problem-solving sessions in the absence of the therapist) so as to enable them to cope effectively with stressors.

The final stage in this therapeutic programme is devoted to solve special problems, if any. By special problem is meant those problems which the family members have not responded to, or have not been able to solve through their own weekly sessions. The family members are taught a wide variety of behavioural techniques (Mueser and Bellack, 1989) to solve special problems, depending upon the nature of the problems. For example, cognitive-behavioural restructuring techniques for depression, social skills training for social inadequacy, token economy for enhancing daily activity, relaxation and/or desensitisation, or flooding for anxiety, and so on. It is desirable that the whole family members get involved in implementing these strategies.

In a well-controlled study Falloon (1984), and Falloon, Boyd, McGill, Ranzani, Moss, Gilderman, and Simpson (1985) found that schizophrenic patients who received family treatment experienced fewer major exacerbations in schizophrenic symptoms as well as episodes of depression. These patients required, as was found after 9-month and at a 2-year follow-up, fewer emergency crisis sessions than did patients who received individual therapy. Behavioural family therapy not only helps to lower ambient stress which the patient encounters but also helps in reducing the amount of neuroleptic medication (Falloon and Pederson, 1985) which the patient requires to control triggering of and to prevent aggravation of symptoms.

In sum : Relatives are educated to understand and respect both positive and negative symptoms. They are guided to see the illness in terms of the disease model; guilt, shame, blame, and misconceptions are discouraged. Constructive problem-solving is emphasised.

Therapeutic Community

Another development of social therapy is Therapeutic Community / Therapeutic Milieu. Main, Britger, Bion, Dewar, Foulkes, Davidson (1946) were the first to use the term "Therapeutic Community" as a treatment modality. This concept was later popularised by psychiatrist Maxwell Jones (1953). Main (1946) substituted the concept of the hospital as a therapeutic institution, with a framework of social reality. Such a framework provides opportunities for attaining better social insight and for expressing and modifying emotional drives as per the demands of real life. In this treatment method the focus is the community in which the patient and his relatives reside. The reasons for this point of view are not hard to find. Community psychiatry hypothesizes that individual psychopathology is inextricably bound up with psycho-pathology within the family group. According to this view it is not possible to treat one member of the family without helping the other members. Community Psychiatry regards mental health as a public health issue. It not only concerns itself with problems of prevention, also seeks to provide service for treatment employing group psychotherapy. It may also employ therapeutically useful group interactions of all kinds, such as those provided by work, play and education. Also, there is provision for use of medication (prescribed by psychiatrist) for the relief of specific target symptom whenever necessary.

In therapeutic milieu, as a general principle the whole responsibility for managing the ward is spread onto all who have any function therein (Hamilton, 1976). Management of the ward includes both general activities and therapeutic programme. Thus it aims that the hierarchy of authority is flattened and patients are helped to become responsible for their behaviour and activity. Regular meetings are held in the ward to plan ward activities as well as to evaluate the progress of the activities already assigned. This covers not only the maintenance of the ward, but domestic problems as well (Hamilton, 1976). Also, social and recreational activities are organised and finally the therapeutic regime is considered. This starts with the consideration of the problems of the individual members of the ward, which thereby makes the wards meeting a form of group therapy.

The outcome of such therapeutic programme has not been consistent. Thus, *e.g.*, Letemendia, Harris, and Williams (1967) reported that compared to traditional ward set-up, therapeutic community did not reveal any significant outcome. Madew, Singer *et al.* (1966) on the contrary, found significantly better discharge rates following community therapeutic programme. In the latter study all the patients in their community were not suffering from schizophrenia. Hence, not known whether outcome would have been same had the patients been all schizophrenics. However, such a system, as a therapeutic mode is in vogue in some of the hospitals in India, as mentioned earlier (*e.g.*, Kalyansundaram and Verghese, 2000) in this chapter.

Therapeutic community programme has its own limitations. In spite of all its efforts and enthusiasms, it is not possible to eliminate the hierarchy completely (Hamilton, 1976). Thus *e.g.*, as Hamilton (1976) stated, when the therapist announces to the members of the ward, especially to new comer that "We are all here to tackle our problems of living together" (Hamilton, 1976), sometimes he is being asked by some of the members of the ward, "how long have you been here, and why have you not settled your problems so far" (Hamilton, 1976) ? etc. such comments, in other words, create some sort of lack of confidence in the members about the efficacy of such programming, and secondly, intelligent patients understand that the therapist is different from the rest of the members though the therapist presumes a role as if he is one of the ward members. This is very much apparent when some of the patients ask the therapist 'How is it that you are paid to do so, and we are not' (Hamilton, 1976) etc. However, such a programming may work well with patients having borderline intelligence. Another great difficulty in community principle is that, in general, wards include patients suffering from many different disorders. In these circumstances, it is very difficult to bring the schizophrenics into full cooperation because of their epathy and withdrawal (Hamilton, 1976). Thirdly, community principle is not applicable into the acutely ill patients. Finally, it may not be too harsh to mention that even today, particularly in India these are only ideals toward which some hospital administrations strive; the realities of hospital environment are far different.

The hospital professional team should expand into the real world of the community. To provide genuine continuity of care they should develop techniques for milieu therapy, thoughtfully integrated with work and social rehabilitation.

In sum : The overall objectives of a therapeutic community are to promote a total environment in which patients are encouraged to communicate easily with one another.This would develop confidence in them. They are thus prepared for life outside the hospital by being allowed to participate in decisions about their welfare.

Evaluation of Therapies

Outcome of any therapeutic intervention should be judged depending upon its meaningfulness to the patients and the percentage of patients that show relief of symptoms, but not depending upon statistical significance only. Many reported studies have shown statistical significance with acceptable level of confidence but a scrutiny of the procedures employed in those studies do show serious methodological limitations. Researchers often fail to employ rigorous methodology (Hartman, Roper and Gelfand, 1977; Eysenck, 1985; Rachman and Wilson, 1983) and thus outcome research for different modes of therapies appears to be full of confusion and controversies. Under the circumstances, comparison of therapies become meaningless, especially when a well-executed therapy is compared with a well-planned but poorly executed one. Therapy should be patient-oriented and its evaluation should be based on social validity (Wolf, 1978).

Discovery of pharmacological therapy (1950s) in schizophrenia has served to highlight the social problems of these patients. There has been a widespread use of neuroleptic drugs in the treatment of schizophrenia. But there too, lots of differences in the research findings are evident. Some authors are of the opinion that neuroleptic drugs have a potent effect on both the positve and negative symptoms of schizophrenia (Goldberg, 1985; Meltezer, 1985), while others (Anderson and Olsen, 1982; Angrist, Rotrosen, and Gershon, 1980; Carlson, 1986; Falloon *et al.,* 1983) reported that these drugs appear less effective in treating negative symptoms (also called prodormal or residual symptoms). Positive symptoms include (Baldessarini, 1985) delusions, hallucinations, incoherence, loose associations, agitated and/or grossly distorted behaviour, and disordered thinking. Negative symptoms include withdrawal, lack of initiative in maintaining personal hygiene, grooming, bunted affect, poverty of speech, apathy, poor judgement, and psychomotor retardation (Meltezer, 1985). Again, it has been evident that these medications cannot help in improving the social competence of patients who have never had developed adequate social skills, or who have lost use of such skills because of disuse for long time (Diamond, 1985). Even impoverished quality of such patient's life experience cannot be improved by these medications (Lehman, 1983). These drugs seem to be effective in reducing acute excitement or withdrawal syndrome but even then they impose debilitating side effects (Johnson, 1985; Van Puttern, and May, 1978). Furthermore, medication appears to have failed in reducing the incidence of relapse. Thus, *e.g.,* Hogarty, Schooler, Ulrich, Mussare, Ferro, and Herson (1979) reported that 40% of treated schizophrenic patients show an exacerbation of symptoms within 1-year follow-up duration. This rate shows an increase, as high as that of 75% (Talbott, 1981) over 3 years following discharge from a psychiatric hospital. Also, rate of relapse is reported to be high among those patients who initially do respond positively to such psychotropic medication (Hogarty *et al.,* 1979). This has led to very poor community adjustment (Goldstorm, and Mandersheid, 1981; Sylph, Ross, and Kedward, 1978) as well as to social rejection of patients (Kirk and Therrien, 1975).

Pharmacotherapy for children, unfortunately has not been uniformly effective (Cameron *et al.,* 1998); outcome studies of drug treatments have been disappointing (Jensen, Ryan and Prien, 1992). This rather has paved ways for research into psychosocial interventions. Efficacy of pharmacotherapy with regard to course and prognosis of schizophrenia illness has been discussed later (Chapter X) in this book.

Direct analysis, a dramatic technique developed by Rosen (1947, 1953) had been reported to be highly successful with schizophrenic patients. This is an intense and extremely active verbal approach which involves deep, immediate interpretations of the patient's primary process, and is accompanied, if needed, by direct physical activity. Bookhammer, Meyers, Schober, and Piotrowski (1966) in an effort to evaluate systematically the efficacy of this technique selected 14 first-break schizophrenic patients (age ranged 15-35 years) from consecutive admissions to psychiatry unit of Philadelphia General Hospital. Comparable control patients received 'usual treatment'. After about 5-5½ years follow-up period the authors failed to demonstrate any significant difference between patients receiving direct analysis (57% improved) with other controls (67% improved). However, because of the deficiencies noted in Rosen's study no specific conclusions could be drawn about its efficacy. Some such deficiencies are – no mention was made of the frequency and duration of the technique employed. No standardised measure was used to assess the outcome. What type of treatment received by the control groups was not mentioned. According to Fromm-Reichmann (1952) the primary purpose of direct analytic method is not to cure schizophrenics, but rather, to 'help them to emerge quickly from acute psychotic episodes'. To reduce quickly acute psychotic episodes drug treatment is most effective. The latter is likely to make the patient amenable to psychotherapy, if at all the therapist considers the patient suitable for psychotherapy.

At the Massachusetts Mental Health Centre Grinspoon, Ewalt, and Shader (1967) demonstrated the effects of long-term psychoanalytically oriented psychotherapy on chronic schizophrenic patients, with and without drugs. Twenty experimental subjects were selected from among a group of 41 single male (aged 16-35 years). They were all hospitalised at the Boston State Hospital for over 3 years, the remaining 21 patients acted as controls. At first all the patients were placed upon a placebo regimen. Thirteen weeks later half of the patients were given Thioridazine, and the rest half continued to receive placebo. Both the groups received individual psychotherapy twice a week for 2 or more years. Behavioural assessments were done by nurses, social workers, the therapist, and senior residents. Those patients receiving psychotherapy along with drug showed slight but significantly greater improvement. Difference between the two groups tended to disappear when placebo was substituted for thioridazine during a 3 month period, at the end of the study.

In general, however, classical psychoanalysis has been seldom advised as treatment of choice for people with schizophrenia and similar other illnesses (*e.g.,* autism). Patients with such disorder have not been profited effectively because of their cognitive disturbances (*e.g.,* McNeil, 1970) as well as social withdrawal (Gomes-Schwartz, 1984). Some times parents of such children / patients have been advised to undergo psychoanalysis but there too results have not been much encouraging throughout (Eisenberg, 1956; Sullivan, 1976).

May (1968) in a comparative study of 5 treatment methods in schizophrenia at the Camarillo State Hospital selected randomly 220 first admission schizophrenics (aged 16 to 48 years). They had no history of epilepsy and addiction. They were randomly assigned to different methods of treatment, *viz.,* psychotherapy, psychotherapy with drug, only drug, and ECT. On the average psychotherapy patients were seen 2 hours/ week till they were either released or declared failure of treatment at the end of 1 year. May reported that for first admission schizophrenics in the middle prognosis range, individual psychotherapy of an "ego supportive, reality defining" type was an ineffective method of treatment when compared to drugs. May opined that psychotherapy alone, in schizophrenics, is not the treatment of choice, because an adjunct of drug with psychotherapy showed better results compared to psychotherapy alone. May's conclusion is also open to criticism since no follow-up has been reported. Moreover, psychotherapy given was too brief (Grinspoon, 1969; Leavitt, 1968; Michels, 1969), too non-intensive (Hamilton, 1979; Wexler, 1968), and the therapists were lacking in skills (Leavitt, 1968; Rosen, 1969).

Several authors concluded that addition of psychotherapy, active milieu, and other modern treatment methods did not significantly improve or even alter, in a 2-year period, the outcome of hospitalised chronic schizophrenics. This conclusion, however, is confused, since the study lacked a control group in the same setting which did not receive psychotherapy. Furthermore, the pair of patients were not "matched" before the study and then assigned randomly to the treatment group (Cole, 1967). Also, therapists' motivation for participating in this study as well as their skills were not assessed. Karno and O'Grady (1969), and Karno and Vandenbos (1970) reported that patients receiving psychotherapy by experienced therapist spent significantly less time in the hospital after 1-year than drug-treated controls.

Rogers (1969) client–centered psychotherapy claimed that psychotherapy for schizophrenic patients can produce measurable differences from control patients. Rogers was of the opinion that its effectiveness depends upon the following characteristic of the therapeutic relationship. Congruence – genuineness – the therapist responds as a real person. Empathy – the therapist senses and expresses the client's felt needs. Unconditional positive regard – the therapist expresses a warm and positive acceptance towards his client.

The results of a study designed and conducted under Roger's direction at the Mendota State Hospital failed to report any satisfactory outcome. Eight "more chronic" (hospitalised over 8 months), 8 "more acute" (hospitalised less than 8 months), and 8 normal volunteers were selected randomly to receive client centered therapy from 8 therapists. The subjects were matched according to age, sex, socio-economic status, and chronicity. The experimental subjects were seen twice a week in 50-minute session till the termination (several months to 2½ years) of treatment. Blind raters rated before beginning, every 3 months during, and immediately after termination and 1-year following termination. Several tests like MMPI, TAT, Rorschach etc. were used. Some of the major findings of this study were that schizophrenic patients receiving psychotherapy showed a slightly better rate of release from hospital and this differential was maintained a year after termination (Rogers, Gendlin, Kiessler, and Traux, 1967). None of the other measures showed any significant difference from the controls.

However, a major contaminating factor in this study is that the schizophrenic controls received drugs as a regular part of their "usual hospital" treatment, while the psychotherapy patients received medication "only in emergencies", *i.e.,* in a completely uncontrolled, irregular and unknown fashion. Therefore, it is difficult to be sure, in restrospect, how drugs affected the findings of this study. Moreover, the rating instrument used to evaluate the psychotherapeutic relationship was too idiosyncratic, as viewed by Vaccaro, 1967. However, this study requires special mention since it was the first to state that psychotherapy for schizophrenic patients can produce measurable differences from control patients and that its effectiveness depends upon the establishment of a therapeutic relationship characterised by empathy and congruence.

In sum: The conventional psychotherapies with its unhurried pace and detailed exploration are expensive and time consuming. Each session runs about 40-50 minutes and the number of sessions require for each patient ranges, on an average, 2-3 years period if not more, since conventional therapies, especially the Freudian approach emphasizes on resolution of unconscious conflicts and development of insight (though not mostly applicable to psychotics). It is acceptable only to those who are wealthy and also have leisure time to spend for it. Strictly speaking it is not geared for handling emergency situations (crisis). For these reasons brief psychotherapy has received the attention of mental health workers. As a treatment form brief psychotherapy had its origin since 1920s (Ferenczi, 1926). In contrast to long-term psychotherapy brief psychotherapy quickly focuses on specific and critical problems to be solved so as to aid the patient to acquire self-knowledge about his inabilities to cope with the difficulties. Therefore, brief psychotherapy has enjoyed a recent surge of interest (Barten, 1969; Aguilera, Messick, and Farrelle, 1970).

Unlike conventional methods, in brief psychotherapy the therapist systematically probes all facets of the patient's situation relating to the problem for which the patient seeks help. After the first interview the therapist formulates theory about the patient's problems. In subsequent sessions (usually not more than 10) the therapist does not allow digressions and focuses only on issues that have direct bearing onto the patient's present problems. The therapist helps the patient acquiring self-knowledge into his problems and then to translate these knowledge into action.

Of course not all patients benefit from such treatment. Those who are likely to be benefited can be identified based on several characteristics. These are, *e.g.,* crisis is of recent onset (Bellak and Small, 1965; Gotteschalk, Mayerson, and Gittlies, 1967; Straker, 1968; Wolberg, 1965) previous adjustment satisfactory (Gillman, 1965; Sifneos, 1967), stable environment in which the patient functions (Pumpian-Mindian, 1953), and that the extent of precipitating stress is not overwhelming (Alexander, 1944; Sarvis, Dewees, Johnson, 1958). Brief psychotherapy is unlikely to give satisfactory outcome in paranoid schizophrenics, and in patients with long-standing psychiatric illness (Wolberg, 1965).

Milieu therapy originally designed by Bettelheim and Sylvester (1948) aimed to demonstrate that reorganisation of the institutional ward would foster group interactions (Osmond, 1957) by removing debilitating effects of long-term hospitalisation (Wing, 1979). Outcome research employing milieu therapy is yet inconclusive. Greenblatt, Solomon and Evans (1965) conducted intensive milieu therapy on chronic schizophrenic patients at the Boston

State Hospital and reported that milieu therapy indicated positive effects. Similar was the trend of findings of Hamilton (1963). But in a latter study there appears to have number of unexplained areas (*e.g.*, the study mentioned that there were stimulating environment, but no mention is made about the components of stimulating environment) which make replication of such studies difficult. In contrast, Clompi (1983), and Goldberg and Rubin (1984) reported that certain patients do not improve after milieu therapy rather react poorly to an overstimulating environment. Sanders, Smith and Weissman (1967) at the Philadelphia State Hospital treated chronic schizophrenic patients employing milieu therapy and reported that this technique account for therapeutic effect. But negative outcomes have been reported by others (*e.g.*, Hemsley, 1978; Schooler and Spohn, 1982). However, some of these early studies gave impetus for restructuring milieu therapy in a systematic manner and also to include principles of behaviour modification and social learning skills in such intervention programme. In another study Paul and Lentz (1977) compared social learning (response cost, time-out, shaping, prompting etc.), milieu therapy (Communication, problem solving etc.), and traditional therapies (chemotherapy, psychotherapy) and reported that milieu therapy was superior to traditional custodial care in hospital but social learning therapy was found superior to both milieu therapy, and traditional hospital care. Even after 18 months follow-up social learning therapy was found to have a significant longer maintenance.

Research evidences show that there is a number of prerequisites for healthy involvement in group psychotherapy, the most basic of these is a non-psychotic disorder. Though some studies reported success with schizophrenic patients (Kanas, 1985), group psychotherapy, in general, is reported to be less successful with severely psychotic patients (Bednar and Lawlis, 1991). This is probable due to their difficulty in establishing interpersonal relationships as well as in bringing forth deep-rooted feeling (insight) of the patients.

There is very little evidence on the efficacy of existential therapeutic modalites in the treatment of schizophrenia (Biswanger, 1965).

Serok and Zemet (1983) treated 9 experimental and 8 control subjects over a period of 2½ months applying Gestalt Therapy and reported a significant difference in reality differentiation and perception for treatment subjects in comparison to their pre-treatment phase and also the control group. However, subjects were also treated simultaneously with variety of other techniques. Moreover, to assess outcome of this therapy the authors employed the Rorschach test which is not free from subjectivity in scoring. The authors though claimed that a number of disturbed behaviour diminished overtime, they failed to quantify this improvement in behaviour. Furthermore, this therapy may be applicable only with highly communicable patients.

With a conceptual shift in the present understanding of the causes of schizophrenia, there is a noticeable shift in application of its treatment modalities also. Some treatments focus on specific cognitive deficits. It is based on the notion that (Beck *et al.*, 1979) cognitions cause emotional states and various types of psychopathology. Systematic errors, in thinking and perception can be modified through cognitive restructuring, not only in depressed patients, but with other types of psychopathology also.

There are many models of cognitive therapy. Of these the best known three are Ellis' rational-emotive therapy, Beck's cognitive therapy, and Meichenbaum's self-instructional training technique. Therapeutic principles with regard to schizophrenia has been described by Alford and Correia (1994) and meta-cognitive approaches been advocated by Perris and Skagerlind (1994). Cognitive therapy has been employed with schizophrenic patients (Schwartz-Place and Gilmore, 1980; Meichenbaum and Cameron, 1973; Margolis and Shemberg, 1976) but results are as yet far from conclusive. Further research with empirically derived evidences is needed.

The meta-cognitive approach focuses on the interaction between biological and psychological factors with a view to account for how illness may contaminate the view of the patients own self. Coping-strategy enhancement technique has been devised (Tarrier *et al.,* 1990) and outcome reports are found to be favourable. However, many of the studies have not applied well-controlled design that could be the reason for controversies in the existing research reports. Cameron *et al.* (1998) in this regard reported that to maximize the effects of cognitive therapy, the effects of cognitive deficits in the personality development of the patients require a thorough understanding. Despite differences in the approach between the cognitive therapists and behaviour therapists, of late there has developed a kinship between the two.

Cognitive therapies thus utilise behavioural concepts. For example, the covert conditioning model regards private events as covert forms of behaviour that is overtly observed (Homme, 1965). This situation parallels principles of classical and operant conditioning (Kazdin, 1977). It is evident from several research reports that application of direct reinforcement works relatively better as a therapeutic method, for such patients, than those of other methods. In this context, O'Leary and Wilson (1975) long before opined that "reinforcement procedures have been the predominant means of the behavioural treatment of psychotic disorders" (O'Leary and Wilson, 1975). Thereafter a wide range of methods have been employed in controlling different behavioural problems of schizophrenic patients. A good number of behavioural treatment programmes have been proved effective in reducing delusional behaviour (*e.g.,* Patterson and Teigen, 1973; Falloon *et al.,* 1983), hallucinations (*e.g.,* Alford and Turner, 1976; Turner, Herson, and Bellack, 1977), aggressive behaviour (*e.g.,* Falloon *et al.,* 1983; Dalldorf, 1983; Favell, 1983; Mesibov, 1983). The later studies also reported that psychotropic drugs have also been used to control aggression but results of such chemotherapy have been inconsistent especially from the point of view of maintenance of improved behaviour/desired behaviour. Shortcomings in many such studies may be attributed to lack of adequate staff training (Birrell and Henderson, 1986), and lack of consistency among staff and administrative difficulties (Birrell and Henderson, 1986) particularly when such techniques are employed in in-patient set-up. Therapists now believe that behaviour is determine by a broad range of factors (biological, psychological and learning) and hence, the most integrated approach is necessary to achieve a comprehensive treatment outcome. The technique which is mostly in use now is popularly known as 'CBT' (cognitive behaviour therapy). Reported findings though are not free from controversies, in general however, there prevails a belief that compared to cognitive therapy alone, CBT helps to decrease the amount of drug required, and also to increase the interval time between relapses.

While evaluating the effectiveness of child therapy, it has been reported that about half of all treatment studies, over the past 20 years account for behaviour modification and cognitive/behavioural therapies (Kazdin, Bass, Ayers and Rodgers, 1990). Traditional therapies in child psychiatry, *viz.*, family therapy, play therapy and/or combined approaches, have been only infrequently examined (Cameron *et al.*, 1998), while very few studies using controlled clinical trials have looked at psychodynamic psychotherapy (Fonagy and Moran, 1990).

A number of criticisms have been raised regarding application of behaviour therapy to chronic schizophrenics. Some authors, *e.g.*, Davidson (1969) opined that the improvement noted in the patients by the therapists may have been a non-specific effect. This he stated with the argument that it is an old clinical tradition that chronic schizophrenics tend to deteriorate in a stagnant environment so that any change will halt the deterioration and sometimes even reverse it dramatically. In most of the reports made by the behaviour therapists it was noted that the patients received more attention than that they received in the past, and since this was often not adequately controlled for, the improvement claimed by the therapists may have been non-specific one. In reply to Davidson's argument it should be mentioned that though it is likely that chronic schizophrenics will tend to deteriorate in a stagnant environment, it is unethical not to think of ways and means to remove the stagnant condition of the environment where the patients live. Secondly, assuming that the patients have been given more attention than that they had received earlier, it is no wonder that in any therapeutic measure the main target is the patient himself and thereby if the patient shows improvement, it does not nullify the efficacy of the therapeutic technique employed. Thirdly, taking it to be granted, as Davidson pointed out, that the patients had received more attention during behaviour therapy, by this did Davidson mean that in a hospital ward, while applying traditional methods of treatment chronic patients are not given enough attention? Does it mean that the traditional methods of treatment were being employed mechanically as a routine procedure? Actually, so far as the chronic schizophrenics are concerned, it is not a question of a giving more attention; the question, on the contrary, is how to make the patient amenable to a therapeutic situation (receiving his attention) and in this sense, behaviour therapists have helped in achieving the latter, which however, is a basic requirement for any therapeutic measure to be employed. Lastly, even today our existing knowledge about schizophrenia is so to say incomplete. This is more so with regard to the treatment of chronic patients where traditional methods of treatment have reached a plaque. Therefore, many more new attempts are to be made to demonstrate as to how chronic schizophrenics could be helped to overcome their disordered behaviour. In doing so our aim should be to help the therapists in applying, as well as in reframing and re-modelling their techniques with concrete suggestions, if necessary, instead of criticizing a technique in unsound way.

Also, Davidson (1969) pointed out that there has been insufficient distinction between the effects of chronic schizophrenia and the effects of institutionalisation to which such patients are vulnerable. In reply, it may be stated that since the traditional methods of treatment have failed to show full recovery, hence the patient has become chronic. And when chronic, it is a usual procedure that they are put into institutions. Be it, whatever it may, everyone would agree that management of such patients is a great problem because of their non-responsiveness to the environmental stimuli. Behaviour therapists, aim to help such patients in developing the habit of responding to the environment, as far as practicable, at least for such actions as, self-help behaviour.

Again, some criticis are of the opinion that the amount of improvement obtained by behaviour therapeutic methods is limited. So long chronic institutionalised schizophrenics are considered 'hopeless', whatever limited improvement obtained by these methods should be encouraged, especially when traditional methods of treatment have failed to show any further light to improve the conditions of such patients. Nevertheless, behaviour therapists have succeeded in demonstrating that even severely withdrawn patients can be helped to show at least moderate level of improvement.

Over and above, every therapeutic technique has some limitations, and behaviour therapy is no exception to that, though it has a good theoretical foundation and has achieved a reasonable degree of success (Ullmann and Krashner, 1969a,b; Liberman, 1972). However, limitations become more apparent because of inappropriate use of a given technique. One should not be dogmatic either to criticize or to accept a given technique. Clinician should be free to accept a given technique with all its merits and limitations, but should be careful in its application. Only on suitable patients a given technique should be applied of course by a trained professional clinician be it behaviour therapy or any other form of traditional psychotherapy. It is wrong to assume that any patient would show improvement with any form of treatment. In selecting a specific therapeutic technique, the less dogmatic the therapist is, the better is the expected outcome. In case a given patient appears unsuitable for behaviour therapy, the patient should be referred to receive other forms of treatment and viceversa. In this context Hall and Baker (1973) reported that unsuitable choice of patients, staff, and techniques can 'Wreck and Discredit' a complete therapeutic programme. Likewise, over-rigidity in applying behaviour therapeutic techniques may lead to a failure. Therefore, it should be undertaken only by those who have a proper understanding of the theory and practice.

Prior to employing behavioural intervention programme one has to formulate the goals of such intervention in a systematic manner. Of course, modification may be necessary depending upon the severity of the patient and need of the patient to be treated. For example, to begin with a schizophrenic patient having acute symptoms the first goal is to reduce hallucinations, delusions, loose associations and some such others disturbed behaviour. The second goal may be developing social skills and interpersonal skills including problem solving and assertive training. Further steps may involve family training, vocational training, rehabilitation programme etc. For an extensive discussion and review of pertinent articles on several behavioural techniques employed in the treatment of schizophrenia, the interested readers are referred to Curran, Monti and Corrivean (1982), Slazinger (1981), Hagen (1975). A good number of techniques have been employed with a view to reduce the behaviour problems exhibited by persons with schizophrenia. Some of these are time-out from positive reinforcement (Wolf, Risley and Mees, 1964; Cayner and Kiland, 1974), contingent electric shock (Corte, Wolf and Locke,1971; Tate and Baroff, 1966), contingent restraint (Azrin, Besalel and Wisotzek, 1982), and overcorrection (Johnson, Baumeister, Penald, and Inwald, 1982; Matson and Stephens, 1977). Token economy programme has been applied successfully to alter psychotic symptoms in in-patient set-up, particularly for the chronic schizophrenic patients.

Clinicians getting renewed interest in family therapy because of the role of expressive emotion in causing hostility, confusion (Hooley, 1985) and finally leading to relapse (Zubin and Spring, 1977; Anderson, 1983; Goldstein, 1984; Vaughan *et al.,* 1984). Discharged patients sent to live with their relatives (Brown, Bone, Alinson, and Wing, 1966) as well as with those relatives who exhibit expressed emotion had shown a relatively higher rate of relapse than those who lived on their own (Brown *et al.,* 1966) or lived with relatives with low expressed emotion (Vaughan and Leff, 1976). Family therapy helps the patient in reducing stress, in getting boost-up regarding family support as well as in reorienting the family people regarding maintenance of a suitable environment required for the patient (Wong, Massed, Mosk and Liberman, 1986). Hogarty, Anderson, and others (1986) in a controlled study of family therapy, social skills training, and maintenance chemotherapy in the aftercare (2 years study) treatment of schizophrenic patients found that the group on medication alone had the highest relapse rate, while the group that received the combination of family treatment, social skills and medication had shown the lowest relapse rate; only family treatment and medication group, and the social skills training and medication group came in between. In family therapy success has been claimed with family of schizophrenic child. Psychoeducation to reduce 'expressed emotion' brought down the probability of relapse and re-hospitalisation (Leff, Kuipers, Berkowitz, *et al.,* 1992). Likewise, family psychoeducation programme integrated with pharmacotherapy offer a delay in relapse (Rangaswami, 2000) and bring improved social functioning (Goldstein and Miklowitz, 1995). A number of other studies have been reported (*e.g.,* Goldstein, 1984) but most of these show lack of proper controls. Hogarty *et al.'s* (1986) study however, demonstrate the importance of a multimodal therapeutic approach for the schizophrenic patients.

Several methods of psychosocial rehabilitation have been applied successfully to the treatment of schizophrenia, a detailed discussion of which has been made earlier in this chapter. At present, in India too, there is a significant shift in the application of treatment modalities, from the intraindividual to the interindividual sphere of life. Generally, there is a movement towards approaches which are family based, team-oriented, and largely community based. This approach emphasizes independent living (Santos, 1996). However, biases and misconceptions still prevail with regard to psychosocial rehabilitation. Bachrach (1996) is of the opinion that such misconceptions and biases lead to the polarisation of psychosocial services, in the form of 'either/or' approach of treatment. She has defined psychosocial rehabilitation as 'a therapeutic approach that encourages a mentally ill person to develop his or her fullest capacities through learning and environmental supports' (p.293, Bachrach, 1996). Bachrach identified 9 common concepts (described earlier in this chapter) of rehabilitation approach. To remove misconceptions public awareness/education is necessary in the sense that mentally ill persons also have strength which they can utilise, with proper guidance, for independent living. In this context, Bachrach (1996) advocated that "mentally ill individuals be viewed as persons who have strengths in addition to their illnesses and who necessarily respond to their illnesses in distinctive personal ways" (p.31, Bachrach, 1996). Psychosocial rehabilitation model conceptualises (Cameron *et al.,* 1998) the following factors for the treatment of persons with schizophrenia: the integration of multiple services, the continuity of care, and need for long-term intervention. Also, long-term follow-up is necessary to stabilise treatment effects.

Failure of well-controlled studies to demonstrate the effectiveness of psychotherapy stems from an insufficient knowledge about the critical variables which one has to control in the psychotherapeutic process. Secondly, comprehensive treatment revaluation should include dependent variables from biological, social and psychological areas. Thirdly, treatment outcome should be evaluated by those who have no commitments (Weissman, 1984) to the treatments being compared. Fourthly, therapists must be free from biases toward other orientations. Fifthly, standardised techniques should be used by clinician therapists so that variations from one laboratory to other would be minimal. A common mode of research methodology should be framed to evaluate effects of different modes of treatment. Psychotherapy should be rendered by well-trained, well-motivated and experienced therapists.

For the greater benefit of the patients community, therapists require to be long sighted to find common bases of many apparently competing treatment modalities, and also must appreciate the need for improved collaboration in the treatment and management of patients with schizophrenia.

Need for an Integrated Approach

No science is without conflicts and controversies. Mental health, as a field of study, is no exception to it. However, debates promote the extension of knowledge. It is now strongly felt that despite the continuing debate over the usefulness of the concept of schizophrenia and doubts about its validity, psychologists need an adequate framework for psychological formulation of the phenomenon schizophrenia. It is understood that the unfolding of schizophrenia is not a homogeneous affair as early psychiatric doctrine suggests (Kraepelin, 1902). It requires a team work which can be accessible to trained professionals who have a wide range of background apart from psychology. This echoes strongly of the view made by Muijen, Marks, Connolly and others (1992) that the time has come for a convergence between the community care programme and the individual psychosocial interventions. The potential of such an integration is glimpsed in studies of long-term course of schizophrenic disorders within and between cultures.

Treatment of schizophrenia now includes a broad array of therapeutic modalities which are quite different from one another. Individual case study reports though suggest the viability of combining psychotherapy with pharmacotherapy (Beitman, 1991), till 1995, research reports to confirm this impression have not been conclusive (Hollon and Fawcett, 1995). This may be due to the fact that previously psychotherapy of schizophrenia was often practised in the absence of clear guidance (McGlashan, 1983) and even by some less experienced persons, which makes it difficult to measure its efficacy.

Combined treatment may be more effective when significant comorbidity is present in the patients (Rush and Kupfer, 1995). Needless to mention that, as per the report of the National Comorbidity Survey (Kessler, *et al.,* 1994) comorbidity in psychiatric population is now greater compared to earlier belief.

Fenton and Cole in 1995 and even earlier Goldstein (1991) and Marder, Johnson Cronk, Wirshing and Eckman (1991) observed that medication though remain the necessary cornerstone of treatment of schizophrenia, a variety of psychotherapeutic approaches, *viz.,* individual, group, family therapy, social-skills learning, do enhance the treatment outcome. These help the patient and the family members to deal with the initial crisis immediately, to identify the stressors, developing coping mechanisms, relapse prevention, and medication compliance. This might help in reducing dose of medication in the long-term (Cameron *et al.,* 1998).

Outcome studies are often concerned with measuring relapse or re-hospitalisation. In fact, professionals mostly overlook the time/period when treatment has given optimal outcome and when least. The latter, actually has given an idea as to how treatment may complement each other.

Outcome of therapy may be considered using a phase-specific model of illness (Fenton and Cole, 1995; Hogarty *et al.,* 1995). In the acute phase, crisis intervention (to reduce symptoms), family support and psychoeducation are the issues to be addressed. In the maintenance phase, issues like, medication compliance, personal well-being, relationships, social-skills, vocational placements, family burden, relapse prevention are to be addressed. For the chronic nature of the illness, since symptom recurrence is inevitable, focus of attention be on the functional status and quality of life (Cameron *et al.,* 1998) measures.

Evaluation is done mostly by a competitive rather than a collaborative approach; there is a tendency to generalise the outcome research findings, ignoring largely the fact that the illness is heterogeneous. Also, a tendency prevails to measure symptom reduction, relapse and re-hospitalisation, rather than the quality of life (Ostow, 1979; Hollon and Fawcett, 1995), this thus largely ignores the role of 'individualisation' of treatment (Cameron *et al.,* 1998) overtime. Given the multiple treatment needs of schizophrenia, it is advised to measure complementary treatment modalities; this will pave way to research in integrated treatment approach. Of course application of integrated approach requires an attitude of openness on the part of both the physician and other clinical professionals to come out from biases toward other orientations and to embark upon a cooperative venture. Thus, a broader therapeutic programme involving medico-psycho-social treatment strategies must be developed for the treatment of individuals with schizophrenia.

Psychotherapeutic Intervention : Indian Scenario

Psychotherapy to be relevant and meaningful needs to be embedded in the cultural traditions of the patients. Indian psyche has always been sensitive to issues like, 'Karma' (action), 'Dharma' (duty), 'Papa-Punya' (sin and noble deeds), 'Yoga' and 'Moksha' (liberation) and 'Purva-Janma' (re-birth). There is almost inseparable link between the religious and philosophical ideas and psychological thought in the East. Indian culture thus, is deeply rooted in religion and spirituality. Indian patients in general, accept such practices with genuine understanding or with a blind faith, either (Ramprasad, 2003; Rao, 1978a,b).

There has been an ingrained contradiction in Indian patients between the concepts of independence and dependence (Dhairyam, 1961) and in its application in real life. "The Indian culture and philosophy has been unique in its fostering of spiritual independence and growth in the people. This seems to be in direct contrast to their dependence on experts in the material, physical and emotional realm" (Dhairyam, 1961). Again, Indian adolescents and youths are in great contradictions and confusions today, because of Indian traditional values on the one hand, and modern, materialistic Westernised values on the other. Such value conflicts leads to symptoms manifestation. In formulating intervention programmes utmost importance be given to the selection of methods which could be suitable to mitigate such conflicts in the patients of our culture.

Discontentment has been raised by clinicians and academicians (Patel, 2000) on the application of Westernized explanatory concepts of psychotherapy to Indian context. The concern of the Third World countries, in this regard, was raised by Sinha and Holtsman (1984) long back and attempts have also been made for indigenisation of psychotherapy (*e.g.*, Neki, 1973, 1976). A comprehensive review on this is available (Rangaswami, 1996). Andrew, Dias-Saxena and Patel (2000) described the rationale, development and piloting of counselling intervention for general/common mental disorders seen in general health care units in India.

Intervention techniques so far applied in our population may broadly be categorized as analytically oriented psychotherapy (less frequently applied in recent years). Behaviour Therapy, Cognitive Behaviour Therapy including Biofeedback (BFB), Cognitive Therapies, Meditation and Yoga Therapies including Asanas, Guided Somatopsychic Relaxation including PMR, Supportive Psychotherapy (combined with medication), Pharmacotherapy, and Community Rehabilitation programmes. But the present write up is concerned only with those techniques which have been employed on schizophrenic patients in India. Government of India in its National Mental Health Programme (1982) urged the need for community participation in the development of mental health services in the community. Though some efforts have been given, in totality the outcome has not been very promising probably because of lack of infrastructural facilities including specialised manpower, particularly in rural parts of India.

Though there was no structured evidence for the role of cognitive behavioural interventions prior to 1970s for patients with psychosis, the current literature consistently shows that these strategies play important roles in amelioration of psychotic symptoms, such as, hallucinations. A progressive shift is noted in understanding psychopathology and interventions in schizophrenia from completely behavioural and cognitive and thereafter to cognitive-behavioural perspectives (Prasadrao, 2000). Further research is needed to identify such method of treatment which could be patient specific; there is need to assess the cost effectiveness of these interventions and also need to find out the critical components of the treatment (Mitra and Chattopadhyay, 2003). A critical review of the existing literature on the utilization of behavioural and cognitive behavioural strategies to deal with auditory hallucinations in schizophrenia has been given by Prasadrao (2000). Rangaswami (2000) has demonstrated the impact of psychosocial family intervention on first episode Schizophrenics to prevent progression of the illness and also its relapse (detailed earlier in this chapter). In the management of such patients, thus recently there is a shift in emphasis from the intraindividual to interindividual approach in Indian set-up.

Drug treatment is not without unwanted effects and critical controversy (Rickles, 1981). To overcome controversies regarding efficacy of any treatment what is required is to establish treatment outcome predictors (Mitra and Chattopadhyay, 2001, 2003; Mitra, Bandyopadhyay and Chattopadhyay, 2002) which can essentially contribute to identifying factors important for intervention. In a study on 28 OCD patients in India premorbid personality traits are found to be sound predictors for response to treatment with combined behaviour therapy procedures (Sahoo, Gills and Misra, 2002). Client characteristics, *viz.*, age, rigidity, depression and anxiety emerge as two functional units - primary cluster (anxiety, rigidity, and age) and secondary cluster (depressive trait, age and anxiety) for serving sound predictors of response to behaviour therapy in patients with OCD. Similarly, ego functions have been claimed to be reliable predictors for determining therapy outcome in psychotic patients (S. Basu, J. Basu and Bhattacharyya, 2002; J. Basu, S. Basu, and Bhattacharyya, 2004). Ego functions, stressful life events and severity of psychopathology in schizophrenia in Indian patients will be discussed later (Chapter XI).

Ghorpade and Kumar (1988) have given a detailed account of two types of Eastern psychotherapy, *viz.*, Abhidhamma, and Yoga. These authors have also focussed on the need for and role of cultural bound psychotherapy for emotionally disturbed patients in general. Since nothing in particular about applicability of such therapeutic techniques onto schizophrenic patients has been mentioned in the study, further detailing of those techniques appears beyond the scope of this write-up. Interested readers may be referred to Ghorpade and Kumar (1988).

9

CHAPTER

Vocational Training and Rehabilitation

Job-training program is the ultimate goal of most of such training and rehabilitation services. Such services are rendered for the development of, as far as practicable, an economically independent patient. Of course, as a prerequisite for such programme various independent living skills, namely, dressing up properly, maintaining personal hygiene etc. as well as general work habits of the patients are taken into account for their placement. After the patients have received training, initially placement is done on a part-time basis, and that too in a sheltered programme so that close supervision and guidance can be rendered to the patients until the patients deem suitable for permanent / long term assignments. As a part of rehabilitation programme group meetings are held on a regular basis. This is done to provide support, reinforcement and encouragement to the patients. Programmes are arranged in such a way that these do not hamper day treatment facilities (namely, individual / group treatment) in anyway (Liberman, Kuehnel, Phipps, and Cardin, 1984). So long the patient does not show competence he is not considered suitable for promotion to a higher level (Liberman *et al.,* 1984). In the purview of our national economy, the scenario regarding placement in occupation however, is quite different in India. This will be discussed later in this chapter.

A comparative rehabilitation programme for the chronically ill patients should follow certain stages sequentially (Mesibov, Schopler, and Sloan, 1983). The first of these stages may be called a prevocational stage which aims to motivate the patient to develop appropriate work attitudes and later work habits. The second stage involves limited exposure to a number of different work experiences. The next stage is to see how well the patient can adjust in work situation he is assigned to. Depending upon his progress of adjustment and efficiency in work, in the next stage attempts are made to expose the patients gradually to higher pressure of work. Subsequent stage involves assessment as to how far the patient is able to cope with the additional demands (Work-speed, Work-efficiency, and perseverance, etc.) he encounters in higher work assignments. Wages are made contingent upon his quality of job-training skills developed and quality of work completed within the scheduled time. Provided the patient has shown satisfactory performance, decisions are taken to place him in fulltime employment but with close supervision in a sheltered programme or in local business. The next is a transitional stage when the patient may be given employment within the community on a part-time basis. But at this stage too, the patient requires close supervision. The final stage is designated as a stage for continued supervision and follow-up services with a view to evaluate competency developed by the patient(s) in different areas. This is required as a prerequisite for placement of the patient at a higher level of job (Mesibov, Schopler, and Sloan, 1983) within the community.

Levy (1983) introduced a teacheradvocate model to meet the goals in vocational training programmes. The teacher, in this case, is a professionally trained individual who is assigned initial responsibilities to make the patient competent for adequate adjustment in job-sitaution and to encourage the patient to continue the same later on his own (patient's) initiative. Smith and Coleman (1986) reported that teacher-advocate model is effective to increase work productivity.

Of late, a behaviour-oriented day treatment programme (Kuehnel, DeRisi, Liberman, and Mosk, 1984) has been employed in vocational training programme in the West. This programme involves arrangement of educational workshops in an effort to help the patients to reintegrate themselves into the community. In addition to this, Kuehnel *et al.* (1984) had also implemented a credit incentive system which is similar to a token economy programme discussed earlier in this book (Chapter-VIII).

Clinicians would agree that schizophrenic patients are notoriously poor at complying with medication after their release from hospital (Ayd, 1975). Such non-compliance to prescribed drug is due to poor after care attendance, patient and family attitudes concerning the illness, forgetfulness and failure to understand the importance of drug compliance in preventing relapse (Falloon, 1984). Cognitive structuring and use of reinforcers could be used (Falloon, 1984) to increase drug compliance. Boczkowski, Ziechner, and Desanto (1985) compared behavioural psychoeducational and control interventions on medication compliance behaviour of chronically ill schizophrenic patients and found that the behaviourally trained patients were more compliant compared to the other groups. Outcome of this research was measured by pill counts, and self-report methods. Epstein and Gluss (1982) however, questioned the validity of such methods which are often used to assess drug compliance. Using behavioural contracting, other behavioural techniques, Keane, Foy, Nunn, and Rychtarik (1984) reported that alcoholic patients showed increased compliance to treatment and thereafter Keane *et al.* suggested that self-monitoring, and behavioural contracting may be helpful to increase drug compliance in schizophrenic patients.

Drug compliance among schizophrenic patients may improve through patient education. To include family members along with the patient in the educational programme appears worthwhile. Ideally, such educational programme should begin prior to the hospital discharge (Curran, Sutton, Faraone, and Guenette, 1985; Kessler and Waletzky, 1981). Of course it is often found difficult to convince patients and their family members regarding the importance of drug compliance (Shapiro, 1981).

Some of the researchers (*e.g.,* Kessler and Waletzky, 1981) are of the opinion that use of longer-action (3-4 weeks) injectable medication may help in increasing drug compliance in chronic patients. But several attempts, in the Western countries, to evaluate the efficacy of this approach revealed mixed results (Hogarty, Schooler, Ulrich, Mussare, Ferro and Herron, 1979; Kessler and Waletzky, 1981; Simpson and Lee, 1978). Hayness (1979) opined that an integrated approach, *i.e.,* behavioural therapy techniques along with adequate patient supervision including administration of drug, appears to be most effective for increasing drug compliance in chronic patients with schizophrenia. This however, requires a teamwork of professionals.

The aim of rehabilitation is not so much to reduce frustrations and provide satisfaction from social and occupational activities. It aims to make the patient feel that when eventually he leaves hospital he does not mean a loss of security and exposure to the struggle and competition of life. In general patients with minimal symptoms of affective disturbance respond best. In those patients having high degree of affective disturbances, the use of drugs is likely to improve their response to rehabilitation.

A number of other model programmes (*e.g.,* Liberman, Kuehnel, Phipps, and Cardin, 1984) have been instituted with a view to provide services, in a biopsychosocial orientation, to the chronically ill patients.

In sum: The above mentioned research reports provide information that there are two kinds of chronic schizophrenic patients who are likely to benefit from this type of training programme. The first variety consists of patients who have had an acute attack, have made a good improvement, subsequently have been discharged from hospital, and are under supervision. But follow-up shows that instead of continuing to improve they stagnate so much so that may even begin to deteriorate and become apathetic. Family's hopes about the patient is minimal. In such circumstances, it is advisable for the patient to attend the Day Hospital. If his condition demands so, he may be re-admitted so that he can be given a proper programme of activities.

The second variety of patients consists of those who have shown deterioration from neglect owing to previous lack of facilities. An environment which provides a regular routine lacking in variety, and which gives no responsibilities and no worthwhile occupation promotes deterioration. Add to this is the absence of any companionship other than that of other schizophrenics. Such an environment makes the patient more apathetic and withdrawn, so much so that the patient fails to look after himself. Such chronic patients in mental hospital show gross 'institutionalisation'.

Psychosocial Rehabilitation (PSR)

This is a recent concept which has replaced the term psychiatric rehabilitation, the latter refers predominantly to drug prescription and drug compliance, whereas the former refers to the affected person, his family and community as well.

PSR has been defined as 'a therapeutic approach that encourages a mentally ill person to develop his or her fullest capacities through learning and environmental supports' (p. 29,

Bachrach, 1996). There are 9 common concepts (Bachrach, 1996) of rehabilitation approach: a) individualised treatment, b) focus on the environment, c) focus on the patients strength, d) patient involvement, e) restoring hope, f) emphasis on vocational potential, g) comprehensive care, h) continiuity of care, and i) therapeutic alliance. Of these 9 concepts, the continuity of care, the integration of multiple services, and the need for long term intervention are required (Bachrach, 1996, 1998) in the treatment of schizophrenia. Needless to mention that therapeutic relationship is an integral part (Mosher and Burti, 1992) of the model.

Coming to its methods–several methods of PSR have been positively applied. Generally there is a movement towards approaches which are team oriented and community based. Such an approach emphasises the scope of independent living (Santos, 1996; Bachrach, 1996) for the patients.

In India, in this respect efforts have been made to study some priority areas like coping mechanisms of care givers and family burden of disease (Singh, 2002; Chadda, 2003). Another need of the community is to develop packages for the family and care givers attending to the needs of the persons suffering from mental illness including those suffering from dementia.

It is well known that schizophrenia have extraordinary difficulty in establishing and maintaining social relationships. Several studies have focussed on social factors and human interactional variables in exacerbation of or improvement in schizophrenic symptoms. Social under stimulation (Watts and Bennett, 1983), social-poverty of the hospital environment (Wing and Brown, 1961) were found to be associated with clinical poverty in patients. Likewise, expressed emotion of relatives of schizophrenic patients have shown a strong association between expressed emotion of relatives and relapse. Better outcome was seen in 1st admission patients who had contacts with relatives and friends directly through telephone or letters (Buck, 1984).

Attempts to introduce a psychosocial rehabilitation as an intervention strategy in the form of interpersonal interaction have been relatively few in Indian set-up. A study in 1988 (Shailajakumari and Sathyavathi) on Indian patients revealed that interpersonal requirements of schizophrenic patients reflect a high need for inclusion, control and affection. Since Indian family set-up and interaction pattern are different from that of the Western families, a therapeutic strategy involving social interaction be sought for to suit the specific needs of the patients of our culture. In a study on 132 Indian chronic schizophrenic (21-50 years) patients (66 males) with duration of illness between 1-15 years, and educational level averaged at primary school, a pre-post control group procedure was employed with one group of patients receiving the intervention of planned interpersonal interactions, and the matched control group not receiving any such intervention (Sovani and Thatte, 1994). The experimental and control groups of patients were long term in-patients in a residential mental health institution (Mean duration of hospitalisation 8 years). Activities the patients were made involved included introduction of group members, introduction to the concept of a group, rules regarding group activity and a discussion of group days, timings, attendance, etc. in the initial 2 sessions. From the 3rd session onwards the groups were made involved in telling stories, recitation of poems, discussion of current events like sports, election, etc. In addition, games like Forfeits, Antakshari were played. Similarly Quiz Programmes were arranged on simple information like months of the year, animals, birds, famous personalities, etc. Also, playing and listening to music, newspaper reading and discussion on major newspaper items, on hobbies and dreams about the feature were included in the activities. The last session focussed on a discussion of gains from the group and reactions of group members. Activities consisted of 35 minutes sessions twice a week over 5-6 weeks.

A significant change in the task performance of experimental group of patients was noted as a result of exposure to interpersonal interaction in small groups. Only in the area of attention a refractory deficit in chronic schizophrenia, but no change was seen in the areas of motor speed, verbal fluency. But less significant changes were seen in the areas of perceptual motor accuracy ($P < 0.002$) and affective reactivity ($P < 0.005$). Thus, benefits accrued from such intervention strategies appeared to have direct impact in terms of improvement in cognitive abilities (Sovani and Thatte, 1994), better social competence, as well as for better prognosis. Both in the areas of therapy and rehabilitation psychosocial intervention prove to be valuable method.

The rehabilitation unit of NIMHANS Bangalore has been expanding (Kalyansundaram and Verghese, 2000) and comprehensive rehabilitation services are being provided with through teamwork to be mentally ill patients and also to those who are mentally handicapped. Each team as a unit offers services like, occupational therapy, day care programme, vocational rehabilitation, family education services, etc., to the patients and their family members. Thus family could be a unique system of treatment.

The simplicity, easy accessibility and cost-effectiveness make this method more viable, particularly in a country like India, for alleviation of behavioural deficits in schizophrenia.

In sum : This approach believes that patients have strength in spite of their illness and they should be provided with adequate facilities to respond in a desired direction in their social adjustment in distinctive personal ways. It highlights the common base of many apparently distinct treatment modalities, and the need for a collaboration for the greater benefit of the patient.

Comments

Rehabilitation activities in developing countries, particularly in India, very rarely view their modus operandi systematically. This is because (i) for the purpose of rehabilitation mostly in the hospital set up/NGOs, arrangement is made to keep the patient engaged in some sort of occupation training, namely, Weaving, Knitting, etc. Perhaps this effort could best be described as occupational therapy, rather than rehabilitation in strict sense of the term (granting that job-placement is a part of rehabilitation). The aim of rehabilitation is not only to reduce frustration providing occupational activities; it also aims to make the patient feel that eventually when he leaves the hospital, he would be in a position to interact well with others utilising social/emotional cues with confidence and security; (ii) In India, even today, opportunities for job-placement for such patients is very very meagre. So, after receiving training in some occupation, when the patient returns to family, he becomes totally unemployed, which induces further frustration in him. Had the patient been trained to gain psychological strength through family interaction during the course of rehabilitation, he perhaps could tolerate better his pain of remaining unemployed; (iii) There are very few systematic attempts to assess the outcome of the rehabilitation training the patients are provided with; (iv) Such assessment also requires systematic follow-up programme. Follow-up programmes should include training and research both concerning mental health problems in general.

Such being the present scenario of rehabilitation in India, some of the professionals have expressed their great concern and sorrow stating that, in this sense, psychiatric rehabilitation has been an end in itself here, rather than being a means to the end (Ranganathan, Channabasavanna, Murali, Bharathi, and Padankatti, 1996). Of late, however, attempts have been made to change the scenario. Comprehensive rehabilitation services through teamwork the patients are being provided with to cope with difficulties as far as practicable.

10

CHAPTER

Course and Prognosis

The onset of gross schizophrenic disorganisation though often occurs suddenly, careful examination of the patient's developmental history does show that there have been many indications of personality disturbances in earlier years. As early as 1958, in this context O'Neal and Robins, based on a follow-up study reported that children who became schizophrenic later in life had history of having suffered from infectious diseases during the first two years of life. Also, hearing problems, difficulties in locomotion etc. are more frequently reported in such children than those of the normal children. The boys were often reported to have a feminine appearance. The presence of antisocial behaviour antedated the schizophrenic reactions to half of O'Neal and Robins' subjects who were later so diagnosed. Also, they were found to be physically aggressive, incorrigible, and pathological lyers. They had more phobias, feelings of depression, and paranoid trends when compared to normal children. However, these findings, they reported based on children seen in one particular clinic only and therefore, require replications prior to its generalisation.

Formerly the incurable nature and progressive course of schizophrenia were implied in the definition of the disease as such. A favourable outcome was rather considered presumptive evidence of an error in diagnosis. Of course, in recent years too, there has been an increasing recognition that the episodic nature of a psychosis and the occurrence of symptomfree termination may not necessarily exclude its schizophrenic nature. But at the same time some authors (*e.g.*, Kolb, 1973) are of the opinion that even though schizophrenia be regarded as a special type of illness, a permanent disorganisation of personality does not necessarily follow. Therefore, the course of the illness schizophrenia has to be discussed taking in view the different characteristics of it and in doing so, at this juncture, it seems necessary to define some of the terms like, 'phase', 'shift', 'exacerbation', 'process', and 'reactive' (Hamilton, 1976), which are frequently used by researchers. A 'phase' of an illness is followed by a complete return to the premorbid state (Hamilton, 1976), while in a 'shift' there is a partial recovery. Also in the latter there is an acute episode and occurrence of new symptoms. An 'exacerbation' is characterised by a sudden worsening of a clinical state without the appearance of any new symptoms. The words 'process' and 'reactive' have already been discused in detail earlier (Chapter II) in this book and need not be repeated here.

Arnold (1955) based on follow-up studies on 500 schizophrenics over a period of 3-30 years reported phasic course of illness with complete cure in 1.6%, and shifting course in 9.6% of the cases. He also noted a phasic course passing over into a shifting course in 4.0% and phasic course passing over into a process with exacerbations in 3.4% of the cases.

Morrison, Winokur, Crowe, and Claney (1973) followed up 200 schizophrenic patients for 10 years and found that 20% had never been discharged from hospital. Only 8% ever recovered. Most of the recoveries occurred within first two to three years following discharge from hospital and a few after 5 years. Based on 5-year follow-up programme Wing (1966) reported that among first admission, 50% showed satisfactory recovery so much so that they required little attention from rehabilitation or aftercare during these years. One quarter of the patients were found to be still severely ill at the end of the 5 years, and the rest were reported to be handicapped by less severe symptoms.

Kennedy (1963), Mandelbrote and Folkard (1963), Ruesch, Brodsky, and Fischer (1963) reported that chemotherapy enables almost half of first admissions to be discharged within four months, and two-thirds to be discharged within six months, and a large percentage to be discharged within one year. However, discharge is not considered synonymous of cure but rather with control. A patient is released only when his symptoms are sufficiently under control so much so that he can be returned to other forms of treatment, such as out-patient treatment. In a 3-year follow-up study Clark and Mallen (1963) reported that only 11% of the schizophrenics remained symptomfree over this period of time. On the other hand, 72% showed sufficient return or exacerbation of their symptoms as to require re-hospitalisation. From the above, it is evident that the picture concerning the course and progress of this illness is still grim, and more recently attention is being devoted to determine the factors those may be associated with a more favourable prognosis. These factors have been depicted well by Suinn (1975) and Hamilton (1976) long before. Hamilton (1976) proposed that while considering prognosis, three aspects of the illness are to be assessed. These are chances of recovery from the present attack, possibility of recurrence, and probability of deterioration.

Recently in our own laboratory (Mitra and Chattopadhyay, 2001, 2003; Basu, Basu, and Bhattacharyya, 2004) as well as in the laboratory of other Indian researchers (*e.g.*, Sahoo, Gills, and Misra, 2002) some such factors (see Chapter XI) have been determined. Some of these important factors will now be mentioned briefly.

Indices from the Developmental History of the Patient

As already mentioned above, some authors are of the opinion that prior to the onset of acute schizophrenia, some minor abnormalities are generally found to be present in such patients which are usually evident through a careful history taking. To quote Bleuler, "However, whenever we have a thorough case history, it is the exception if we are not able to detect the previous earlier signs of disease whether it be nervous symptoms, character changes or even direct overt schizophrenic manifestations". For example, depression or neurosis may occur prior to the onset of classical schizophrenic illness. Such illnesses, do not last long and are usually followed by apparently complete recovery, though sometimes later a typical schizophrenic may occur. At this juncture, the original illness is often regarded as a manifestation of schizophrenia, but there is, in fact, no way of proving this. In some cases, the onset of the illness is at a definite point of time, but some prodormal symptoms, like depression, anxiety, suspiciousness, lack of concentration, mild hypochondriasis, and restlessness are usually found to be present for days, weeks or months together prior to the appearance of unequivocal schizophrenic symptoms. In some cases, the exact point of onset is uncertain, as because the illness progresses slowly and insidiously. However, caution should be exercised so that one does not equate any and every psychological difficulty noted in a given individual prior to the apparent onset of the schizophrenic illness with that of schizophrenia. As for example, problems of adjustment noted in adolescents. No doubt, adolescence crises become the starting point of future manifestation of schizophrenia in some individuals, but adolescent crises and difficulties are much commoner than schizophrenia in general population, and therefore, it does not seem reasonable to (Hamilton, 1976) attribute all the psychological and behavioural difficulties noted in adolescents as manifestations of pre-schizophrenic illness.

Even today, in a given individual, the effects upon the personality and future adjustment noted in the appearance of a schizophrenic reaction remain equivocal. In some individuals a permanent disorgnisation of personality invariably follows whereas in others, acute and clearly psychogenic schizophrenia may at times disappear (Kolb, 1973) without leaving any injury to the personality. Such a variation in its effects may be attributed to the nature and degree of the illness on the one hand, and on early detection and systematic therapeutic intervention including follow-up, on the other. Thus, *e.g.,* in infants the expectation of social adaptation is minimal if mutism continues until the age of five or so (Kolb, 1973). In some individual the course is intermittent, whereas in some others, the course is continuously progressive.

Age of Onset and Sex

Severe defects are much commoner in the adolescents and young adults than in the middle-aged. Recovery is much less common when the illness begins in adolescence and in early adult life (Suinn, 1975). This is because severe deterioration of personality is likely at the age of onset than the onset of illness around 40 years or more (Hamilton, 1976). Earlier and gradual mode of onset have been associated with poor outcome in Indian research reports as well (*e.g.,* Rangaswami, 2000). Kolb (1973), on the contrary, opined that age of onset is not of prognostic significance except that late age offers a less favourable prognosis. Likewise, sex has no prognostic significance (Kolb, 1973). In a study on Indian adolescents the gender discrimination indicated rates of 18.8% in boys and 22.8% in girls (Bhola and Kapur, 2000). This study, however, was on emotional disturbances in general, and not particularly on schizophrenia. However, the need to study adolescents separately and to understand their unique problems in relation to Indian set up has been emphasised repeatedly by Indian researchers (Prabhu, 1987; Sethi, 1982; Kapur, 1992; Sitholey and Chakraborty, 1992).

Nature of Onset

An acute onset favours a good outcome. The presence of clear-cut precipitating factors is indicative of recovery (Hamilton, 1976). Marked depressive features and the preservation of adequate affective expression indicate a good prognosis. Flattening of affect and incongruity are poor prognostic signs (Hamilton, 1976; Rangaswami, 2000). Patients with a first episode and shorter duration of illness having auditory hallucinations, early wakening, morning depression and guilt are less likely to relapse within one year after hospital discharge (Leff and Wing, 1971).

Holmboe and Astrup (1957) investigated the relationship between different clinical features and prognosis in a series of 255 schizophrenic patients. Likewise, Arnold (1955) correlated clinical features of acute schizophrenia and prognosis. In a later study Vaillant (1966) extracted six factors as favourable indices of prognosis which have been supported by other researchers as well (Rangaswami, 2000). These factors are – an acute onset, presence of a clear precipitating event, presence of confusion, or deterioration, presence of depression, family history of psychotic depression, and a good premorbid adjustment. However, a more comprehensive review of earlier studies has been made by Huston and Pepernick (1958) (for detailed the reader is referred to Suinn, 1975; Hamilton, 1976).

Precipitating Factors

Psychological (*e.g.*, conflicts, mental strain) and physical (*e.g.*, bodily illness) factors have been associated with better outcome (Mayer-Gross *et al.*, 1974).

Types

Acute catatonic illnesses with stormy onset and excitement though have a good prognosis for the attack, there is a high probability of recurrence. Certain catatonic clinical features, *viz.*, stereotypes, negativism, and parakinesis suggest an unfavourable course of the illness. In the simple type with its treacherous and injurious effects on personality, developing in the absence of unusual environmental stress poor prognosis is indicated. Hebephrenic clinical pictures suggest a poor outlook. The course of this type of illness tends to be one of severe regression (Suinn, 1975), although occasionally remissions occur before the final disorganisation of personality. Process schizophrenics show relatively poorer prognostic risks (Stephens and Astrup, 1965) than reactive patients. The outcome of acute paranoid schizophrenia is not as good as acute-catatonic illness, but is relatively better than hebephrenia. Sometimes the question is asked as to whether the paranoid type of schizophrenia ever recovers. In replying this question one has to take into account the definition of the term, an issue which has already been detailed earlier in this book. No doubt, remissions occur in paranoid schizophrenia, but these may be looked upon as social recoveries

(Kolb, 1973); rarely they are to be judged as psychological recoveries, even though during the interval the patient's adjustment is well socialised and no distortions of reality in response to subjective needs is apparent. In general, however, intolerant and bitter attitudes (Kolb, 1973) are indicative of a presence of a malignant process. Regarding pseudoneurotic form, Cattell (cited by Kolb, 1973), based on a follow-up study, reported that 60% of his patients never required hospital treatment. The remaining 40% required hospitalisation periodically. Only one in five developed overt psychotic symptoms and one half of them remitted. Only 10% thus evolved the classical forms of schizophrenia. Cattell followed up these patients for a period of 5-20 years.

Duration of Illness

Long term follow up studies show a wide variability in outcome. In some patients first episode is reported to be followed by a permanent recovery, while in others signs of long-term decline are reported (Crow, MacMillan, Johnson *et al.,* 1986). Duration of illness prior to treatment is also an important predictor of outcome. The number of psychiatric episodes and longer the duration the patients experiences (Rangaswami, 2000), the poorer the outcome. However, psychological variables are good predictors of such heterogeneous outcome.

Physique

Usually a pyknic body build is said to favour recovery whereas the dysplastic physique indicates poor prognosis (Hamilton, 1976). But in a series of 255 acute schizophrenic Holmboe and Astrup (1957) noted schizophrenic defects in 53% of pyknics and in 36% of leptosomes. However, the defects in the latter was much more severe than that in the former.

Intelligence

An I.Q. below the average is usually taken as a poor prognostic index (Suinn, 1975; Hamilton, 1976). Kolb (1973) on the contrary, reported that prognosis is not influenced by the intelligence or previous education of the patient.

Personality

A well-integrated pre-morbid personality is usually associated with recovery or minimal defect, whereas a pre-morbid schizoid personality is considered of a poor prognostic sign (Hamilton, 1976), and this is more so if the psychosis represents an insidious development. The presence of cyclothymic factors in the personality background renders a favourable prognosis. The existence of anxiety and also of an easily ascertained emotional problem makes the prognosis more favourable. If the pre-morbid personality was not strong enough to withstand everyday life routine difficulties, the prognosis is not good (Suinn, 1975). Poor ego functions (Basu, Basu and Bhattacharyya, 2002, 2004), poor pre-morbid adjustment have been associated with poor outcome in Indian research reports as well (*e.g.,* Rangaswami, 2002; Mitra and Chattopadhyay, 2002, 2003; Mitra *et al.,* 2003) (for background information see Chapter V).

Family History

The remitting schizophrenics have been reported to have a greater frequency of relatives with affective disorder than the non-remitting cases (Vaillant, 1966). The latter had a greater incidence of schizophrenia among their relatives than the former. Some other researchers in the West (*e.g.*, Hamilton, 1976) have failed to confirm that family history has a bearing on prognosis. However, for background information on the impact of family history see chapter on etiology.

Community Attitude

Attitude of the parents and sibling, and of the friends and neighbour are crucial in the patient's final adjustment. Thus social recovery is often more dependent on the environment (Hamilton, 1976), than on the clinical features of the patient. Brown, Birley and Wing (1972) in this context reported that great emotional involvement of the members of the family coupled with expressed hostility is strongly associated with symptom relapse. These authors also opined that decline in occupational level, low unskilled work, failure to achieve satisfactory sexual adjustment are indications of poor prognosis.

The patients and their relatives should be persuaded that a job considerably below the pre-morbid level (Hamilton, 1976; Rangaswami, 2000) should be tried after discharge. Lack of employment leads to exacerbation of the symptoms. In Indian culture it is difficult to make sure that each patient after hospital discharge is provided with job opportunities suitable to him, where millions of normals are jobless. However, the parents should be advised to make the patient engaged in some family works in a daily routine basis. He also should be encouraged to get involved in social interaction through games and/or music, etc., if at all he has got no formal occupation. Sometimes, it is noted in our culture that highly emotional relatives having too close contact with patient refrain him from being engaged in routine life activities. This should not be encouraged. Brown *et al.* (1972) in this context suggested that this could be mitigated by ensuring that the patient is not in too close contact with the highly emotional relatives. However, in Indian culture such a separation is likely to cause additional tension in the patient and also may create emotional problem in the parents. Therefore, considering Indian family set-up the parents should be advised to assign the patient a schedule of work in his everyday life programme, if at all he can not be provided with a job outside the family. Parents should be advised to keep an eye onto their patient's regularity in following the schedule he is assigned to, as well as initiative taken by the patient, and motivation and level of perfection he shows gradually overtime. Parents should be in touch with the clinician regarding procedures to be employed in framing and re-framing of the schedule assigned to the patient, when necessary.

Cultural Factors

Overwhelming research evidences suggest that the outcome for people with schizophrenia in Western industrialised countries is markedly inferior to those in the Third World (Lin and Kleinman, 1988). In their study on African an Indian schizophrenic patient living in

Mauritius, Murphy and Rahman (1971) reported that after 12 years follow-up involving 98% of their original sample, 64% reported no further episodes contrasting with 49% in a comparable British Sample followed by after 5 years (Brown, Bone and others, 1966). Such apparent resistance to relapse has been documented in less industrialised countries by Verghese, John and others (1989) in India and Waxler (1979), and Mendis (1986) in Sri Lanka. Leff, Wig, Ghosh, and others (1987) compared first-episode samples in London and Chandigarh (a predominantly Urban area of North India) and found a 9-month relapse rate of between 14% and 18% in Chandigarh compared with 29% in London. This difference, however, did not rest on the use of maintenance neuroleptic drugs (Leff, Wig, Bedi and others, 1990). For further detail the reader is referred to the reports of WHO (1979). Sartorius, Jablensky, Korten *et al.* (1986) in a follow-up (over 2 years) study on a cross-sectional samples over eight countries found that a greater proportion of patients in Agra (India), Cali (Columbia), and Ibadan (Nigeria) had more favourable and less disabling outcomes than the patients in Aarhus (Denmark), London, Prague, and Washington. A further epidemiological study (Sartotius *et al.,* 1986) covering ten countries of first episode patients showed a uniform annual incidence rate (1 per 10,000) but variable 2-year outcome between countries, which once again favoured less industrialised nations. In industrialised countries 40% patients showed a "severe" pattern (more than one episode and incomplete remission) compared with 24% in developing ones. Several hypotheses may be formulated to account for this finding. Firstly, the opportunity to engage in socially valued and varied productive roles may be enhanced in non-industrialised societies where there is opportunity to a more flexible use of labour (WHO, 1979). Interestingly, the pattern of recovery in Moscow paralled that of less industrialised countries in 1983 (Warner, 1983) which perhaps is a reflection on the emphasis on full employment and vocational rehabilitation in the USSR at that time.

However, if full employment is an important factor for showing apparent resistance to relapse, then findings in Indian set-up are likely to be in a different direction than those reported above. This is because at present, the rate of unemployment is quite high in India compared to 1979-1989 when Verghese and others reported their findings. In spite of that the incidence of mental illness in India is relatively less compared to that of the Western Industrialised countries. This leads us to formulate another hypothesis *i.e.,* the role of extended family structure (EFS), which is more common in the Third World. EFS may help to diffuse burden and increase tolerance (Waxler, 1979). A better outcome for patients in EFS compared to Nuclear Family Structure (NFS) was documented by El-Islam (1979) in Qatar on the Persian Gulf. A study of expressed emotion (EE) among the EFS in Chandigarh (Leff, Wig, Bedi, Ghosh and others, 1987, 1990) found a much lower prevalence of high EE (23%) compared to London (47%) which was associated with a short-term rate of relapse. Similarly a lower prevalence of high EE in the EFS of Mexican-American families was reported (Karno, Jenkins, and others, 1987) compared to British and American samples.

Some of the major Indian epidemiological studies done in different parts of India, *viz.*, Uttar Pradesh, Bihar, West Bengal, Gujarat, Tamil Nadu and Pondicherry, and Delhi reveal that the prevalence of schizophrenia is 2.5/1000 and perhaps, it is the only disorder whose prevalence is consistent over time (Ganguly, 2000). Fairly large rural-urban (100/69) differences appeared to exist for schizophrenia. The present scenario of the prevalence and rural-urban ratio may be different, as because, the urban patients mostly consult physician privately, whereas the major percentage of the patients reporting to the out-patient departments of the mental/general hospitals come from the rural areas. Nevertheless, rural-urban difference is a vexed issue, often showing the contradictory results. The rural-urban dichotomy is mostly done on the basis of geographical location at the time of investigation, and with no other criteria for analysing such background. Such a dichotomy remains further unclear if one looks into the considerable movement of population between villages, townships, and cities. May be that urban people cope with stress by attending many recreational activities, and keeping links with village life through regular visits; on the contrary urban people, now-a-days, (particularly urban mansion life) create a 'mini-community (Ganguly, 2000) of their own, as a result of which they don't have any scope for free expression of their stress. The rural people, on the other hand, are more expressive in their community. Also, the Indian tradition of joint family system, though weaning, still prevails in the rural set-up comparatively more, than the urban set-up. As a result, urban children/adolescents live a very capsuled life which causes greater inhibition, suppressed aggression in them, which in turn, gives a feeling of social isolation in them.

Determinants of Outcome Study (Sartotius *et al.*, 1986; Leff *et al.*, 1987) identified social isolation and social support as one of the few strong predictors of outcome. In several of the industrialised societies, many more patients live alone. Thus weak or absent social supports may contribute to poor outcome. In less industrialised countries, on the other hand greater social support and increased opportunity to engage in valid and varied social roles may contribute to a superiority in social functioning. Social functioning has been identifried as a significant variable within cultures (Hogarty, Scholler, Ulrich, and Mussare, 1979). It is unlikely that such cross-cultural differences in outcome are the results of a single factors, *i.e.*, family structure. Such differences in the reported findings of outcome studies represent a more complex clustering of culturally related variables such as, attitudes to mental illness, opportunities for social integration an re-integration, motivation, opportunity, and continuity of stable care and so forth.

McJlashen (1988) in this context opined that "The North America Long-term Follow-up Studies suggest that schizophrenia may be quite malleable to prolonged environmental/psychosocial perturbations. These have negative potential if applied too intensively or ambitiously, but positive potential if applied steadily in a supportive rehabilitative more in a context of stable and supportive community care" (p.538). Cross-cultural comparisons of studies also point to a similar conclusion.

Occasionally one may come across a schizophrenic episode of a mild, transitory nature with no subsequent history of recurrence. In such cases one may have to consider whether favourable outcome be characterised as "social recovery" rather than "cure" (Kolb, 1973) or full recovery. It means, the patient may be able to return to his previous social environment, to his previous occupation, or its equivalent, but with some minor symptoms and signs (*e.g.,* shallowness of affect and shyness (remaining in him as residue of the illness he suffered from). In such cases the attitude of employers, supervisors, and fellow-workers are likely to affect the employment environment of the patient. Sometimes it may happen, especially in urban industrial areas, that the odd behaviour of the chronic schizophrenic is not tolerated. Mass education programme in this framework is required for the benefit of the patients. Finally, the responsibilities taken by the physician/clinical psychologist/therapist concerns is of utmost importance here. The therapist should render individual care and treatment. To quote Bleuler (1950) "Although a certain number of patients become deteriorated with every treatment, and others improve even in apparently severe cases, the treatment will decide in more than one-third of schizophrenic cases whether they can become social man again or not". The more individualised and personalised the care and treatment, the greater the rate of recovery be expected. The importance of socially validating outcome though has been recently recognised (Woods, 1984), it might lack construct validity.

Treatment Strategies

Prognostic statements can never be completely meaningful unless one takes into account the nature of therapy the patient has received. Treatment strategies which are concerned with the control of factors such as drug non-compliance, the dose of neuroleptic drugs, level of stimulation in therapeutic as well as in home environments, extra pyramidal side effects, attention and arousal deficits and the stress of everyday life can reduce the rate of relapse hopefully in most of such patients. Hogarty *et al.* (1986, 1991) reported that the relapse rate of 65% to 70% can be reduced to 40% with the use of antipsychotic medication, and this rate can further be reduced to even less than 20% with the addition of psychosocial intervention strategies. Similar rate of prognosis and relapse prevention rate in chronic Indian schizophrenic patients was evident (Rangaswami, 2002) by applying a meta-system (both medical and psychosocial) intervention approach.

Treatment cost analyses have been conducted in various areas (for a review and discussion see Yates, 1985), but in applied behavioural research it is a relatively new approach. Such analyses are essential when third-party funders or private / Government agencies are interested in a programme's monetary products. A clear picture about the role and involvement of third-party funders or private / Govt. agencies in India has been provided by Kalyansundaram and Verghese (2000) and Ranganathan, Channabasavanna, Murli *et al.* (1996) (see Chapter XI).

In sum : Acute onset, a well integrated personality (with above average intelligence) presence of precipitants, occurrence of benign psychosis in the family, catatonic and affective type are considered signs of good prognosis.

Insidious onset, early age onset, marked schizoid pre-morbid personality (limited intellectual activities), emotional instability, and presence of deteriorated schizophrenic patients in the family etc. are the predictors of poor prognosis.

Clinical relevance of a treatment outcome must focus on assessing the desirable clinical changes produced by certain mode of treatment. Such relevance of change has to be judged in context to the community in which the patient lives. Various measures, with a biopsychosocial orientation are to be employed to obtain cross validity of treatment outcome, rather than to rely on any one measure only.

Within the constraints of the illness, to provide opportunity to engage individuals in varied social roles and stable social interaction, with a view to maximising independence and purposive behaviour as well as to widening the burden of care beyond close family members to the wider but stable and familiar community, what would be required is to constitute a model package programme for the care of the patients with schizophrenia.

11

CHAPTER

Research in Schizophrenia in India: Shifts in Trends Over a Decade

There has been a significant shift in research interest toward cross-cultural, sub-cultural, psychophysiological, and neuropsychological comparisons; also a shift from intraindividual to interindividual approach (Sovani and Thatte, 1994) in the management and recovery of schizophrenia is noted in recent research.

Emphasis on standardised approaches to diagnosis and assessment, embodied in the DSM and ICD Nosology, has stressed features that are culturally invariant (American Psychiatric Association, 1994). Although features like neurocognitive deficits, and brain abnormalities appear culturally invariant, many features, such as cultural differences in presentation, severity, course, and medication effects, and the effects of family interaction patterns do show substantial variance with culture. These have been detailed in the previous chapters (IV & V) of this book. The present chapter is an update and interim summary on the recent shifts in trends in research in India on schizophrenia.

Psychophysiological Variables

Psychophysiological research has been relatively less in number during the period covered in this write-up compared to the previous decades. Of the various indices employed in such research, namely, heart rate, blood pressure, EEG evoked potentials, etc.,. GSR has been employed extensively by the researchers in assessing stress related problems (Chattopadhyay *et al.,* 1980, 1982a,b,c; Mukhopadhyay *et al.,* 1994). Sophisticated laboratory facilities are essential in this type of research, which of course is costly. Also, methodology employed in different laboratories requires standardisation so that discrepancies in the results be avoided. Interestingly the concept of LIV ('Law of Initial Values'), a crucial and significant basic concept of psychophysiological research is found to require revision by both the Indian (Mukhopadhyay and Chattopadhyay, 1995) and Western researchers (Bernstein, 1973). Indepth research is necessary on this issue in Indian set-up.

Ego Functions and Stressful Life Events

Ego functions and stressful life events of schizophrenia have been associated with severity of psychopathologies (Basu, 1993; Basu and Basu, 1996; Basu and Banerjee, 1998; Basu, Bhattacharyya and Basu, 2000; Basu, Basu and Bhattacharyya, 1999a,b; 2002; 2004). In contrast to Bellack's original work these authors have found a non-linear trend, *i.e.* dysfunction of ego in different clusters. For example, reality testing and judgement factors of ego functions constitute a cluster for psychotic patients, whereas drive control, defensive functioning, stimulus barrier, thought process and autonomous functioning formed a cluster for patients with GAD. Patients with paranoid schizophrenia and normals of our culture did not show any difference in adaptive regression function of the ego (Basu and Basu, 1996), which requires clarification. Again, object relation of the ego function, unlike those of the West, does not give any clear picture in context to patients of our culture; these findings emphasize the need for cross-cultural investigations.

In a latter study (2004) these authors reported that object relation has a special position in the process of paranoid schizophrenia. This (object relation) was the only ego function, of all the 12 ego functions these authors tested using adapted version of Bellack's (1989) Ego Function Assessment – M-Scale, which appeared to have a significant contribution to all the three indices of psychopathology, *viz.*, psychoticism, anxiety, and depression, these authors employed onto their patients. Disturbed object relations in the psychotics has been explained in terms of split or fusion of self-object representation (Kernberg, 1967). The present results thus have a significant therapeutic implication. These authors investigated 30 women and 30 men (mean age 30.13 years) who attended a clinic of Kolkata, India. Since the patients investigated formed a very small section (selected patients were all Bengali only) of the whole Indian population, this points out the need for further research to see the nature of ego functions in such patients of different sub-culture and culture.

Emotions Processing and Recognition

Deficit in emotion recognition has been found to be a characteristic feature of schizophrenia pathology (Mandal, Jain, Haque-Nizamie, Weiss and Schneider, 1999). Schizophrenic patients with positive symptoms have shown a recognition deficit in negative emotions, but not for positive or neutral facial expressions. This may suggest (Mandal *et al.,* 1999) that schizophrenia patients with positive symptoms suffer from some kind of interpersonal difficulties in which they tend to see others happy because of their own style of coping. The style of functioning renders it possible for them to keep arousal-provoking perceptual cues from entering into subjective awareness. Brief visual stimuli enter into a cognitive storage system of large capacity but of short duration (Iconic Image, Neisser, 1967). Schizophrenic's icons are intact but integration of iconic storage into more complex cognitive operations may be deficient. However, many such interpretations, particularly with schizophrenia, is still speculative in nature. More studies especially with meta-analysis of earlier findings and a comparison of studies that used differential deficit designs are required to permit definitive conclusion to be drawn. A critical review on facial expressions of emotion in schizophrenia has been given in Indian cultural context by Mandal, Pandey and Prasad (1998), and Mandal *et al.* (2002).

Emotion processing in schizophrenia has been measured cross-culturally (Habel, Gur, Mandal, Salloum, Gur, and Schneider, 2000) to see whether ethnic background could be associated with it. Although some variation in performance was observed among cultures, similarities were more prominent than differences. Such emotion impairment as these authors (Habel *et al.,* 2000) opined, however, is supportive of a common neurobiological bias in schizophrenia. But small differences in affective impairments with respect to emotional valence probably reflect the influence of culture and demographic variability among the sample investigated. However, replication of these on larger and more diverse sample and combining them with structural and functional imaging will help to know more about neurobiological phenomenon of affective symptoms in schizophrenia, and also about psychopathology and psychophysiology of patients with schizophrenia.

Neuropsychological Variables

On neuropsychological (NPL) perspective lateral transfer deficit (Mandal and Singh, 1993; Tiwari and Mandal, 1998) was considered to be a trait marker in schizophrenia. Deficits in interhemispheric (bilateral) transfer in schizophrenia have been examined both with structural and functional measures. But earlier studies shed little light on whether such bilateral transfer deficit is differentially associated as a trait characteristic of schizophrenia irrespective of the sub-types, or is contingent upon the stage of illness (acute vs remitted), and nature and duration of treatment received. In a later study (Biswas, Haque-Nizamie, Pandey and Mandal, 1996) it was found that even after successful treatment with drugs for 6 months bilateral transfer deficit persists in patients. Also, Indian researchers are of the opinion that lateral performance is less overtly expressed in actual hand preference of patients with schizophrenia (Mandal and Singh, 1993), though right ear advantage and normal lateralisation pattern emerge when acuteness subsides (Shukla, Behera and Mandal, 1993).

Bender Visuo-Motor-Gestalt Test was used, in NPL perspective to determine predominant lobe functions in schizophrenia (Mukhopadhyay, Mukherjee, Chowdhury, Gupta, Basu and Dutta, 1999), and NPL findings have also been utilised in the psychosocial intervention programme in connection with autistic children (Tarafdar, Mukhopadhyay and Basu, 2004).

Impact of SES in Symptom Manifestation

In rural population of India, preponderance of hallucinatory themes of magic and religion (Jadutona, Witchcraft, Evil Spirit) is noted, particularly in less-educated females (Sharma and Agnihotri, 1986) no matter whether the patient hails from North India or Eastern India (Sharma and Agnihotri, 1986). Findings reported in Indian literature, in general, give an impression that poorly educated and those with lower SES report hallucinatory contents centered around witchcraft, magic and evil spirits, whereas educated and those with higher SES relate their content of delusions to telepathy, mode being media transmission (Kala and

Wig, 1982). Fear of some supernatural power is common in Indian patients. Such fear is due to (a) internal insecurity of loosing some object of dependency, (b) fear of punishment to be imposed by the supernatural power because of personal guilt feelings, *e.g.*, sex guilt; whereas for Western patients such fear, if present, is due to suppression of aggression. In rural population of Rajasthan, India, possession syndrome is reported (Kapur, 1987). Three syndromes based on sex guilt, commonly reported in Indian culture are 'Dhat' (seminal loss) (Singh, 1985), 'Koro' (dysphoric penile erection) (Chowdhury, 1992), and 'Jhinjhini' (numbness, fear of paralysis and impending death) (Nandi, Banerjee, Saha, Sen and Bhattacharyya, 1992).

Co-existence of other psychiatric morbidity with Dhat Discharge needs special mentioning. Depression, both like that of neurotic or psychotic is seen to be commonly associated with this problem along with anxiety and hypochondriasis. Such patients usually respond well with anti-depressants (Bandyopadhyay, 1999). Eclectic approach is required for its management (Kapur, 1987); relatively less number of studies on such phenomenon has been reported in the recent years.

Culture Context and Schizophrenic Symptomatology: Home Role

Patients with schizophrenia in developing countries like India, Colombia, and Nigeria are less likely to remain incapacitated by the disorder for long term than those who have schizophrenia in developed countries such as the United States, Great Britain. In developing countries patients with schizophrenia, for example, are more likely to be cared for at home by a broad network of family members who share responsibility for the individual. In contrast, in developed countries, it is less likely that the person with schizophrenia lives with family or that his/her immediate family has other family members nearby who share in the care (Jablensky, 1989). Caring for a family member with schizophrenia is a huge burden. When this burden is shouldered by only a few persons, there can be tremendous conflicts in the family which may exacerbate the symptoms of the patients with schizophrenia. Family involvement with the patients, on the contrary, in India, was found effective in reducing relapse following hospital discharge (Rangaswami, 2000). Accordingly, Indian researchers (*e.g.*, Rangaswami, 2000) have advocated the impact of psychoeducational family intervention on 1st episode schizophrenics to prevent progress of the disease and also its relapse. Of course, a shift in emphasis from the intraindividual to interindividual approach, in the management of such patients, particularly with regard to families of schizophrenia, has been evident in Indian research since 1970s (Sathyavathi, 1974, 1977).

Schizophrenic Symptomatology: Culture Specificity

In symptom manifestation of schizophrenia wide cross-cultural and sub-cultural variations have been reported. Auditory hallucinations occur more frequently in Western schizophrenic patients, whereas visual hallucinations are common in outside Western cultures. Indian patients were reported to experience more of delusions of bodily control and being poisoned (Kala and Wig, 1982) than the Western patients. Involvement of family members in aggressive and persecutory themes in Indian patients could be a refelction of their process of socialisation where in high premium is placed on obedience to elders and aggression receives hardly any encouragement. May be that as Suhail states, repressed hostility/aggression reappears in the form of delusions of persecution (Suhail, 2000).

Interestingly, research findings reveal that people endeavour to keep their culture intact even after migrating to other cultures. For *e.g.,* delusions of ghost possession, which is uncommon in Britain but common in South-Asian countries, has also been reported in the Asians living in the U.K. (Hale and Pinniti, 1994; Bose, 1997). Indian schizophrenic patients living in Britain experienced persecutory delusions (being attacked, harmed, poisoned) while White patients had shown greater themes of telepathic communication. This shows that the White patients believe in extra sensory perception of the power of their own mind, whereas the British-Indians perceive power in external sources (Suhail, 2000). Rapid social change due to industrialisation though has brought some significant change in the contents of delusions over the decades in both Indian (Sharma and Agnihotri, 1986) and Western culture (Suhail, 2000), there is evidence that indigenous beliefs continue to be retained even amongst educated patients (Bhattacharyya, 1986).

Cross-cultural comparisons of hallucinations and delusions have mostly been made by collecting research findings reported from other countries. Such comparisons lack empirical evidences because of methodological differences. Suhail's (2000) study is free from such limitation. But major weakness of this study is its retrospective design. Nevertheless, this is very important study which depicts that one's cultural values and expectations affect the way the distress is perceived and expressed. Apart from inherent cultural values, shared cultural values are important in the sense that sharing of two cultures at the same time may have a demanding impact on one's mental health. Analysis of such contents are essential in the treatment of these patients.

Research on Psychotherapy, Psychoeducation and Vocational Rehabilitation in Schizophrenia: A Combined Approach

Pharmacotherapy is effective in treating acute symptoms but not in removing the residual cognitive and social deficits (Penn and Mueser, 1996) altogether. Psychoeducation and vocational rehabilitation approach combined with maintenance pharmacotherapy have reduced (Rangaswami, 2000) the risk of relapse and improved social-adjustment and quality of life of the patients. This study highlights that for the patients with bio-psychosocial etiology, combined pharmacotherapy and psychosocial interventions increases the functional capacity to a greater extent. The rehabilitation unit of the NIMHANS, Bangalore, has been expanding (Kalyansundaram and Verghese, 2000) where comprehensive rehabilitative services are being provided with through teamwork. Family ward is a unique system at the NIMHANS which has to be implemented by specialists working in different parts of the country.

12

CHAPTER

Future Directions of Research in Schizophrenia in India and Policy Implementation

Research studies should afford a large arena where both unique and familiar behaviour pathologies can be examined for the light they shed on etiology. Cross-cultural and sub-cultural research to compare interrelationship among biological and environmental variables is needed. To achieve this what we need is standardised approaches to diagnoses and assessment, an issue which has been mentioned by Ley (1970; cited by Ganguly, 2000) long before. Ley opined that personal preferences in ways of describing patients lower the validity of assessments (might even lead to develop 'diagnostic steroetypes') (Ley, 1970). Questionnaires and schedules used for screening out symptom-free individuals and detecting suspected cases are sometimes improvised by individual team members. Errors are likely to creeping in here leading to false negatives (Ganguly, 2000). Such errors are likely to be more in field studies.

Secondly, to evaluate psychological status completely on the basis of self-rating indices would be subject to falsification for various reasons. Because the use of questionnaire/ inventories rests mainly upon what wilder has called the "Inventory Promise". That is, the underlying assumptions are that the subjects are always motivate to describe their feelings exactly. In practice, however, we see that subjects, especially patients, show lack of motivation to read the items carefully, understand clearly and to fill in the forms properly.

Thirdly, though there is a tremendous development in publishing variety of psychological tests to suit the needs of contemporary Indian society, the concepts however, have been frequently borrowed from the Western Psychological Literature. Of late, the self-report measures, often use examples from Indian social set up, and in this way the content is contextualised to some extent. Though the problem of cultural bias is partly overcome, in this way, conceptual mapping remains problematic so far as understanding the presence of the phenomenon in the culture and its distribution are concerned (Srivastava, and Misra, 1996; Srivastava, Tripathi, and Misra, 1996).

Fourthly, a subjective psychological test can be misused in the absence of any monitoring system and lack of knowledge about the principles and problems of psychological assessment at large. At the same time it is impossible to develop a test that can measure the same construct for groups with diverse cultural backgrounds (Misra, Sahoo, and Puhan, 1999). One possible way to obviate this difficulty is to use some objective measures, *viz.,* psychophysiological, neuropsychological (NPL) etc., where the experimenter is not at all dependent on the subjects verbatim, nor the subject can manipulate his answers in anyway. Puhan and his associates have constructed a number of tests involving a projective inventory approach (Puhan, 1995) to assess aggression, dependence proneness, social responsibility etc. They have demonstrated a low correlation of these measures with social desirability as compared to the correlation between self-report measures and social desirability. But in projective tests also interrater reliability has to be assessed which again demands more expertise.

In a study, Suhail (2000) reported that a sizable proportion of the Asian respondents complained about difficulty in understanding the concept behind each item of a questionnaire test. This could be the reason for obtaining inconsistencies in the reported findings, *e.g.,* anxiety, revealed through questionnaire methods as opposed to those obtained through psychophysiological measure mostly show contradictions (Sanyal, Chattopadhyay and Biswas, 1998; Mukhopadhyay and Chattopadhyay, 2000; Chakraborty, Saha, Mukhopadhyay, Chattopadhyay and Biswas, 2001). Furthermore, adequate knowledge about Ss autonomic vis-à-vis biological stability and central capacity for arousal modulation required in life-adjustment, can best be understood through indirect measures, like, GSR, EMG, EEG etc. (Mukhopadhyay, De, Chattopadhyay and Biswas, 1996). Electrophysiological measures were reported to be better indicators of biological stability, *e.g.,* CNS arousal, than subjective reports (Mohanty, Das, Mukundan and Jamuna, 1993a,b). To assess treatment outcome we need parallel tests, which are not mostly available. But use of objective measures can help to obviate such problems related to repeated measures (subjective). Likewise, training outcome can be measured in unbiased way through objective tests. In a pre- post-design on 274 (230 males) athletes Khan and Mohan (1992) assessed the effects of training at the institute of Sports Training, Patiala. They have emphasised the need for employing objective measures to validate the results (Saha, Saha, Mukhopadhyay and Chattopadhyay, 2001; Chattopadhyay, Saha, and Saha, 1994). If such be the situation with normals, patient population could surely be assessed better through objective measures.

Fifthly, psychological tests developed mostly by academic psychologists, but their validity is determined largely by practising clinical psychologists; a balance between scientific vigour and clinical utility is often difficult to achieve (Thapa, 2000). However, NPL methods have helped to overcome some such problem to a certain extent (Chattopadhyay, 1998). NPL tests may be described as objective-subjective, whereas psychophysiological measures may best be designated as objective-objective. It is possible to have a standardized laboratory methodology, like International 10-20 System in EEG recording, throughout the country to avoid subjectivity totally. However, brain scan and MRI would be better indicator compared to traditional EEG measures to study lobe functions and different symptomatology.

Studies should be undertaken to ascertain the psychometric properties of tests employed independent of test constructors. Such an exercise would enhance the credibility of test scores so that our predictions are found dependable. The assessment of intelligence, *e.g.*, in India requires altogether a different orientation to make an authentic appraisal of intellectual function (Srivastava, Tripathi, and Misra, 1996). Systematic training like that of apprenticeship in learning is necessary for the diagnosticians to have a shift in focus from absolute dependency onto questionnaire measures to that of indirect objective measures for better reliability of obtained findings through quick and easy elimination of the errors, which contaminate data, particularly with psychiatric patients. Such a shift, however, must not mean that in general, the reliability of standardized questionnaires is in question.

Attempts must be made to integrate laboratory models of intervention with reality oriented models. There are mainly three models of therapeutic intervention. Clinical model, community model and social action model. Social action model is perhaps impractical in our country at the moment. Methods of community intervention have taken four forms: crisis intervention, consultation, mental health education, and utilization of para professionals, particularly for the socially disadvantaged group.

Successful implementation of rehabilitation programmes in the community requires primarily three measures – involvement of community agencies, utilization of community support, and adequate training for mental health professionals. For adequate training multifarious issues related to the patients' needs and problems are to be focussed.

In India multifarious social problems, like, unemployment, poverty, illiteracy, stigma and professional pessimism pose great challenges to any rehabilitation worker. Need to be aware of available community resources (*e.g.*, immediate availability of treatment facilities) and limitations (*e.g.*, believing spirituality, witchcraft etc.), and readiness to deliver health services even in the remote corner of the rural areas (WHO, 1979) have been emphasized by Indian researchers long before (Reddy, Channabasavanna, Gouridevi, Doss, Prabhu, Sheriff, Kaliaperumal and Reddamma, 1986). Barring sporadic attempts, no systematic effort has been made in India to make use of community resources in the field of mental health. In some mental hospitals and of late some school and college students have been involved in giving entertainments or related recreational activities. Even these meagre activities are rarely documented (Ranganathan and Parthasarathi, 1982; Ranganathan, Reddy, Sheriff, Parthasarathi and Kaliaperumal, 1991).

Ranganathan, Channabasavanna, Murli, Bharathi, and Padankatti (1996) have clearly depicted the nature of agencies came forward to offer help for resource utilization in the community services. Of the 236 community agencies 30.5% of business and commercial organizations (did not extend their services) and more than 50% of Government agencies did not provide necessary help. Welfare agencies (for disabled students and non-students volunteer) extended their help without any reservation. Reasons for such resistance to offer help were fear, anxieties, and false belief and stigma related to mental patients, even after their recovery from such illness (Ranganathan *et al.,* 1996). This shows the necessity to educate our people related to the sensitivity to the patient's needs and problems. In a primary care setting in Goa the prevalence of Common Mental Disorders (CMD) (Equivalent to the Neuroses) was reported to be 46% which was strongly associated with females, economic problems and disability. Mostly multiple drugs, injectable vitamins and Benzodiazepines are the methods of treatments as Indian patients, in general, expect such methods of treatment instead of counselling/psychotherapy (Patel, 1996, 2000). To expand psychological treatment, Andrew, Dias-Saxena and Patel (2000) developed and standardized technique of counselling. Unfortunately nearly half of the patients attended only one session, which shows that these people need to be aware of the benefit of such treatments first prior to its application.

Community Mental Health

The National Mental Health Programme of India (Government of India, 1982) has emphasized the need for community participation in the development of mental health services in the country. This can be done through collaboration with sectors like education, social welfare etc.

This aims to make our general population aware about identification and utilization of the resources for scientific treatment of mental illness through mental health professionals. This can be done only through change of attitude of public through utilization of the impact of interaction of the mental health professionals with the community.

Rural Development

India is a country mostly populated with rural people and agriculture is the main vocation for them. Owing to unavoidable consequences of modernization, Westernisation, urbanization, and industrialization, traditional life style of the villagers are changing and thereby the gap between city and village in most of the areas has decreased. Still village population has lack of resources and due to poverty they live under impoverished conditions. These problems have drawn the attention of our professionals (Patel, Pereira, Continho, R. Fernandez, J. Fernandez, and Mann, 1998) particularly of clinical psychologists, and attempts have been made to bring some change in the value system and attitude of people living in villages (Chakraborty, 1991).

Government of India decided to focus on bringing about alround development of the villages and a variety of programme were launched. These programmes were unsuccessful mainly because of their failure to change mental make-up of rural masses. The failure of our planning efforts in inducing an urge for improvement and change in behaviour is not necessarily a matter of economic opportunities and lack of resources only, but it requires significant changes in the behavioural style and strategies of the villagers. They show lot of resistance to accept innovation and progress (Tiwari, Srivastava, and Tripathi, 2002).

A concerted efforts of the mental health professionals, planners, specially policy makers, along with teachers, voluntary workers, socio-religious and political leaders, police personnel, guardians be made in implementing a successful programme. That is, a team spirit is indispensable in psychosocial rehabilitation. This will definitely pave way for improving quality of life of people disturbed due to mental health problems.

Bibliography

ABRAMOWTIZ, I.A., and COURSEY, R.D. (1989). Impact of an educational support group of family participants who take care of their schizophrenic relatives. *J. Consult. Clin. Psychol.*, 57, 232-236.

ACKERNECHT, E.H. (1968). A short history of psychiatry, 2nd edition ed. New York, Hafner Publishing Company.

ADEOYE, L.T. (1955). The role of cultural factors in paranoid psychosis among the Yourba Tribes. *J. Ment. Sc.*, 101, 237.

AGUILERA, D.C., MESSICK, J.M., and FARRELLE, M.S. (1970). *Crisis intervention: theory and methodology.* St. Louis : Mosby.

AI-ISSA, I. (1995). The illusion of reality or the reality of illusion : Hallucinations and culture. *Brit. Jl. Psychiat.*, 166, 366-373.

AKHTAR, S. (1988). Four culture-bound psychiatric syndrome in India. Int.*Jl. Soc. Psychiat.*, 34, 70-74.

ALANEN, Y.O. (1958). The mothers of Schizophrenia patients. *Acta. Psychiat. Neurol. Second.*, 33, Suppl., 124-263.

ALANEN, Y.O. (1966). The family in the pathogenesis of Schizophrenia and neurotic disorders. *Acta. Psychiat. Second.*, 33, Suppl., 189.

ALEXANDER, F. (1944). The indications for psychoanalytic therapy. *Bull New York, Acad. Med.*, 20, 319-332.

ALFORD, B.A., and CORREIA, C.J. (1994). Cognitive therapy in schizophrenia : Theory and empirical status. *Behav. Therap.*, 25, 17-33.

ALFORD, G.S., and TURNER, S.M. (1976). Stimulus interference and conditioned inhibition of auditory hallucinations. *J. Beha. Ther. & Exptl. Psychiat.*, 7, 155-160.

ALTSCHUL, S. (1988). Childhood bereavement and its aftermath. Madison, C.T.: International Universities Press.

AMERICAN PSYCHIATRIC ASSOCIATION (1984). Medical and legal problems in psychiatric coding under the DSM and ICD systems. *Am. J. Psychiatry*, 141, 418-420.

AMERICAN PSYCHIATRIC ASSOCIATION (1987). Diagnostic and statistical manual of mental disorders (3rd ed revised), Washington, D.C. APA.

AMERICAN PSYCHIATRIC ASSOCIATION (1994). (4th ed), Diagnostic and Statistical Manual of Mental Disorders, American Psychiatric Press, Washington, D.C. APA.

AMERICAN PSYCHIATRIC ASSOCIATION (2000). Diagnostic and statistical manual of mental disorders (4th ed. Text revision), Washington, D.C., APA.

AMERICAN PSYCHIATRIC ASSOCIATION (2005). Diagnostic and statistical manual of mental disorders (DSM-IV-TR). First Indian edition. Jaypee Brothers, Medical Publishers Ltd., New Delhi.

ANDERSON, C. (1983). A psycho-educational model of family treatment for Schizophrenia. In H. STIERLIN, L.C. WYNNE, & M. WICHSCHING (Eds.), *Psycho-social intervention in Schizophrenia*, New York Sringer Publishing Co.

ANDERSON, E.W. and MALLINSON, W.P. (1941). Psychogenic episodes in the course of major psychoses. *J. Ment.* Sc., 87, 383-281.

ANDERSEN, N.C. and OLSEN, S. (1982). Negative vs Positive Schizophrenia : Definition and Validation. *Arch. Gen. Psychiat.*, 39, 789-794.

ANDREW, G., DIAS-SAXENA, F., and PATEL, V. (2000). The development of a counselling treatment for common mental disorders in general health care settings. *Ind. J. Clin. Psychol.*, 27(1), 72-79.

ANGRIST, B., ROTROSEN, J., and GERSHON, S. (1980). *Differential effects of neurolytics on negative versus positive symptoms in Schizophrenia Psychopharmacol.*, 72, 17-19.

APPLETON, W.S. (1974). Mistreatment of patients' families by psychiatrists. *Amer. J. Psychiat.*, 131, 655-657.

ARIETI, S. (1955). Interpretation of Schizophrenia, New York, Rober Brunner.

ARIETI, S. (1959). Schizophrenia : The manifest symptomatology, the psychodynamic and formal mechanisms. In Ariets, S. (ed) *American Handbook of Psychiatry*, vol.1, New York.

ARNOLD, O.H. (1955). *Schizophrener prozers and Schizophrene Symptom Gesetze* (Schizophrenic process and Schizophrenic Symptom Laws), Viena : Maudrich.

ARTISS, K.L. (1966). Paranoid thinking in everyday life. *Arch. Gen. Psychiat.*, 14, 89-93.

ASTRUP, C. (1957). "Experimentelle Unter such Vher diestivu nagender hoheven Nerventatigueit lies anuten Und Subchronischen Schizophreinen" (experimental investigations of the disorders of higher nervous activity in acute and sub-chronic Schizophrenic). *Psychiat. Neurol. U. Med. Psychol. Lpz.*, 9, 33.

AWAD, A.G. (1995). Quality of life issues in medicated schizophrenic patients. In C.L. Shriqui, H.M. Nasrallah (eds) *Contemporary issues in the treatment of schizophrenia*, Washington, D.C. : American Psychiatric Press.

AX, A.F., and BAMFORD, J.L. (1970). The GSR recovery limb in chronic Schizophrenia. *Psychophysiol.*, 7, 145-147.

AX, A.F., BAMFORD, J.L., BECKETT, P.G., FRETZ, N.F. and GOTTLIEB, J.S. (1970). Autonomic conditioning in chronic schizophrenia. *J. Abn. Psychol.*, 76, 140.

AYD, F.J. (1975). The depot fluphenazines : A reappraisal after 10 years' clinical experience. *Amer. J. Psychiat.*, 132, 491-500.

AYD, Jr F.J., BLACKWELL, B. (1970). Discoveries in biological psychiatry (eds), Philadelphia, J.B. Lippincott.

AYDIN, N., DANE, S., OZTURK, I., USLU, C., GUMUSTEKIN, K., and KIRPINAR, I. (2001). Left ear (right temporal hemisphere) advantage and left temporal hemispheric dysfunction in schizophrenia. *Percept. Mot. Skills*, 93(1), 230-238.

AYLLON, T. and AZRIN, N.H. (1968). *The loner economy : A motivational system for therapy a rehabilitation.* Appleton-Century-Crofts, New York.

AYLLON, T. and MICHAEL,J. (1959). The psychiatric nurse as a behavioural engineer. *J. Exp. Omal. Behav.*, 2, 323.

AZRIN, N.H., BESALEL, V.A. and WISTOZEK,J.E. (1982). Treatment of self injury by a reinforcement plus interruption procedure. *Analysis and Intervention in Developmental Disabilities*, 2, 105-113.

BACHRACH, L.L. (1996). Psychosocial rehabilitation and psychiatry: What are the boundaries? *Canad.J. Psychiat.* 41, 28-33.

BAGSHAW, M.H. and BENZIES, S. (1968). Multiple weakness of the orienting reaction and their dissociation after in monkeys. *Exptl. Neurol.*, 20, 175-187.

BAGSHAW, M.H. and KIMBLE, D. (1972). Bimodal EDR Orienting Response characteristics of limbic leisoned monkeys, correlates with Schizophrenic patients. *Paper presented to Society for Psychophysiologcial Res.*, Boston, Mass, October.

BAGSHAW, M.H., KIMBLE, D.P. and PRIBRAM, K.H. (1965). The GSR monkeys during orienting and habituation and after ablation of the inppocampus, and infero-temporal cortex. *Neuropsychologia*, 3, 111-119.

BAHRAMALI, H., LIM, L.C., RENNIE, C., MEARES, R. and GORDON, E. (2001). ERPS associated with and without an orienting reflex in patients with schizophrenia. *Int.J. Neuroscience*, 108(3-4), 163-174.

BAKER, R. (1975). Behavioural techniques in the treatment of Schizophrenia. In *New Perspectives in Schizophrenia* (ed. FORREST, A. and AFFLICK,J.) Edinburgh : Chur-chill, Liningstone.

BALDESSARINI, R.J. (1985). Drugs and the treatment of psychiatric disorders. In A.G. Gilman, L.S. Goodman, T.W. Rall, and F. Murad (Eds.) *The Pharmacological basis of therapeutics* (7th ed), New York : Macmillan.

BANDYOPADHYAY, G.K. (1999). Anxiety in patients with dhat Syndrome. *Psychol. Res.Jr.*, 23 (1 & 2), 29-35.

BARTEN, H.H. (1969). The coming age of the brief psychotherapies. In Bellak, L. and Barten, H.H. (Eds.). *Progress in Community Mental Health*, vol.1, New York : Grune and Strattn.

BASU, J. (1993). Applicability of ego function assessment scale a guided interview schedule on Shizophrenics, neurotics and normals : A preliminary report. *Psychol. studies*, 38(3), 119-224.

BASU,J. and BANERJEE, M. (1998). Adaptation of the English version of the Ego function assessment scale (modified) by Bellack for Indian adults. *Ind.J. Clin. Psychol.*, 25(1), 57-65.

BASU,J. and BASU, S. (1996). Ego function profile of male psychiatric patients in comparison to normals. *Psychol. Studies*, 41(1&2), 16-22.

BASU, J., BASU, S., and BHATTACHARYA, S. (2004). Ego functions in relation to stressful life events and indices of psychopathology in paranoid schizophrenia. *Psychol. Rep.*, 95, 1248-1252.

BASU, S., BASU, J. and BHATTACHARYA, S. (1999a). Stressful life events and psychiatric disorders. *Psychol. Res.Jr.*, 23(1&2), 21-27.

BASU, S., BASU, J. and BHATTACHARYA, S. (1999b). Ego function and their relation to psychyopathologies. *Ind.J. Clin. Psychol.*, 26(1), 82-87.

BASU, S., BASU, J. and BHATTACHARYA, S. (2002). Ego functions : A comparative study. *Ind.J. Clin. Psychol.*, 29(2), 104-109.

BASU, S., BHATTACHARYA, S. and BASU, J. (2000). A factor analytic study of ego functions assessment. *J. Person. Clin. Studies*, 16(2), 132-136.

BATESON, G. (1972). *Steps to an ecology of mind.* New York : Ballantine.

BATESON, G., JACKSON, D.D., HALEY, J., and WEAK, L.J. (1956). Towards a theory of Schizophrenia. *Behav. Sci.*, 1, 251-264.

BEARD, J.H., PROPST, R. and MALAMED, T.J. (1982). The Fountain House Model of Psychiatric Fountain Rehabilitation. *Psychosoc. Rehab.* J., 5, 47-53.

BECK, A.T., RUSH, A.J., SHAW, B.F., and EMERY, G. (1979). Cognitive therapy of depression, New York, Guildford.

BEDNAR, R.L. and LAWLIS, G.F. (1991). Empirial research in group psychotherapy. In Bergin, A.E. and Garfield, S.L. (Eds.). *Handbook of Psychotherapy and Behaviour Change : An empirical analysis*, New York : Wiley.

BEITMAN, B.D. (1991). Medications during psychotherapy. Case studies of the reciprocal relationship between psychotherapy process and medication use. In B.D. Beitman, G.L. Klerman (Eds.), *Integrating Pharmacotherapy and Psychotherapy*, Washington, D.C., American Psychiatric Press.

BEKHTEREV, Y.M. (1912). die Auwendung der methods der motorishen Assoziations reflexe fur Anfdecfung der Simulation. Z. *Gesemte. Neurol. Psychiat.*, 13, 183.

BELL, D.S. (1965). Comparison of amphetamine psychosis and Schizophrenia. *Brit. J. Psychiatry.*, 111, 701-299, 422.

BELLAK, L. (1948). Dementia Praecox. *The decades work and present states :* A review and evaluation. New York : Grune.

BELLAK, L. (1958). *Schizophrenia : a review of the syndrome.* New York : Logos press.

BELLACK, L. (1970). The validity and usefulness of the concept of the Schizophrenic Syndrome. In R. Cancre (Ed.) *The Schizophrenic Reaction.* New York : Bruner/Mazel.

BELLACK, L. (1989). Ego function assessment : A manual, New York, Consulting Psychologists Press.

BELLACK, A.S., HERSEN, M. and KAZDIN, P. (1984). An examination of the efficacy of social training for chronic Schizophrenic patients. *Hospital and Community Psychiat.*, 35, 1023-1028.

BELLACK, A.S., TURNER, S.H., HERSEN, M. and LUBER, R.F. (1984). An examination of the efficacy of social skills training for chronic Schizophrenic patients. Hospital and Community Psychiat., 35, 1023-1028.

BELLAK, L. and SMALL, L. (1965). Emergency psychotherapy and brief psychotherapy, New York: Grune and Stratter.

BENDER, L. (1953). Childhood Schizophrenia. *Psychiat. Quart.*, 27, 663-681.

BENNETT, D. (1970). The value of work in psychiatric rehabilitation. *Soc. Psychiat.*, 5, 224-232.

BENNETT, D. and WING, J.K. (1963). *Sheltered workshops for the psychiatrically, in Trends in the Mental Services* (Ed. FREEMAN, H., and FAZNDALE, J.) Chap. 27, Oxford, Pergamon.

BENTALL, R.P., HADDOCK, G. and SLADE, P.D. (1994). Cognitive therapy for persistent auditory hallucinations : From theory to therapy. *Beha. Ther.*, 25, 51-66.

BENTON, M.K., and SCHROEDER, H.E. (1990). Social skills training with schizophrenics : a meta-analytic evaluation. *J. Consult. Clin. Psychol.*, 58, 741-747.

BERGER, H. (1938). Das electroencephalogram Das menchen Malle an der Saale, Bechdruckerei Das Waisenhauses. *Nova Acta. Leopoldina*, 6, 139.

BERNHEIM, K.F. and LEWINE, R.R.J. (1979). *Schizophrenia : Symptoms, causes, treatments*, New York : W.W. Norton.

BERNSTEIN, A.S. (1968). The orienting response and direction of stimulus change, *Psychmon. Sc.*, 12, 127-128.

BERNSTEIN, A.S. (1969). To what does the orienting response respond? *Psycho-physiol.*, 6, 338-350.

BERNSTEIN, A.S. (1970). Phasic electrodermal orienting response in chronic Schizophrenics : II. Response to auditing signals of varying intensity. *J. Alen. Psychol.*, 75, 146-156.

BERNSTEIN, A.S. (1973). To what does orienting response respond? *Psychophysiol.*, 10, 338-350.

BERNSTEIN, A.S. and TAYLOR, K.W. (1978). The interaction of stimulus information with potential stimulus significance in eliciting the skin conductance orienting response. *Paper presented at the N.A.T.O. Conference on Orienting.* Amsterdam.

BERZE, J. (1914). *Primary insufficiency of psychic activity.* Uienna, Deuticke.

BERZE, J. and GRUHLE, H.W. (1929). *Psychologic der Schizophrenie* (Psychology of Schizophrenia), Berlin : Springer.

BETTELHEIM, B. and SYLVESTER, E. (1948). A therapeutic milieu. *Amer. J. Orthopsychiat.*, 18, 191-206.

BHASHKARAN, K. (1959). A psychiatric study of Schizophrenic reaction patterns in an Indian mental hospital. *Int. J. Soc. Psychiat.*, 5, 41.

BHASKARAN, K. (1963). A psychiatric study of paranoid Schizophrenics in an Indian mental hospital. *Psych. Quart.*, 37, 334.

BHASKARAN, K. and SAXENA, B.M. (1970). Some aspects of Schizophrenia in the two sexes. *Ind. J. Psychiat.*, 12, 177-184.

BHATIA, M.S. and MALIK, S.C. (1991). Dhat syndrome : A useful diagnostic entity in Indian culture. *Brit. J. Psychiat.*, 159, 691-695.

BHOLA, P., and KAPUR, M. (2000). Prevalence of emotional disturbances in Indian adolescent girls. *Ind. J. Clin. Psychol.*, 27(2), 217-222.

BILDER, R., LIPSCHUTE-BROCH, L., REITER, G. *et al.* (1992). Intellectual deficits in first-episode schizophrenia : Evidence for progressive deterioration. *Schizo. Bull.*, 18, 437-448.

BILDER, R.M., GOLDMAN, R.S., ROBINSON, D. *et al.* (2000). Neuropsychology of first-episode schizophrenia : Initial characterisation and clinical correlates. *Amer. J. Psychiat.*, 157, 549-559.

BHATTACHARYA, J.P. (1986). Psychalgia : Ethno-Psychiatric knowledge in Bengal. *Foreign and Comparative Studies.* South Asian Series, No.11, New York, Syracuse University.

BIGELOW, L.B., NUSRALLLAH, H.A. and RAUCHER, F.P. (1983). Corpus callosum thickness in chronic schizophrenia. *Brit. J. Psychiat.*, 142, 284-287.

BIRRELL, J., and HENDERSON, M. (1986). The psychological approach. In C. Hume and I. Pullen (Eds.) *Rehabilitation in Psychiatry*, New York : Churchill-Livingstone.

BISWANGER, L. (1965). Existential analysis, psychiatry, Schizophrenia. *J. Existential Psychiat.*, 1, 157-165.

BISWAS, P.K. (1983). Characteristics of Autonomic responses in psychiatric patients and normal subjects. *Ph.D. Thesis*, Calcutta University.

BISWAS, A.K., HAQUE-NIZAMIE, S., PANDEY, R., and MANDAL, M.K. (1996). Bilateral transfer deficit in schizophrenia : a trait marker. *Psychiat. Res.*, 64, 115-120.

BLACKWELL, B. (1963). Hypersensitive crises due to monoamine-oxidase inhibitors. *Lancet.*, 2, 848.

BLEULER, E. (1911). *Demention praecox oder die Gruppe der Schizophrenien.* Leipzig:Deuticke.

BLEULER, E. (1913). Artistic thinking. *Amer. J. Insanity*, 69, 873.

BLEULER, E.P. (1924). Text book of psychiatry (Trans. BRILL, A.A.) New York: Macmillan (Reissued by Dover Publications, London, 1951).

BLEULER, M. (1943). "Die Spatschizophrenen Krankheitabilder (the late Schizophrenic Clinical Pictures), *Fortscher. Neurol. Psychiat.*, 15, 259.

BLEULER, E. (1950). *Demention Praecox or the group of Schizophrenics.* Transl. By Joseph Zinkin, International University Press, Inc.

BLEULER, E. (1950b). *Demention Praecox.* International University Press, New York.

BOCZKOWSKI, J.A., ZIECHNER, A., and DESANTO, N. (1985). Neuroleptic Compliance among Chronic Schizophrenic Outpatients : An intervention outcome repnt. *J. Consult. Clin.* Psychol., 53, 666-671.

BOND, E. (1954). Results of psychiatric treatment with a control series. *Amer. J. Psychiat.*, 110-561.

BOSE, R. (1997). Psychiatric and the popular concept of possession among the Bangladeshi in London. *Int. J. Soc. Psychiat.*, 43, 11-15.

BOSTOW, D.E. and BAILEY, J.B. (1969). Modifications of severe disruptic and aggressive behaviour using brief time-out and reinforcement procedures. *J. Appl. Beha. Anal.*, 2, 31-57.

BOOK, J. (1953). A genetic and neuropsychiatric investigation of a North Swedish Population with special regard to Schizophrenia and mental deficiency. *Acta. Genet.*, 4(1), 133, 145.

BOOKHAMMER, R.S., MEYERS, R.W., SCHOBER, C.C., and PIO TROWSKI, A.Z. (1966). A five year follow-up study of Schizophrenics treated by Rosen's "direct analysis", compared with controls. *Amer. J. Psychiat.*, 123, 602-604.

BOWLBY, J. (1980). Attachment and loss (vol.3), New York, Basic.

BRADSHAW, W.H. (1993). Coping-skills training versus a problem-solving approach with schizophrenic patients. *Schiz. Bull.*, 10, 418-419.

BRENNER, H.D. (1994). Cognitive therapy with schizophrenic patients : Conceptual basis, present state and future direction. *Acta. Psychiat. Scandi.*, 90 (suppl. 384), 108-115.

BRENNER, H.D., HODEL, B., RODER, V., and CORRIGAN, P. (1992). Treatment of cognitive dysfunctions and behavioural deficits in schizophrenia. *Schizo. Bull.*, 18, 21-26.

BRENNER, H.D., RODER, V., HODEL, B., KIENZIC, N. *et al.* (1995). Integrated psychological therapy for schizophrenic patients. *Bern. Switzerland* : Hogrefe and Huber.

BRILL, A. (1913). Publouto or hysteria among Peary's Eskimos. *J. New Ment. Dis.*, 40, 514.

BROADBENT, D.E. (1958). *Perception and communication.* New York : Pergamon Press.

BROEN, W.E.J. (1968). *Schizophrenia : research and theory,* New York : Academic.

BROOTA, A. (1991). Kinesthetic perception in Schizophrenics. *J. Pers. Clin. Psychol.*, 7(1), 77-82.

BROOTA, A., KAUR, H., and BATRA, S. (1988). Perception of time in Schizophrenics. *J. Pers. Clin. Psychol.*, 4(1), 69-73.

BROOTA, A. and PANT, N. (1989). Perceptual regression in Schizophrenia. *J. Pers. Clin. Psychol.*, 5(1), 29-33.

BROWN, C.W., BONE, M., ALISON, B., and WING, J.K. (1966). Schizophrenia and Social Care, Mandsley Monograph No.17, London, Oxford University Press.

BROWN, G.W., BIRLEY, J.L.T. and WING, J.K. (1972). Influence of family life on the course of Schizophrenic disorders : A replication. *Brit. J. Psychiat.*,121, 241-258.

BROWN, G.W., MONCK, E.M., CARSTAIRS, G.M. and WING, J.K. (1962). Influence of family life on the course of Schizophrenic illness. *Brit. J. Soc. Prevent. Med.*, 16, 55-68.

BRYDEN, M.P. (1982). *Laterality : functional asymmetry in the intact brain.* Academic Press, New York.

BUCHSBAUM, M.S. (1975). Averaged evoked response augmenting / reducing in Schizophrenia and affective disorders. In : Freedman, D.K., ed. *Biology of the major psychoses.* Raven Press, New York, pp. 129-142.

BUCHSBAUM, M.S. (1977). The middle evoked response components and Schizophrenia. *Schzo. Bull.*, 3, 93-104.

BUCHSBAUM, M.S., INGUAR, D.H., KESSLER, R. *et al.* (1982). Cereloral glucography with position tomography. *Arch. Gen. Psychiat.*, 39, 251.

BUCK, R. (1984). Communication of emotion. New York, Guilford Press.

BURNHAM, D.L., GLADSTONE, A.L. and GIBSON, R.W. (1969). *Schizophrenia and the Need Feer Dibmma.* New York, International University Press.

BURROW, T. (1928). The basis of group analysis. *Brit. J. Med. Psychol.*, 8, 198-206.

BUSS, A.H. (1966). *Psychopathology,* New York : Wibey.

CACIOPPO, J.T. and GARDNER, W.T. (1999). Emotion. *Annu. Rev. Psychol.*, 50, 372-385.

CALLAWAY, E. (1975). *Brain electrical potentials and individual psychological differences.* New York, Grune & Stratter, Inc.

CALLAWAY, E., JONES, R.T., and LAYNE, R.S. (1965). Evoked responses and segmented set of Schizophrenia. *Arch. Gen. Psychiat.*, 12, 83-89.

CALLAWAY, E., and STONE, G. (1960). Re-evaluating the focus of attention. In L. Uaar, and J.G. Miller (Eds.) *Drugs and Behaviour,* New York : Wiley, pp. 393-398.

CALLAWAY, E., TUETING, P., and KOSLOW, S.H. (1978). Eds., *Event-related brain potentials in man.* Academic Press, New York.

CAMERON, N. (1939). Schizophrenic thinking in a problem – solving situation. *J. Ment. Sci.*, 85, 1012.

CAMERON, N. (1944). Experimental analysing Schizophrenic thinking. In *Language and thought in Schizophrenia* (ed.) KASANIN, J. Berkeley, University of California Press.

CAMERON, N. (1947). *The psychology of the behaviour disorders*, Boston : Houghton, Mifflies.

CAMERON, P., ENNIS, J. and DEADMAN, J. (1998). Standards and guidelines for the psychotherapies, University of Toronto Press, Toronto.

CARLSSON, A. (1978). Antipsychotic drugs, neurotransmitters and schizophrenia. *Amer. J. Psychiat.*, 135, 164.

CARLSSON, A. and LINDQUIST, M. (1983). Effect of chloropromazine or haloperidol or formation of 3-methoxy tyramine and novmetanephrive in mouse brain. *Acta. Pharmacologia*, 20, 140-144.

CARLSON, N.R. (1986). *Physiology of behaviour* (3rd ed.), Boston : Allyn & Bacon.

CAROTHERS, J.C. (1947). A study of mental derangement in Africans and an attempt to explain its peculiarities more specially in relation to African attitude of Life. *J. Ment. Sci.*, 93, 548.

CAROTHERS, J.C. (1948). A study of mental derangement in African and an attempt to explain its peculiarities, more especially in relation to the African attitude to life. *Psychiat.*, 11, 47.

CARR, E.G., and LOVAAS, O.I. (1983). Contingent electric shock as a treatment for severe behaviour problems. In S. Axelord and J. Apsche (Eds.), *The effects of punishment on human behaviour*, New York, Academic Press.

CARSTAIRS, G.M., and KAPUR, R.L. (1976). The great universe of Kota : Stress, change and mental disorder in an Indian village. University of California Press, Barkeley.

CAYNER, J.J. and KILAND, J.R. (1974). Use of brief time out with three Schizophrenic patients. *J. Beha. Ther. & Exptl. Psychiat.*, 5, 141-143.

CHADDA, R.K. (2003). A survey of burden and coping strategies of patients with mental disorders. *Project Report* ICMR, IHBAS, Delhi.

CHAKRABORTY, A. (1991). Culture, colonialism and psychiatry. *Lancet*, 337, 1204-1207.

CHAKRABORTY, S., SAHA, S., MUKHOPADHYAY, P., and CHATTOPADHYAY, P.K. (2001). Swimming and anxiety amelioration in children : A study using self-report and psychophysiological indices. *Bang. J. Sports Sci.*, 1(1), 44-53.

CHAKRAVORTY, A. (1966). Visual hallucination. *Ind. J. Psychiat.*, 8(1), 21-25.

CHAPMAN, J. and McGHIE, A. (1962). A comparative study of disordered attention in Schizophrenia. *J. Ment. Sci.*, 108, 487-500.

CHATTERJEE, R.G., CHATTERJEE (CHATTOPADHYAY), P.K. and BHATTACHARYYA, A.K. (1978). Time estimation in psychotics and neurotics : An experimental study. *Psychologia*, 21(4), 237-240.

CHATTERJEA, R.G., CHATTOPADHYAY, P.K., BHATTACHARYYA, A.K., and BISWAS, P.K. (1979). Linear estimation in psychotics and neurotics : An experimental study. *Cal. Rev.*, 4(4), 19-21.

CHATTERJEA, R.G., CHATTOPADHYAY, P.K., and BISWAS, P.K. (1980). Estimation of Task-oriented time in the psychotics. Psychologia, 23(3), 1889-1892.

CHATTERJEA, R.G., CHATTOPADHYAY, P.K., BISWAS, P.K., BHATTACHARYYA, A.K. and ROY, R. (1979). Reaction time in Schizophrenia and Normals. *Psychological Studies*, 24(2), 79-81.

CHATTERJEA, R.G., CHATTOPADHYAY, P.K., ROY, A.R., BHATTACHARYYA, A.K. and BISWAS, P.K. (1980). Role of trait anxiety and induced arousal on two-flash threshold of Schizophrenics. *Psychologia*, 23(2), 101-104.

CHATTERJEA, R.G., CHATTOPADHYAY, P.K., ROY, A.R., BISWAS, P.K., BHATTACHARYYA, A.K., and BASU, A.K. (1980). Role of trait anxiety and induced arousal in two-flash threshold of neurotic patients. *Psychol. Repnts.*, 46, 231-234.

CHATTOPADHYAY, P.K. (1981). Bilateral skin-resistance response in anxiety. *Ind.J. Clin. Psychol.*, 8(1), 29-34.

CHATTOPADHYAY, P.K. (1983). Bilateral E.E.G. evoked responses in anxiety. *Ind.J. Clin. Psychol.*, 10(1), 151-157.

CHATTOPADHYAY, P.K. (1998). Assessment of cognitive potentialities : A neuro-psychological approach. In A. Sen and A. Sen (Eds), *Challenges of contemporary changes : A psychological perspective on future of human society*, New Age International Publishers, New Delhi, pp. 73-92.

CHATTOPADHYAY, P.K., BANDHYOPADHYAY, S., BASU, A.K., BRAHAMA-CHARI, R.N. and GHOSH, A.K. (1989). Premortised anxiety, and status of blood cortisol and prolactin in erophageal and laryngeal cancer patients. *J. Psychol. Res.*, 33(1), 46-53.

CHATTOPADHYAY, P.K. and BISWAS, P.K. (1983). Characteristics of galvanic skin response in Anrins patients and normal subjects. *Ind.J. Clin. Psychol.*, 10(1), 159-164.

CHATTOPADHYAY, P.K., BISWAS, P.K. and BASU, A.K. (1980). Time estimation in psychiatric patients and normal subjects. *Ind.J. Clin. Psychol.*, 7, 43-46.

CHATTOPADHYAY, P.K., BISWAS, P.K. and CHATTORAJ, M. (1982). The Personality Questionnaire (PQ) : its applicability on education Bengalee psychotic patients. *Ind.J. Clin. Psychol.*, 9(2), 137-140.

CHATTOPADHYAY, P.K., BISWAS, P.K., CHATTORAJ, M. and BASU, A.K. (1979). State and trait anxiety in psychotic, somatic, and psychosomatic patients and normal subjects. *Ind.J. Clin. Psychol.*, 6, 221-223.

CHATTOPADHYAY, P.K., BISWAS, P.K., CHATTORAJ, M., and BHATTACHARYA, A.K. (1990). Psychoticism, neuroticism, and extroversion in educated Bengalee adults. *Manas*, 37(1-2), 41-44.

CHATTOPADHYAY, A.K., BISWAS, P.K. and MITRA, A. (1982). Estimation of the oriented time in Schizophrenics, anxious neurotics and normals. *Ind.J. Clin. Psychol.*, 9(1), 19-23.

CHATTOPADHYAY, P.K., BOND, A.J., and LADER, M.H. (1975). Characteristics of galvanic skin response in anxiety states. *J. Psychiat. Res.*, 12, 265-270.

CHATTOPADHYAY, A.K., COOKE, E., TOONE, B. and LADER, M.H. (1980). Habituation of physiological responses in anxiety. *Biol. Psychiat.*, 15(5), 711-723.

CHATTOPADHYAY, P.K., and DAS, M. (1983). Stressful life events and psychopathological episodes. *Ind.J. Clin. Psychol.*, 10(2), 227-231.

CHATTOPADHYAY, P.K. and DASGUPTA, S. (1992). Trait anxiety, neuroticism, and extraversion in long and short sleeper children. *Bang. J. Psychiat.*, 13, 1-5.

CHATTOPADHYAY, P.K., DASGUPTA, S. and GHOSH, K.K. (1982a). Cortisol and morbid anxiety. *Ind. Psy.*, 1(2), 10-15.

CHATTOPADHYAY, P.K., DASGUPTA, S., and GHOSH, N.K. (1982b). Measurement of anxiety in psychiatric patients : An interdisciplinary approach. *J. Psychol. Res.*, 26(3), 121-127.

CHATTOPADHYAY, P.K., DASGUPTA, S. and LAHA, H. (1982c). Physiological and psychological aspects of anxiety in psychiatric patients and normal subjects. *Ind. J. Psychiat.*, 159-163.

CHATTOPADHYAY, P.K., DE, S. and BISWAS, D. (1993). Impact of parental deprivation on cognitive functioning. *Ind. J. Clin. Psychol.*, 20(2), 63-68.

CHATTOPADHYAY, P.K., MAJUMDAR, A. and BASU, A.K. (1982). Habituation of electrodermal responses in tension headache suffers and non-tension headache controls. *Ind. J. Psychiat.*, 24(1), 61-65.

CHATTOPADHYAY, P.K., MALLICK, N. and SPIELBERGER, C.D. (1984). Adaptation of the state-trait inventory for Bengalee students. In : SPIELBERGER, C. *et al. (eds.), Cross cultural anxiety*, vol.3, Cl.10, Hemisphere Publishing Company, New York, London.

CHATTOPADHYAY, P.K., ROY, A.R., BISWAS, P.K. and BHATTACHARYYA, A.K. (1980). Habituation of alpha attenuation responses in depressed and normal subjects. *Ind. J. Clin. Psychol.*, 22, 151-155.

CHATTOPADHYAY, P.K., SAHA, S., and SAHA, S. (1994). Recent trends in research on psychological aspects of games and sports in India : A critical review. *Soc. Sci. Int.*, 10(2), 51-60.

CHATTOPADHYAY, P.K., SAHAY, R. and BISWAS, P.K. (1979). Accuracy in linear estimation : A study with three different lengths. *Ca. Rev.*, 5(1&2), 101-102.

CHAUHAN, S., JAIN, R.K., and KUMAR, A. (1983). Delusions in the psychodynamics of functional psychotic disorders. *Ind. J. Clin. Psychol.*, 10, 293-298.

CHEN, C.H., HUNG, C.C., WEI, F.C. and KOONG, F.J. (2001). Debrisoquine-4-hydroxylase (cyP 2 D6) genetic polymorphisms and susceptibility to schizophrenia in Chinese patients from Taiwan. *Psychiatr. Genet.*, 11(3), 153-155.

CHIARELLO, C. (1988). Lateralisation of lexical processes in the normal brain : A review of visual half-field research. In : A. Whitaker (ed.) *Contemporary reviews in neuropsychology*, Springer, New York.

CHOWDHURY, A.N. (1992). Koro Social Response (Urban) : A longitudinal study of North Bengal Koro Epidemic. *Ind. J. Psychiat.*, 34, 36-52.

CLADRIGE, G. (1978). Animal models of Schizophrenia. The care for LSD-25, *Schizo. Bull.*, 4, 186-209.

CLARK, J. and MALLEN, B. (1963). A follow-up study of Schizophrenia and depression in young adults. *Brit. J. Psychiat.*, 109, 491.

CLAUSEN, J.A. (1966). Family structure, socialisation, and personality. In Hoffman, L. and Hoffman, M. (eds.) *Review of United Development Research*, vol. II, New York: Russell Sage.

CLAUSEN, J.A. and KOHN, M.L. (1959). Relation of Schizophrenia to social structure of a small city. In Paramanick, B. (ed.) *Epidemiology of Mental Disorders*, Washington, D.C., AAAS.

CLAUSEN, J.N. (1966). Family structure, socialisation and personality. In Hoffman, L., and Hoffman, M. (eds.) *Review of Child Development Research,* vol. II, New York : Russell Sage.

CLOMPI, L. (1983). How to improve the treatment of Schizophrenia : A multicausal illness concept and its therapeutic consequences. In H. Stierlin, L.C., Wynne, and M. Wirsching (Eds.) *Psychosocial intervention in Schizophrenia.* New York, Springer-Verlag.

COLE, J.O. (1967). A lack of controls. *Int. J. Psychiat.*, 4(2), 129-131.

CONNELL, P.R. (1958). Amphetamine psychosic, Mandsley Monograph, No.5, London: Oxford University Press.

CONRAD, K. (1958a). Die beginnende Schizophrenie. Versuchejeiser Gestalt Analyse des Wahns (Commencing Schizophrenia : An attempt at a Gestalt Analysis of Delusion). Stuttgart, Thieme.

CONRAD, K. (1958b). "Uber Begriffund Wesender Apophanie" (On the concept and esscence of apophamy, in Mehrdimensionale Dignostik Und Therapie. Festschrift Zum 70. Geburtsteg Ernst Kretschmen), Stuttgart, Thieme.

COOPER, J.M. (1933). Mental disease situation in certain cultures. *J. Aben. Soc. Psychol.*, 29, 10.

COOPER, J.C. (1970). Use of a procedure for standardising psychiatric diagnosis In: *Psychiatric Epidemiology*, ed. Ahere, E.H., and Wing, J.K. London : Oxford University Press.

CORRIGAN, P.W. (1991). Social-skills training in adult psychiatic populations : A meta-analysis. *J. Behav. Ther. & Exptl. Psychiat.*, 22, 203-210.

CORTE, H.E., WOLF, M.M. and LOCKE, B.J. (1971). A comparison of procedures for eliminating self-injuries behaviour of retarded adolescents. *J. Appl. Beha. Analysis*, 4, 201-213.

COX, M.D., and KLINGE, V. (1976). Treatment and management of a case of self-injuries. *Beha. Res. And Ther.*, 14, 382-385.

CRANDELL, D.L. and DOHRENWEND, B.P. (1967). Some relations among psychiatric symptoms, organic illness and social class. *Amer. J. Psychiat.*, 123, 1527.

CRIDER, A. (1979). Schizophrenia: A biophysiological perspective. Hillsdale NJ: Lawrence Erlbaum.

CROMWELL, R.L. (1987). Argument concerning schizophrenia : The left hemisphere drains the swamp. In : Glass, A. (Ed.), *Individual differences in Hemispheric Specialisation. Plenum Press,* New York.

CROMWELL, R.L. and HELD, J.M. (1969). Alpha blocking latency and reaction time in Schizophrenics and normals. *Percept. Mot. Skills*, 29, 195-201.

CROW, J.J. (1982). Biological basis of mental disorders: The case of viral aetiology. In NAMBA, M. and KAIYA, H. (eds.) *Psychology of Schizophrenia*, New York, Pergamon Press.

CROW, T.J., MACMILLAN, J.F., JOHNSON, A.C. *et al.* (1986). The Northwich Park study of first-episode of schizophrenia : II. A randomised controlled trial of prophylactic treatment. *Brit. J. Psychiat.*, 148, 126-127.

CURRAN, J.P., MONTI, P.M. and CORRIVEAU, D.P. (1982). Treatment of Schizophrenia. In A.S. Bellack, M. Hersen, and A.E. Kazdin (Eds.) International Handbook of Behaviour Modification, New York: Plenum.

CURRAN, J.P., SUTTON, R.G., FARAONE, S.U. and GUENETTE, S. (1985). Inpatient approach: In A.S. Bellack, M. Hersen and A.E. Kazdin (eds.) *International Handbook of Behaviour Modification*, New York: Plenum.

DALLDORF, J.S. (1983). Medical needs of the adolescents. In E. Schopler and G.B. Mesibow (Eds.) *Autism in adolescents and adults*, New York, Plenum.

DASGUPTA, S. (1984). A study of anxiety: Unpublished Ph.D. thesis, University of Calcutta.

DASGUPTA, S., CHATTOPADHYAY, P.K. and GHOSH, K. (1983). Arousal in psychiatric patients: An interdisciplinary approach. *Ind. J. Clin. Psychol.*, 10, 233-238.

DAVID, A.S. (1990). Insight and Psychosis. *Brit. J. Psychiat.*, 156, 798-808.

DAVIDSON, G.C. (1969). Appraisal of behaviour modification techniques with adults in industrial settings. In *Behaviour Therapy : Appraisal and Status* (Ed.) FRANKS, C.M., New York: McGraw Hill.

DAVIDSON, M.A., McINNES, R.G. and PARNELL, R.W. (1957). The distribution of personality traits in seven year-old children : a combined psychological, psychiatric and somatotype study. *Brit. J. Edu. Psychol.*, 27, 48-61.

DAVIS, J.M. (1975). Critique of single amine theories: Evidence for a influence in the major mental illness. In : Freedman, D.K., ed. *Biology of the Major Psychoses.* Raven Press, New York, pp. 333-342.

DEUTSCH, A., and MUNICH, R. (1996). Psychotherapy with the severely and persistently mentally ill. In S. Soreff (ed.), *Handbook for the treatment of seriously mentally ill.* Toronto : Hogrefe and Huber.

DEUTSCH, H. (1945). *The psychology* : Gunne & Stralter, New York.

DEUTSCH, M. and DAVIS, K.I. (1983). Schizophrenia : a review of diagnostic and biological issues: II Biological issues. *Hosp. Comm. Psychiatry*, 34, 423.

DHAIRYAM, D. (1961). Research and need for development of psychotherapy. Menon, T.K. (ed.) *Recent Trends in Psychotherapy*, Orient-Longman.

DIAMOND, R. (1985) Drugs and the quality of life. The patients point of view. *J. Clin. Psychol.*, 46, 29-35.

DIEM, O. (1903). "Die einfach demente Form der Dementia Praecox (Dementia Simplex)" (the simple demented form of dementia praecox (dementia simplex). *Arch. Psychiat. Nerven Kr.*, 37, 111.

DIXON, L.B., and LEHMAN, A.F. (1995). Family intervention for schizophrenia. *Schizo. Bull.*, 21, 631-643.

DOHRENWEND, B.F., and DOHRENWEND, B.S. (1969). Social status and psycho-logical disorder : a casual inquiry. New York: Wiley.

DOUGLASS, R.J. (1972). Parlevian conditioning and the brain. In : Beakes, R.A. and Halliday, M.S., eds. *Inhibition and Learning.* Academic Press, London.

DRAKE, R.E. and SEDENER, L.I. (1986). The adverse effects of intensive treatment of chronic schizophrenia. *Comp. Psychiat.*, 27, 313-326.

DUMERMUTH, G. (1971). Electronic data processing in pediatric ERG – research. *Neuropediatric*, 2, 349-357.

DYKMAN, R.A., REESE, W.G., GALBRECHT, C.R., ACKERMAN, P.T. and SUNDERMAN, R.S. (1968). Autonomic responses in psychiatric patients. *Annl. N.Y. Acad. Sci.*, 147, 237-303.

EDELBERG, R. (1970). The information content of the recovery limb of the electrodermal responses. *Psychophysiol.*, 6, 527-539.

EGETH, H. (1967). Selective attention, *Psychol. Bull.*, 67, 41-57.

EISENBERG, L. (1956). The autistic child in adolescence. *Amer. J. Psychiat.*, 112, 607-612.

EKDAWI, M.Y. (1972). The Netherne Resettlement Unit : results of 10 years. *Brit. j. Psychiat..*, 121, 417-424.

EKMAN, P. (1982). Emotion in the human face. Cambridge University Press, New York.

EKMAN, P., FRIESEN, W.V. (1986). A new pan-cultural facial expression of emotion. *Mol. Emot.*, 10, 159-168.

EL-ISLAM, M.F. (1979). A better outlook for Schizophrenics living in extended families. *Brit. J. Psychiat.*, **135**, 343-347.

ELKES, J. (1961). Schizophrenic disorder in valuation to level of neural organisation: the need for some conceptual points of reference. In Folch, P.J. (ed.) *The Chemical Pathology of the Nervous System*, London, Pergamon.

ELLINGSON, R.J. (1954). The incidence of ERG abnormally among patients with mental disorders of apparently non-organic origin. *Amer. J. Psychiatr.* 111, 263-275.

ELLIS, A. (1973). Rational-emotive therapy. In R.J. Corsini (Ed.) *Current psychotherapies*, Itasca, IL : Peacock Publishers.

ELSÄSSER, G., and GRÜNEWALD, H.W. (1953). "Schizophrene order Schizophrenica psychosen Hirntraumatikern" (Schizophrenic and Schizophrenia – live psychoses in patients with brain injury). *Brit. J. Psychiat.* 190, 134.

EPSTEIN, L.H. and CLUSS, P.A. (1982). A behavioural medicine perspective on adherence to long-term medical rements. *J. Consult. Clin. Psychol.*, 50, 950-971.

ERNST, K. (1956). Geordnete Familienverhal tuisse Spaterer Schizophrener in Lichteeiner Naclunter Such Organisation. *Arch. Psychiat. Nervenkr.*, 194, 255-263, 303.

EVANS, A.S., BULLARD, D.M. and SOLOMON, M.H. (1961). The family as a potential resource in the rehabilitation of the chronic Schizophrenic patients : A study of 60 patients and their families. *Amer. J. Psychiat.*, 117, 1075-1083.

EYSENCK, H.J. (1976). Psychoticism as a dimension of personality, Hodder and Stonghton, London.

EYSENCK, H.J. (1985). Studying the effects of psychotherapy. In R.N. Gaind (Ed.), *Current themes in psychiatry*, vol.4, Medical and Scientific Books, New York.

EYSENCK, S.B.G. and McGURK, B.J. (1980). Impulsiveness and venture someness in a detection centre population. *Psychol. Rep.*, 47, 299-306.

FAIRBAIRN, W.R.D. (1952). *Psychoanalytic studies of the personality.* Tarvistock Publications, London, Routbdge & Kegan Paul.

FAIRWEATHER, G.W. (1964). *Social psychology in treating mental illness : an experimental approach*, New York, Wiley.

FALLOON, I.R.H. (1984). Developing and maintaining adherence to long term long-taking regiments. *Schizo. Bull.*, 10, 412-417.

FALLOON, I.R.H., BOYD, J.L. and McGILL, C.W. (1984). *Family care of Schizophrenia.* New York.

FALLOON, I.R.H., BOYD, J.L., McGILL, C.W., RANZANI, J., MOSS, H.B., GILDERMAN, A.M. and SIMPSON, G.M. (1985). Family management in the prevention of morbidity of Schizophrenia: Clinical outcome of a two years longitudinal study. *Arch. Gen. Psychiat.*, 42, 887-896.

FALLOON, I.R.H., FLANAGAN, S., FOY, R., LUKOFF, D., NARDER, S. and WITTLIN, B. (1983). Treatment of Schizophrenia, In C.E. Walker (ed.), *The handbook of clinical psychology : theory, research and practice*, Homewood, II, Dow-Jones-Irwin.

FALLOON, I.R.H. and PEDERSON, J. (1985). Family management in the prevention of morbidity of Schizophrenia : The adjustment of the family. *Brit. J. Psychiat.*, 147, 156-163.

FARIS, R.E.L. (1934). Cultural isolation and the Schizophrenic personality. *Amer. J. Social*, 40, 155-164.

FARIS, R.E.L. (1969). Cultural isolation and the Schizophrenic personality, 1434, 40, 155-164. Reprinted in Buss, A.H. and Buss, E. (Eds.). *Thesis of Schizophrenia*, New York: Atherton.

FARONE, S.V. and TSUANG, M.T. (1985). Quantitative models of the genetic transmission of Schizophrenia. *Psychol. Bull.*, 98, 41-66.

FAVELL, J.E. (1983). The management of aggressive behaviour. In E. Schopher and G.B. Mesibow (Eds.), *Autism in adolescents and adults*, New York, Plenum.

FAVELL, J.E., McGIMSEY, J.E. and JONES, M.L. (1978). The use of physical restraint in the treatment of self-injury and as positive reinforcement. *J. Appl. Beha. Anal.*, II, 225-241.

FEDERN, P. (1952). *Ego psychology and the psychoses.* London : Image.

FEINBERG, I., BRAUM, M., KORESKO, R.L. and GOTTLIEB, F. (1969). Stage 4 sleep in Schizophrenia. *Arch. Gen. Psychiat.*, 21, 262-266.

FENTON, W.S., and COLE, S.A. (1995). Psychological therapies of schizophrenia : Individual, group, and family. In : G.O. Gabbard (Ed.), *Treatments of Psychiatric Disorders*, Washington, D.C., American Psychiatrics Association.

FENZ, W.D. and VELNER, J. (1970). Physiological concomitants of behaviour indexes in Schizophrenia. *J. Abn. Psychol.*, 76, 27-35.

FERENCZI, S. (1926). Further contributions to the theory and technique of psycho-analysis. London, Hogarth.

FERSTER, C.B. (1961). Positive reinforcement and behavioural deficits of children. *Child Development*, 32, 437-456.

FERSTER, C.B. and DEMYER, M.K. (1962). A method for experimental analysis of the behaviour of children. *Amer. J. Orthopsychiatry*, 32, 89-98.

FEUCHTWANGER, E. and MAYER-GROSS, W. (1938). Brain injury and Schizophrenia. *Schweif. Arch. Neurol. Psychiat.*, 41(17), 301.

FINK, M. (1973). The electrodermal in clinical psychiatry. In : Mendels, J., ed., *Biological Psychiatry*, John Wiley and Sons, New York, pp. 331-344.

FISH, F.J. (1958). Classification of Schizophrenia. *Brit. J. Psychiat.*, 104, 944.

FISH, F.J. (1962). Schizophrenia: Bristol, Wright.

FLANIGAN, S., GABRIELI, E.R. and MacLEAN, P.P. (1957). Cerebral charges revealed by radioautography with S35-labeled I-methiomine. *Arch. Neurol. Psychiat.*, 77, 588-594.

FKOR-HENRY, P. (1969). Psychosis and temporal lobe epilepsy : a controlled investigation. *Epilepsia*, 10, 363-395.

FLOR-HENRY, P. (1976). Lateralised temporal limbic dysfunction and psychopathology. *Arnals. New York, Acad. Sci.*, 280, 777-793.

FLOR-HENRY, P. (1978). The undergone psychoses : A reflection of literalised dysfunction of the limbic system. In : LIVINGSTON, K.E. and HORNYKIEWICZ, O., eds., *The continuing evolution of the limbic system concept.* New York, Plenum Press, pp. 389-404.

FONAGY, P., and MORAN, G.S. (1990). Studies on the efficacy of child psychoanalysis. *J. Consult. Clin. Psychol.*, 58, 684-695.

FONBERG, E. (1972). Control of emotional behaviour through the hypothalamus and amygdaloid complex. In : *Physiology, Emotion and Psychosomatic Illnesses*, CIBA Foundation Symposium, Holland, Academic Science Publishers, pp. 131-161.

FORREST, F., GEIER, C., SNOW, H., and STEINBACK, M. (1964). Drug maintenance problems of rehabilitated mental patients : The current drug dosage "merry-go-round". *Amer. J. Psychiat.*, 121, 33.

FOXX, R.M. and LIVESAY, J. (1984). Maintenance of response suppression following over correction: a 10-year retrospective examination of eight cases. *Analysis of Intervention in developmental Disabilities*, 4, 65-69.

FOXX, R.M., McMORROW, M.J., BITTLE, R.G. and BECHTEL, D.R. (1986). The successful treatment of a finally-diagnosed included contingent electric shock. *Beha. Ther.*, 17, 170-186.

FRANZEN, G. and INGUAR, D.H. (1975a). Abnormal distortion of cerebral activity in chronic Schizophrenics. *J. Psychiat. Res.*, 12, 199-214.

FRANZEN, G., and INGUAR, D.H. (1975b). Absence of activation of frontal structures during psychological testing of chronic Schizophrenics. *J. Neurol. Nemosung, and Psychiat.*, 38, 1027-1032.

FREEMAN, W. (1953). Level of achievement after lobotomy : A study of one thousand cases. *Amer. J. Psychiat.*, 110, 269.

FREEMAN, T., CAMERON, J.L. and McGHIE, A. (1958). Chronic Schizophrenics – London : Tavistock.

FREEMAN, A., SIMON, K., BEUTLER, L. and ARKOWITZ, H. (1989). Comprehensive handbook of cognitive theory. New York, Plenum.

FREUD, S. (1896). 'Weitere Bernernungen ulcer die Abwehr – Neuropsychosen'. In Strachey, J. (Ed.). *Interpretation of dreams*, George Allen & Unwin Ltd., London, 1982.

FREUD, S. (1914a). *The Psychopathology of Everyday Life.* New York : MacMillan.

FREUD, S. (1914b). On narcissim an introduction. In collected papers, vol. IV, London: Hogarth Press (First Published in 1914).

FREUD, S (1924). "Certain neurotic mechanisms in jealousy, paranoia, and homosexuality", in collected papers, vol.II, London, Hogarth Press.

FREUD, S. (1924). "Psychoanalytic notes upon an autobiographical account of a case of paranoia", in Collected Papers, vol.III, London : Hogarth Press.

FRIEDE, R. (1966). The histochemical architectures of Ammon's Horn as related to its selective ability. *Acta. Neuropathologica*, 6, 1-13.

FRIEDHOFF, A.J. and VAN WINKLE, E. (1953). Conversion of dopamine to 3,4-dimethoxyphenyl acetic acid in Schizophrenic patients. *Nature*, 199, 1271-1272.

FRITH, C.D., STEVENS, M., JOHNSTONE, E.C. and CROW, T.I. (1979). Skin conductance responsivity during acute episodes of Schizophrenia as a predictor of symptomatic improvement. *Psychol. Med.*, 8, 1-6.

FROMM-REICHMAN, F. (1948). A twin study of individuals infantile autism. In M. Ruller and E. Schloper (eds.) *Autism : A reappraisal of concepts and treatments*, New York: Plenum Press, pp. 219-241.

FROMM-REICHMAN, F. (1952). Some aspects of psychoanalytic psychotherapy with Schizophrenics, In : Brody, E.B. and Redlich, F.C. (eds.) Psychotherapy with Schizophrenics. New York : International Universities Press, Inc.

FROMM-REICHMAN, F. (1954). Psychotherapy of Schizophrenia. *Amer. J. Psychiat.*, 111, 410-419.

FRUCHITWANGER, E. and MAYER-GROSS, W. (1938). "Hirnverletzumy and Schizophrenia" (brain injury and schizophrenia). *Schweiz. Arch. Neurol. Psychiat.*, 41, 17.

FUXE, K. (1965). Evidence for the existence of monoamine neurons in the central nervous system. IV. Distribution of monoamine nerve terminals in the central nervous system. *Acta. Psychol. Scandinarica*, 64, 37-84.

GABBARD, G.D. (1999). Schizophrenia: In G.D. Gabbard (ed.) *Psychodynamic Psychiatry in Clinical Practice*, Washington, D.C., APA.

GANGULY, D. (2000). Epidemiological findings on prevalence of mental disorders in India. *Ind. J. Psychiat.*, 42(1), 14-20.

GARMEZY, N. (1966). The prediction of performance in Schizophrenia. In Hoch, P.H. and Zubin, J. (Eds.). *Psychopathology and Schizophrenia*, New York, Grune and Straltin, pp. 129-181.

GENSISTS, D.M., RAGLAND, J.D., GUR, R.C., and GUR, R.E. (1997). Neuropsychological model of schizophrenia : A longitudinal study. *Schiz. Res.*, 24, 289-298.

GERARD, D.L. and HOUSTON, L.G. (1953). Family setting and the social etiology of Schizophrenia. *Psychiat. Quarterly*, 27, 90-101.

GESCHWIND, A. and GALABURDA, A.M. (1985). Cerebral lateralisation : Biological mechanism, associations, and pathology : A hypothesis and a program for research. *Arch. Neurol.*, 2, 428-459.

GEVINS, A.S., ZEITLIN, G.M., DOYLE, J.C., YINGLING, C.D., SCHAFFER, R.E., CALLAWAY, E. and YEAGER, C.L. (1979). Electro encephalogram correlates of higher cortisol functions. *Science*, 203, 665-668.

GHORPADE, M.B., and KUMAR, V. (1988). Introduction to modern psychotherapy. *Himalaya Publishing House*, Mumbai.

GILLIES, H. (1949). The Schizophrenic disorders. In : *Modern Practice in Psychological Medicine*, ed., J.R. Rees, London, Hurper, pp. 272, 315.

GILLMAN, R.D. (1965). Brief psychotherapy : a psychoanalytic view. *Amer. J. Psychiat.*, 122, 601-611.

GOLDBERG, A. and RUBIN, B. (1984). Recovery of patients during periods of supposed neglect. *Brit. J. Med. Psychol.*, 37, 266-272.

GOLDBERG, S.C. (1985). Negative and deficit symptoms in Schizophrenia do respond to neuroleptics. *Schizo. Bull.*, 11, 453-456.

GOLDSTEIN, A. (1984). Psychological skill training : *structured learning technique*, New York, Pergamon Press.

GOLDSTEIN, K. (1939). The significance of special mental tests for diagnosis and prognosis in Schizophrenia. *Amer. J. Psychiat.*, 96, 575

GOLDSTEIN, K. (1944). Methodological approach to the study of Schizophrenic thought disorders. In *Language and Thought in Schizophrenia* (ed.) KASANIN, J.S., Berkeley : University of California Press.

GOLDSTEIN, M.J. (1991). Schizophrenia and family therapy. In : B. Beitman, and G.L. Klerman (Eds.), *Integrating Pharmacotherapy and Psychotherapy*, Washington, D.C., American Psychiatric Association.

GOLDSTEIN, M.J., ACKER, C.S., CROCKETT, J.J. and RIDDLE, J.J. (1966). Psychophysiological reactions to films by chronic Schizophrenics : I. Effects of drug status. *J. Aben. Psychol.*, 91, 335-344.

GOLDSTEIN, M.J., and MILKLOWITZ, D.J. (1995). Effectiveness of psycho-educational family therapy in the treatment of schizophrenic disorders. *J. Marital and Family Ther.*, 21, 361-376.

GOLDSTEIN, N.J., RODNICK, E.H., EVANS, J.R., PHILIP, R.A. *et al.* (1978). Drug and family therapy in the aftercare of acute schizophrenics. *Arch. Gen. Psychiat.*, 35, 1169-1177.

GOLDSTEIN, W. (1978). Toward an integrated theory of Schizophrenia. *Schizo. Bull.*, 4, 426-436.

GOLDSTROM, I. and MANDERSHEID, R. (1981). The chronically mentally ill. A descriptive analysis from the uniform data instrument. *Community Support Services*, 2, 4-9.

GOMES-SCHWARTZ, B. (1984). Individual psychotherapy of Schizophrenia. In A.S. Bellack (Ed.), *Schizophrenia*, Orland, FL : Grune and Stratton.

GOTTESMAN, I.I., McGUFFIN, P. and FARMER, A.E. (1987). Clinical genetics as clues to the "real" genetics of Schizophrenia. *Schze. Bull.*, 13, 23-47.

GOTTESMAN, I.I. and SHIELDS, J. (1982). *Schizophrenia : epigenetic puzzle.* Cambridge University Press, Cambridge.

GOTTLIEB, G.S., FROHMAN, C.E. and BECKETT, P.G.S. (1969). A theory of neuronal malfunction in Schizophrenia. *Amer. J. Psychiat.*, 126, 149-156.

GOTTESCHALK, L.A., MAYERSON, P. and GOTTLIEB, A.A. (1967). Prediction and evaluation of outcome in an emergency brief psychotherapy clinic. *J. Nerv. Ment. Dis.*, 144, 77-96.

GOVERNMENT OF INDIA (1982). National Mental Health Programme for India. Ministry of Health and Family Welfare, New Delhi.

GRAHAM, F.K. and CLIFTON, R.K. (1966). Heart rate change as a component of the orienting response. *Psychol. Bull.*, 65, 305-370.

GREEN, M.F., SATZ, P., SMITH, C. and NELSON, L. (1989). Is there atypical handedness in schizophrenia? *J. Abn. Psychol.*, 98, 57-61.

GREENBLATT, M. (1944). Age and electroencephalographic abnormality in neuro-psychiatric patients : A study of 593 cases. *Amer. J. Psychiat.*, 101, 82-90.

GREENBLATT, M., SOLOMON, M., and EVANS, A.S. (1965). *Drugs and social therapy of chronic Schizophrenia.* Springfield, II : Charles C. Thomas.

GRINKER, R.R., WERBLE, B. and DRYE, R.C. (1988). *The borderline syndrome : A behavioural study of ego functions.* New York : Basic Books, Inc.

GRINSPOON, L. (1969). The utility of psychotherapy with Schizophrenia. *Int. J. Psychiat.*, 8(4), 727-729.

GRINSPOON, L., EWALT, J.R., and SHADER, R. (1967). Long term treatment of chronic Schizophrenia. *Int. J. Psychiat.*, 4(2), 116-128.

GRUEN, P.H., SECHER, E.J., ALTMAN, R., LANGER, G., TABRIZI, M.A. and HALPERN, F.S. (1978). Relation to plasma prolactin to clinical response in Schizophrenic patients. *Arch. Gen. Psychiat.*, 35, 1222-1227.

GRUNTHAL, E. (1936). On the psychoses of epilepsy. *Z. ges. Neurol. Psychiat.*, 154, 395-470.

GRUZELIER, J.H. (1973). Bilateral asymmetry of skin conductance orienting activity and levels in Schizophrenia. *Biol. Psychiat.*, 1, 21-41.

GRUZELIER, J.H. (1978). Propranolol acts to modulate autonomic orienting habituation processes in Schizophrenia. In : Roberts, E., and Amacher, P., eds., *Propranolol and Schizophrenia*, vol.99, A.R. Liss, Inc., New York; pp. 99-118.

GRUZELIER, J.H. (1987). Cerebral laterality and schizophrenia. In : Glass, A. (Ed.,) *Individual differences in hemispheric specialisation*, Plenum Press, New York.

GRUZELIER, J.H. (1990). Brain localisation and neuropsychology in schizophrenia : Syndrome and neurodevelopmental implications. In : Hafner, H., and Gattaz, W.F. (Eds.), *Search for the cause of schizophrenia*, vol.2, Springer-Verlag, Berlin, pp. 301-320.

GRUZELIER, J.H. and VENABLES, P.H. (1972). Skin conductance orienting activity in a heterogegeous sample of Schizophrenics. *J. Ment. Dis.*, 155, 227-228.

GRUZELIER, J.H., and VENABLES, P.H. (1973). Skin conductance responses to tones with and without attentional significance to Schizophrenic and non-Schizophrenic psychiatric patients. *Neuropsychologia*, 11, 221-230.

GRUZELIER, J.H. and VENABLES, P.H. (1975a). Relations between 2-flash threshold discrimination and electrodermal activity, re-examined in Schizophrenics and normals. *J. Psychiat.* Res., 12, 73-85.

GRUZELIER, J.H. and VENABLES, P.H. (1975b). Evidence of high and low levels of physiological arousal in Schizophrenia. *Psychophysiol.*, 12, 66-73.

GUENTHER, W., DANOS, P., GODET, J.L., GUILBERT, E., BREITLING, D., and RODNOT, P. (1988). Bilateral brain dysfunction during motor activity in Type-II schizophrenia measured by EEG mapping. *Biol. Psychiat.*, 23, 295-311.

GUESS, D., HELMSTETTER, E., TURNBULL, H.R., and KNOWLTON, S. (1987). Use of aversive procedures with persons who are disabled : A historical review and critical analysis TASH Monograph Series, No.2, Seattle, TASH.

GUNDERSON, J.G., FRANK, A.F., KATZ, H.M., VANNICELLI, M.L., FROSCH, J.B., and KNAPP, P.H. (1984). Effects of psychotherapy in schizophrenia : II. Comparative outcome of two forms of treatment. *Schiz. Bull.*, 10, 564-598.

GUPTA, A. (1993). Differential hemisphere processing of information in schizophrenia. *J. Psychiat. Res.*, 27, 79-88.

GUPTA, A., and SACHDEVA, A. (1991). Information processing strategies employed by paranoid and non-paranoid schizophrenia : A laterality study. *Ind. J. Psychiat.*, 33, 307-308.

GUR, R.E. (1977). Motoric laterality in balance in Schizophrenia. *Arch. Gen. Psychiat.*, 34, 33-37.

GUR, R.E. (1978). Left hemisphere dysfunction and left hemisphere overactivation in Schizophrenia. *J. Abn. Psychol.*, 87, 226-238.

GUR, R.E. (1979). Cognitive concomitants of hemispheric dysfunction in schizophrenia. *Arch. Gen. Psychiat.*, 36, 269-279.

GUREJE, O. (1988). Sensorimotor laterality in schizophrenia : which features transcend cultural influences? *Acta. Psychiat. Scand.*, 77, 188-193.

HABEL, UTE, GUR, R.C., MANDAL, M.K., SALLOUM, J.B., GUR, R.E., and SCHNEIDER, F. (2000). Emotional processing in schizophrenia across cultures : Standardised measures of discrimination and experience. *Schizo. Res.*, 42, 57-66.

HAGEN, R.L. (1975). Behavioural therapies and the treatment of Schizophrenics. *Schizo. Bull.*, 1, 70-96.

HALE, A.S., and PINNITI, N.R. (1994). Excorcism – Resistant. Ghost possession treated with clopenthixol. *Brit. J. Psychiat.*, 165, 396-398.

HALL, J. and BAKER, R. (1973). Token economy systems : Breakdown and control. *Beha. Ther. Res., Ther.*, 11, 253-263.

HALL, R.V. and HALL, M.C. (1980). *How to planned ignoring.* Lawrence, Ks : H&H – Enterprise.

HAMILTON, L.A. (Tr.) (1968). May's conclusions are found to be generally confirmed by clinical experience. *Int. J. Psychiat.*, 8(4), 730-733.

HAMILTON, M. (1976). Fishe's Schizophrenia. Bristol. John Wright & Sons.

HAMILTON , V. (1963). Size constancy and curve responsiveness in psychosis. *Brit. J. Psychol.*, 54, 25-39.

HAMILTON, V. (1979). Information processing aspects of neurotic anxiety and the schizophrenia. In: Warburton Hamilton (ed.), *Human stress and cognition*, Wiley, New York.

HANFMANN and KASANIN, J.S. (1942). *Conceptual thinking in Schizophrenia*, New York Nervous and Mental Diseases, Publ. 316.

HARACZ, J.L. (1982). The dopamine hypothesis : an overview of studies with Schizophrenic patients. *Schige. Bull.*, 8, 438-469.

HARE, R.D. (1972). Dissociation of conditioned electrodermal and cardiovascular response in psychopaths. *Presented at the Society for Psychophysiological Res.*, October.

HARE, R.D. (1973). Psychopathy : In Venables, P.H., and Christic, M.J., eds. *Research in Psychophysiology*, Wiley, London, pp. 325-348.

HARPER, R.G., WIENS, A.N. and MATARAZZO, J.D. (1978). *Nonverbal communication : The State of the Art.* New York, John Wiley.

HARTMANN, D.F., ROPER, B.L. and GELFAND, D.M. (1977). In B.B. Lahey and A.K. Kazdin (Eds.) *Advances in Clinical Child Psychology* (pp. 1-46), New York, Plenum Press.

HARVEY, P.D. (1983). Speech competence in and Schizophrenic psychoses : The association between clinically rated though disorder and cohesion and reference performance. *J. Abn. Psychol.*, 92, 368-377.

HASSOL, L., MARGARET, A. and CAMERON, N. (1952). The production of language distraction through personalised distraction. *J. Psychol.*, 33, 289.

HAYNESS, R.B. (1979). Strategies to improve compliance with referral, appointments and prescribed medical regimens. In R.B. Hayness, D.W. Taylor and D.L. Sackett (Eds.), *Compliance in Health Care*, Baltimore : Johns Hophins Univ. Press.

HEATH, R.G., and KRUPP, I.M. (1968). Schizophrenia as a special biologic disease. *Amer. J. Psychiat.*, 124, 1019-1024.

HEIDEGGER, M. (1953). *Seim and Zeit (being and time)*, Pfuthigen : Nerve.

HEIN, P.L., GREEN, R.L. and WILSON, W.P. (1962). Latency and duration of photically elicited arousal response in the electroencephalogram of patients with chronic regressive Schizophrenia. *J. Nev. Ment. Dis.*, 135, 361-364.

HEMSLEY, D.R. (1978). Limitations of operant procedures in the modification of Schizophrenic functioning. The possible relevance of studies of cognitive disturbance. *Beha. Anal. And Mod.*, 2, 165-173.

HENDERSON, D.K. and GILLESPIE, R.D. (1950). *Text Book of Psychiatry*, London, O.U.P.

HESTON, L.L. (1970). *The genetics of Schizophrenia and Schizoid disease science*, 167, 249-259.

HILL, D. (1956). *Electroencephalography*, London, Mcdonal.

HILLBOM, E. (1960). Psychiatric disorders in Foster Home – reared children of Schizophrenic mothers. *Brit. J. Psychiat.*, 112, 819-825.

HOCH, P.H., and POLATIN, P. (1949). Pseudoneurotic forms of Schizophrenia. *Psychiat. Quart.*, 23, 248-296.

HOGARTY, G.E., ANDERSON, C.M., REISS, D.J., KORNBLITH, S.J., GREENWALD, P.D., JAVNA, C.D., MADONIA, M.J. and EPICS Schizophrenia Research Group (1986). Family psycho education, social skill training, and maintenance chemotherapy in the aftercare treatment of Schizophrenia : I. One year effects of a controlled study on relapse and expressed emotion.. *Arch. Gen. Psychiat.*, 43, 633-642.

HOGARTY, G.E., ANDERSON, C.M., REISS, D.J., KORNBLITH, S.J., GREENWALD, P.D., ULRICH, R., and CARTER, M. (1991). Family psychoeducation, social skill training, and maintenance chemotherapy in the aftercare treatment of schizophrenia : II : two-year effects of a controlled study on relapse and adjustment. *Arch. Gen. Psychiat.*, 48, 340-341.

HOGARTY, G.E., GOLDBERG, S.C., and SCHOOLER, N.R. *et al.* (1984). Drugs and sociotherapy in the aftercare of schizophrenia patients III : Adjustment of non-relapsed patients. *Arch. Gen. Psychiat.*, 31, 609-625.

HOGARTY, G.E., KORNBLITH, S.J., GREENWALD, D., DIBARRY, A.L., COOLEY, S., FLESHER, S., REISS, D., *et al.* (1995). Personal therapy : A disorder relevant psychotherapy for schizophrenia. *Schizo. Bull.*, 21, 379-393.

HOGARTY, G.E., SCHOOLER, N.R., ULRICH, R., MUSSARE, E. and others (1979). Fluphenazine and social therapy in the aftercare of Schizophrenic patients. *Arch. Gen. Psychiat.*, 36, 1283-1294.

HOLLINGSHED, A.B., and REDLICH, I.C. (1958). *Social class and mental illness: A community study,* New York : Wiley.

HOLLON, H.D., and FAWCETT, J. (1995). Depression : combined medication and psychotherapy : In : G.O. Gobbard (Ed.), *Treatment of Psychiatric Disorders,* Washington, D.C., American Psychiatric Association.

HOLMBOE, R., and ASTRUP, C. (1957). A fellow-up study of 255 patients and acute Schizophrenia and Schizophrenic from psychoses. *Acta. Psychiat. Second.*, 23, 248.

HOLMOSTEDT, B. (1967). Historical survey. In Efren, D.H., Holmsted, B. and Klina, N.S. (eds.) *Ethnophin mallelogic search for psychoactive drugs.* Public Health Service Publication No. 1645, U.S. Govt. Printing Office, Washington, D.C.

HOLTZMAN, P.S. (1987). Recent studies of psychophysiology in Schizophrenia. *Schze. Bull.*, 13, 49-75.

HOMER, A.L., and PETERSON, L. (1980). Differential reinforcement of other behaviour: A preferred response elimination procedure. *Beha. Ther.*, 11, 449-471.

HOMME, L.E. (1965). Perspective in Psychology : Controls of Coverants, the operants of the mind. *Psychol. Recd.*, 24, 501-511.

HOOLEY, J.H. (1985). Expressed emotions : A review of the critical literature. *Clin. Psychol. Rev.*, 5, 119-139.

HORVATH, T. and MEARES (1979). The sensory filter in Schizophrenia : A study of habituation, arousal and the dopamine hypothesis. *Brit. J. Psychiat.*, 134, 139-145.

HOUTHAN, J.P. (1975). Visual work recognition and autonomic responsivity of Schizophrenic patients. *ISAS Catalogue of Selected Documents in Psychology*, 5, 105.

HURST, L. (1951). Genetics of Schizophrenia : reply to Pastore. *Psychol. Bull.*, 48, 402.

HUSTON, P. and PEPERNIC, M. (1958). Prognosis in Schizophrenia. In L. Bellan (Ed.) Schizophrenia: *A review of the syndrome.* New York : Logos Press.

HUXLEY, A. (1959). *The doors of perception and heaven and hell.* Penguin Press.

IKUTA, A. (1974). Somatosensory evoked potentials (SGP) in normal subjects, Schizophrenics and epileptics, Fukvoka. *Acta. Medica*, 65, 1010-1019.

ISAACS, W., THOMAS, J. and GOLDDIAMOND, I. (1960). Application of operant conditioning to reinstate verbal behaviour in psychotics. *J. Speech and Hearing Dis.*, 25, 8.

ISHIKAWA, K. (1968). On the visual evoked responses in paired light flashes in Schizophrenics. *Korume. Med.* J., 15, 157-167.

ITIL, T.M. (1979). Qualitative and quantitative EEG findings in Schizophrenia. *Schizophrenia Bulletin*, 3, 61-79.

ITIL, T.M., SALETU, B. and DAVIS, S. (1972). EEG findings in chronic Schizophrenics based on digital computer period analysis and analog power spectra. *Biol. Pscyhiat.*, 5, 1-13.

ITIL, T., SIMEON, J. and COFFIN, C. (1976). Qualitative and quantitative EG in psychotic children. *Dis. Nerv. Syst.*, 37, 247-252.

ITIL, M.T., HSU, W., SALETU, B. and MEDNICK, S.A. (1974). Computer ERG and auditory evoked potential investigation in children at high rise for Schizophrenia. *Amer. J. Psychiat.*, 131, 892-900.

ITIL, T.M., SALETU, B. and DAVIS, S. (1972). EEG findings in chronic Schizophrenics based on digital computer period analysis and analog power spectra. *Biol. Psychiat.*, 5, 1-13.

ITIL, T., SIMEON, J. and COFFIN, C. (1976). Qualitative and quantitative ERG in psychotic children. *Dis. Nerv. Syst.*, 37, 247-252.

ITIL, M.T., HSU, W., SALETU, B. and MEDNICK, S.A. (1974). Computer ERG, and auditory evoked potential investigation in children at high rise for Schizophrenia. *Amer. J. Psychiat.*, 131, 892-900.

ITIL, T.M., SALETU, B. and DAVIS, S. (1972). EEG findings in chronic Schizophrenics based on digital computer period analysis and analog power spectra. *Biol. Psychiat.*, 5, 1-13.

ITIL, T.M., SIMEON, J. and COFFIN, C. (1976). Qualitative and quantitative EEG in Psychotic Children. *Dis. New Syst.*, 37, 247-252.

JABLENSKY, P. (1989). Epidemiology and cross-cultural aspects of schizophrenia. *Psychiat. Annals*, 19, 516-524.

JACKSON, D. (1960). *The etiology of Schizophrenia.* New York : Basic Books.

JACO, E.G. (1954). The social isolation hypothesis in Schizophrenia. *Amer. Sociological Res.*, 19, 567-577.

JACO, E.G. (1960). *The social epidemiology of mental disorders.* New York : Russell, Sage Foundation.

JAHAN, M., HAQUE-NIZAMIE, S., NIZAMIE, A., and KHALIQUE, A. (2002). Efficacy of Luria Nebraska Neuropsychological battery in identifying cognitive deficit in epileptic patients. *Ind. J. Clin. Psychol.*, 29(2), 132-138.

JAMES, A.L. and BARRY, R.J. (1980). A review of psychophysiology in early onset psychosis. *Schze. Bull.*, 6, 506-525.

JASPER, K. (1910). "Eifersuch tswahn Ein Beitrag Zur Frage 'Entwicklungeiner Person lichkeit order Prozess" (Delusions of Jealousy. A contribution of the question 'development of a personality of process). *Z. gerNeurol. Psychiat.*, L, 567.

JENSEN, P.S., RAYAN, N.D., and PRIEN, R. (1992). Psychopharmacology of child and adolescent major depression : Present status and future directions. *J. Child and Adolescent Psychopharma*, 2, 31-45.

JOHN, J.P., KHANNA, S., MUKUNDAN, C.R. and REDDY, S. (2001). Relation between psychopathological dimensions and performance of frontal lobe tests in schizophrenia. *Ind. J. Psychol. Med.*, 24(2), 19-26.

JOHNSON, D.A.W. (1985). Antipsychotic medication : Clinical guidelines for maintenance therapy. *J. Clin. Psychiat.*, 46, 6-15.

JOHNSON, J. and KOEGEL, R.L. (1982). Behavioural assessment and curriculum development. In T.L. Koegel, A. Reincover, and A.L. Egel (Eds.) *Educating and Understanding Artistic Children Houston*, TX : College, Hill Press.

JOHNSON, W.L., BAUMEISTER, A.A., PENLAND, M.J. and INWALD, C. (1982). Experimental analysis of injurious, stereotypic, and collateral behaviour of retarded persons: effects of over correction and reinforcement of alternative responding. *Analysis of Intervention of Development Disabilities*, 2, 41-46.

JONES, M. (1953). *The therapeutic community : a new treatment method in psychiatry*. Basic Books, New York.

JUNG, C.G. (1909). The psychology of dementia praecox. *Trans. Brit. Nerve. & Ment. Dis. Monogr.* No.3, New York.

KALA, A.K. and WIG, N.N. (1978). Delusions manifested by India paranoid psychotics. *Ind. J. Psychiat.*, 20, 227.

KALA, A.K. and WIG, N.N. (1982). Delusions across culture. *J. Soc. Psychiat.*, 28, 185-193.

KALLMANN, F. (1946). The genetic theory of Schizophrenia : An analysis of 691 twin index families. *Amer. J. Psychiat.*, 103, 309.

KALLMANN, F., FALEK, A., HURZELER, M. and ERLENMEYER-KIBLING, L. (1964). The developmental aspects of children with two Schizophrenic parents. In P. Solomon and B. Glueck (Eds.), *Recent Research on Schizophrenia Psychiat. Res. Rep.* 19, Washington, D.C., APA.

KALLMAN, F.J. (1930). *The genetics of Schizophrenia*, New York; Augustin.

KALLMANN, L. (1953). *Heredity in health and mental disorder.* New York : Norton.

KALYANSUNDARAM, S. and VERGHESE, M. (2000). *Innovations in psychiatric rehabilitation.* In : S. Kalyansundaram and M. Verghese (Eds.) The Richmond Fellowship Society (India), Bangalore.

KANE, J.M., RIFKIN, A., WOERNER, M., and REARDON, G. (1982). Low dose neuropleptics in outpatient schizophrenics. *Psychopharmacol. Bull.*, 18, 20-21.

KANFER, F.H. (1985). Target selection for clinical change programs. *Behavioural Assessment*, 7, 7-20.

KANAS, N. (1985). Inpatient and outpatient group therapy for Schizophrenic patients. *Amer. J. Psychother.*, 39(3), 431-439.

KANTOR, R.E., WALLNER, J.M. and WINDER, C.L. (1953). Process and reactive Schizophrenia. *J. Consult. Psychol.*, 17, 157-162.

KAPUR, M. (1992). School mental health in India : In S. Malhotra, A. Malhotra, V.K. Verma (Eds.), *Child mental health in India*, New Delhi, Macmillan, India.

KAPUR, M. (2001). Mental health, illness, and therapy. In : Pandey, J. (ed.) *Psychology in India Revisited: Personality and Health Psychology*, vol.2, ICSSR, Sage Publication, New Delhi, India.

KAPUR, R.L. (1987). Commentory on culture bound syndromes and international disease classification. *Cul. Med. Psychiat.*, 11, 43-48.

KARNO, M., JENKINS, J.H., DeLA SELVA, A., SANTANA, F., TELLES, C., LOPEZ, S,. and MINTZ, J. (1987). Expressed emotion and Schizophrenic outcome among Mexican-American Families. *J. Nerv. Ment. Dist.*, 175, 143-151.

KARON, B.P. and O'GRADY, P. (1969). Intellectual test charges in Schizophrenic patients in the first six months of treatment. *Psychother : Theory, Res., and Practice*, 6, 88-96.

KARON, B.P. and VANDENBOS, G.R. (1970). Experience; medicating and the effectiveness of psychotherapy with Schizophrenics : A note on Qrs-May and Tuma's conclusions. *Brit. J. Psychiat.*, 116(533), 427-428.

KARON, B.P. and VANDENBOS, G.R. (1981). Psychotherapy of schizophrenia : the treatment of childs. New York, Jason Aronson.

KAY, D.W.K. and ROTH, M. (1961). Environmental and hereditary factors in the Schizophrenics of old age. *J. Ment. Sci.*, 107, 649-686.

KAZDIN, A.E. (1977). Assessing the clinical or applied significance of behaviour charges through validation. *Beha. Mod.*, 1, 427-452.

KAZDIN, A.E. (1978). *History of behaviour modification : Experimental foundations of contemporary research.* Baltimore : University Press.

KAZDIN, A.E., BASS, D., AYERS, W.A., and RODGERS, A. (1990). Empirical and clinical focus of child and adolescent psychotherapy research. *J. Consult. Clin. Psychol.*, 58, 729-740.

KEANE, T.M., FOY, D.W., NUNN, B. and RYCHTARIK, R.G. (1984). Antapanse compliance in alcoholic veterans. *J. Clin. Psychol.*, 40, 340-344.

KENNEDY, J. (1963). Special message on mental illness and mental retardation. *Amer. Psychol.*, 18, 280.

KERNBERG, O.E. (1967). Borderline personality organisation. *J. Amer. Psychoanal. Assoc.*

KESSLER, K.A. and WALETZKY, J.P. (1981). Clinical use of antipsychotics. *Amer. J. Psychiat.*, 138, 202-209.

KIESSLER, R.C., McGONAGLE, K.A., SHANYANA, Z., and NELSON, C.B. *et al.* (1994). Life time and 12-months prevalence of DSM-III-R psychiatric disorders in the United States : Results from National Comorbidity Survey. *Arch. Gen. Psychiat.*, 51, 8-19.

KETY, S.S., ROSENTHAL, D., WENDER, P.H. and SCHULSINGER, F. (1968). The types of prevalence of mental illness in the biological and adaptive families of adopted Schizophrenics. *Int. J. Psychiat.*, 1, 409-446.

KHAN, H.A., and MOHAN, J. (1992). A study of the effect of special sports training on some psychological attributes of athletes. *Sports Sci.* J., 95(1), 1-10.

KIEV, A. (1972). *Trans cultural psychiatry.* New York, Free Press.

KILLAM, E.K., KILLAM, K.F., and SHAW, T. (1957). The effects of psychotherapeutic compounds on central afferent and limble pathways. *Annals. N.Y. Acad. Sc.*, 64, 784-804.

KIMURA, D. (1961). Cerebral dominance and the perception of verbal stimuli. *Can. J. Psychol.*, 15, 166-191.

KIND, H. (1966). The psychogenesis of Schizophrenia : A review of the literature. *Brit. J. Psychiat.*, 112, 333-362.

KIRK, S.A. and THERRIEN, M.E. (1975). Community mental health and the fate of former hospitalised patients. *Psychiat.*, 38, 209-217.

KIRMAYER, L.J. (1989). Cultural variations in the response to psychiatric disorders and emotional distress. *Soc. Sc. Med.*, 29, 327-339.

KLEIN, M. (1952). *Developments in Psycho-Analysis* (Rivere Joan). London : Hogarth.

KLEINMUNTZ, B. (1974). *Essentials of abnormal psychology.* Harper and Row, New York.

KLEIST, K. (1913). Involutional paranoia. *Allg. 2. Psychiat.*, 70.1. – 248, 247.

KLEIST, K. (1914). Aphasige and Geistekrankheit (aphasia and mental illness). *Munch. Med. Weshr.*, 61, 8.

KLEIST, K. (1921). Autochthonous psychoses of degeneration. *Z. Ges. Neurol. Psychiat.*, 69, 1.-215, 298.

KLEIST, K. (1923). "Die Auffasung der Schizophrenienals systemurankheiter (Heredo-degenerationen)" (the concept of the Schizophrenias as system diseases (Heredodegenerations). *Klin. Wschr.*, 1, 962.

KLEIST, K. (1927). Gegenhalten (motorischer negativismus), Zwangagrifen und Thalamus opticus" (opposition (motor negativism), forced grasping and the optic thalamus), *Mschr. Psychiat. Neurol.*, 65, 317.

KLEIST, K. (1960). Schizophrenic symptoms and cerebral pathology. *J. Ment. Sci.*, 106, 246.

KLERMAN, G.L. (1984). Ideology and science in the individual psychotherapy of schizophrenia. *Schiz. Bull.*, 10, 608-611.

KLOPFER, B. (1946). *The Forschach technique.* New York : World Book Co., p.317.

KOBASA, S.C. (1979). Stressful life events, personality, and health : An inquiry into hardiness. *J. Par. & Soc. Psychol.*, 37(1), 1-11.

KOHN, M.S. and CLAUSEN, J.A. (1955). A social isolation and Schizophrenia. *Amer. Social Rev.*, 20, 265-273.

KOLB, L.C. (1968). Noyes modern clinical psychiatry (7th ed.), Saunders, Philadelphia.

KOLB, L.C. (1973). Modern clinical psychiatry, 8th Edition, W.B. Saunders Company, London, Toronto.

KOLLE, K. (1931). Die Primiare Verrucktheit (Primary madness (paranoia)). Leipzig: Thieme.

KOWALSKI, P.A., DALEY, G.D., and GRIPP, R.P. (1976). Token economy : Who responds how? *Beha. Res. Ther.*, 14, 372-374.

KRAEPELIN, E. (1902). Clinical Psychiatry : A text book for students and physicians. Translated by A.R. Defendorf, 6th ed. of Lehrbuch Der Psychiatric., MacMillan, New York.

KRAEPELIN, E. (1909). Psychiatry, 8th edition, Leipzig : Thieme, pp. 297, 548.

KRAEPELIN, E. (1913). *Psychiatric, ein Lehrbuchfur Studierende und Artzte* (Psychiatry, a text book for students and practitioners), 8th ed., vol.3, Leipzig : Barth.

KRAEPELIN, E. (1919). Dementia praecox and paraphrenia (trans. BARCLAY, R.M.) Edinburgh : Livingstone.

KRAEPELIN, E. (1921). Manic depressive insanity and paranoia (trans. Barelay, R.M.) Edinburgh, Livingstone.

KRAKOWSKI, M., VOLAVKA, J., and BRIZER, D. (1986). Psychopathology and violence : A review of literature. *Comprehensive Psychiat.*, 27, 131-148.

KRETSCHMER, E. (1952). Psycique and character (Trans. SPORT, W.J.H.), London Kegan Paul, Trench and Trubner.

KRISTOFFERSON, M.W. (1967). Shifting attention between modalities : A comparison of Schizophrenics and normals. *J. Abn. Psychol.*, 72, 382-394.

KUBA, M. (1975). A psychopathological and socio-cultural psychiatric study in the possession syndrome. *Trans. Cult. Psychiat. Res. Rev.*, 12, 24.

KUEHNEL, T.G., DERISI, W.J., LIBERMAN, R.P. and MOSK, M.D. (1984). Treatment strategies that promote deinstitutionalisation of chronic mental patients. In W.P. Christian, G.T. Hannah, and D.T.J., Glahn (Eds.), *Programming effective human services : Strategies for institutional charge and client transition.* New York : Plenum.

LAING, R.D. (1960). *The dividend self. An existential study in sanity and madness.* London: Tavintock Publications.

LAING, R.D. (1967). *The politics of experience*, New York, Ballantine Books.

LAING, R.D. (1970). The divided self : an existential study of sanity and madness, New York : Pantheon.

LAING, R.D. and ESTERSON, A. (1970). *Sanity, madness and the family*, Middlesex, Penguin, England.

LAM, D.H. (1991). Psychosocial family intervention in schizophrenia : A review of empirical studies. *Psychol. Med.*, 21, 423-441.

LAMBO, T.A. (1955). The role of cultural factors in paranoid psychosis among Yoruba trile. *J. Ment. Sc.*, 101, 239.

LANDAN, S.G., BUCHSBAUM M.S., CARPENTER, W., STRAUSS, J. and SACKS, M. (1975). Schizophrenia and stimulus intensity control. *Arch. Gen. Psychiat.*, 32, 1299-1245.

LANG, P.J., and BUSS, A. (1965). Psychological deficit in Schizophrenia. II. Interference and activation. *J. Abn. Psychol.*, 70, 77-106.

LANGFELDT, G. (1937). The prognosis in Schizophrenia, and the factors influencing the course of the disease. *Acta. Psychiat. Neurol. Scand.*, Suppl. 13-203, 308-309, 483.

LAPOUSE, R., MONK, M.A. and TERRIS, M. (1956). The drift hypothesis and socio-economic differentials in Schizophrenia. *American Journal of Public Health*, 46, 978-986.

LAQUEUR, H., DUSSIK, K., LaBURT, H., and McLAUGHLIN, W. (1962). *Tactical and strategical considerations in the use of insulin therapy – a joint mental hospital study.* N.Y. Academy of Medicine, No.2.

LATEMENDIA, F.J., HARRIS, A.D., and WILLIAMS, P.J. (1967). The clinical effects on a population of chronic Schizophrenic patients or administrative changes in hospital *Brit. J. Psychiat.*, 113, 959-971.

LAUBSCHER, B. (1937). *Sex, custom and psychopathology*, London, Roulbedge and Kegan Paul.

LEAVITT, M. (1968). It is in the degree of differences, perhaps where the surprise lie. In: May, P.R.A. Treatment of Schizophrenia : A comparative study of five treatment methods. *Amer. J. Psychother.*, 21(4), 845-847.

LEFF, J.P. (1974). Culture and the differentiation of emotional states. *Transenl. Psychiat. Res. Rev.*, 11, 122.

LEFF, J., KUIPERS, L., BERKOWITZ, R., ELECRLEIN-VRIES, R., and STURGEON, D. (1992). A controlled trial; of social intervention in the families of schizophrenia patients. ***Brit. J. Psychiat.***, 141, 121-134.

LEFF, J., KUIPERS, L., BERKOWITZ, R., and STURGEON, D. (1985). A controlled trial of social intervention in the families of Schizophrenic patients : Two year follow-up. *Brit. J. Psychiat.*, 146, 594-600.

LEFF, J., and VAUGHAN, C.J. (1985). *Expressed emotion in families.* New York : Guilford.

LEFF, J.P., and WING, J.K. (1971). Trial of maintenance therapy in Schizophrenia. *Brit. Med.* J., 3, 599-604.

LEFF, J., WIG, N., BEDI, H., MENON , D.K., KUIPERS, L., KORTEN, A., EMBERG, G., DAY, R., SARTORIUS, N., and JABLEWSKY, A. (1990). Relatives' expressed emotion and the course of Schizophrenia in Chandigarh. *Brit. J. Psychiat.*, 156, 351-356.

LEFF, J., WIG, N., GHOSH, A., BEDI, H., MENON, D.K., KUIPERS, L., KORTEN, A., EMBERG, G., DAY, R., SARTORIUS, N. and JABLENSKY, A. (1987). Expressed emotion and schizophrenia in North India III : Influence of relatives' expressed emotion on the course of schizophrenia in Chandigarh. *Brit. J. Psychiat.*, 151, 166-173.

LEHMAN, A. (1983). The well-being of chronic mental patients. *Arch. Gen. Psychiat.*, 40, 369-373.

LEIGHTON, A.H. (1959). *My name is legion*, New York : Basic Books.

LEIGHTON, A.H. (1969). A comparative study of psychiatric disorder in Nigeria and rural North America. In Plog, S.C. and Edgerten, R.B. (Eds.), *Changing perspectives in mental illness*, New York : Helt, Rinehart and Winston.

LEIGHTON, D.C., HARDING, J.S., MACKLIN, D.B., MACMILLAN, A.M., and LEIGHTON, A.H. (1963). *The Character of Danger*, New York : Basic Books.

LEONHARD, K. (1960). The atypical psychosis and Kleist's views on endogenous psychosis. In H.W. Gruhle, R. Jung and W. Mayer-Gross, and M. Müller (Eds.) *Psychiatric der Gegenwart.* Vol.II, Springer, Berlin.

LEONHARD, K. (1961). Cycloid psychoses – Endogenous psychoses which are neither schizophrenic nor manic depressives. *J. Ment. Sci.*, 107, 633.

LEONHARD, K. (1936). *Die Defekt Schizophrenen Krankheits bilder* (the clinical pictures in Schizophrenic defect states), Leipzig, Thieme.

LEONHARD, K. (1959). *Aufteilung der endogenen psychosen* (Classification of the endogenon psychoses) (2nd ed), Berlin : Academic Verlag.

LETEMENDIA, F.J., HARRIS, A.D., and WILLIAMS, P.J. (1967). The clinical effects on a population of chronic Schizophrenic patients or administrative changes in hospital. *Brit. J. Psychiat.*, 113, 939-971.

LEVINE, R.A. (1963). Behaviourism in psychological anthropology. In Wepman, J.M. and Heine, R.W. (Eds.) *Concepts of Personality*, Chicago : Aldine and Atherton.

LEVIT, A.L., SUTTON, S. and ZUBIN, J. (1973). Evoked potential correlates of information processing in psychiatric patients. *Psychol. Med.*, 3, 487-494.

LEVY, S. (1983). School doesn't last forever : What then? Some vocational alternatives. In E.S. Schopler and G.B. Mesibev (Eds.), *Autism in adolescents and adults*, New York, Plenum.

LEWINE, R.R.J., WATT, N.F., PRENTKY, R.A. and FRYER, J.H. (1980). Childhood social competence in functionally disordered psychiatric patients and normals. *J. Abn. Psychol.*, 89, 132-138.

LEWIS, A. (1934). Melancholia : A Clinical Survey of Depressive States. *Brit.J. Psychiatry.*, 80, 277.

LEWIS, A. (1950). Psychological medicine. In : *A Text Book of the Practice of Medicine*, F.W. Price (ed.), Section XX, 8th ed. H.M.S.O., London.

LEWIS, N.D.C. (1960). History of the nosology and evolution of the concepts of Schizophrenia. In : Hoch, P.H., Zubin, J. (Eds.) *Psychopathology of Schizophrenia*, New York, Grune and Stratten, pp. 1-18.

LIBERMAN, R.P. (1972). Behavioural modification of Schizophrenia : A review. *Schizophrenia Bull.*, 6, 37-48.

LIBERMAN, R.P. (1981). Managing resistance to behavioural family therapy. In A.S. Gurman (ed.) *Questions and answers in the practice of family therapy*, vol.1, New York: Brunner / Maze.

LIBERMAN, R.P., and CORRIGAN, P.W. (1993). Designing new psychosocial treatments for schizophrenia. *Psychiatry*, 56, 238-249.

LIBERMAN, R.P., KUEHNEL, T.G., PHIPPS, C.C. and CARDIN, V.A. (1984). *Resource book for psychiatric rehabilitation : Elements of Service for the mentally ill.* Barkeley, CA : Regents of the University of California.

LIBERMAN, R.P., TEIGEN, J., PATTERSON, R. and BAKER, V. (1973). Reducing delusional speech in chronic paranoid Schizophrenics. *J. Appl.. Beha. Analysis*, 6, 57-64.

LIDDLE, P.F., and MORRIS, D.L. (1991). Schizophrenia syndromes and frontal lobe performance. *Brit. J. Psychiat.*, 158, 340-345.

LIDZ, T., CORNELISON, A.R., TERRY, D. and FLECK, S. (1958). The intra familial environment of the Schizophrenic patient VI. The Transmission of Irritionality. *Arch. Neurol. Psychiat.* (Chicago), 79, 305.

LIDZ, T., FLECK, S. and CORNELISON, A.R. (1965). *Schizophrenia and the family*, New York, International Universities Press.

LIFSHITZ, K. (1978). Event related potentials in psychiatric patients and control subjects during varied arousal (Abstract) In Tuetting, P., Callaway, E., and Koslow, S.H. (eds.) *Event related brain potentials in man*, New York : Academic Press, p.620.

LIFSHITZ, K., SUSSWEIN, S. and LEE, K. (1979). Auditory evoked potentials and psychopathology, In : Begleiter, H., ed. *Brain potentials and behaviour*, Plenum Press, New York, pp. 419-436.

LIN, K. and KLEINMAN, A.M. (1988). Psychopathology and clinical course of Schizophrenia: A cross-cultural perspective. *Schizo. Bull.*, 14, 555-568.

LOCKHART, R.A. and LIEBERMAN, V. (1979). Information content of the electrodermal orienting vespouse. In Kimel, H.D., Vanolest, E.H., and Orieboke, J.F. (Eds.), *The orienting reflex in human*, Erlbaum Associates, Pub. Hilledale, New Jersey.

LOMBROSO, C. (1911). Crime: Its causes and remedies. *Little*, Brown, Boston.

LOVAAS, O.I., KOEGEL, R., SIMMONS, J.Q., and LONG, J.S. (1973). Some generalisation and follow-up measures on autistic children in behaviour therapy. *J. Appl. Beha. Analysis*, 6, 131-166.

LOVAAS, O.I., FREITAG, G., GOLD, V.J. and KASSORIA, I.C. (1965). Experimental studies in childhood Schizophrenia : Analysis of self-destructive behaviour. *J. Exptt. Child Psychol.*, 2, 67-84.

LOVIBOND, S.H. (1954). The object – sorting test and conceptual thinking in Schizophrenia. *Aust. J. Psychol.*, 6, 52, 266.

LUCAS, C.J., and COLLINS, J.C. (1962). A socioclinical study of delusions in Schizophrenia. *J. Ment. Sc.*, 108, 747.

LYNN, R. (1963). Russian theory and research in Schizophrenia. *Psychol. Bull.*, 60, 486-498.

MacKAY, A.V.P., BIRD, E.D., and SPOKES, E.G. (1980). Dopamine receptors and Schizophrenia : Drug effect or illness? *Lancet*, 2, 915-916.

MacKINNON, P.C.B. (1969). The palmar anhidrotic response to stress in Schizophrenic patients and in control groups. *J. Psychiat. Res.*, 7, 1-8.

MacLEAN, P.D. (1968). Ammon's Horn : A continuing dilemma : Forwarded to S.R.Y.: Cajal. *The structure of Ammon's Horn.* Translated by L.M. Kraft, Spring Field, 111 : Charles C. Thomas, pp. V-XIX.

MacLEAN, P.D. (1973). Man's limbic brain and the psychoses. In : Boag, T.J. and Campcell, D. (Eds.), *A Triune concept of the brain and behaviour*, Toronto University of Toronto Press.

MacLEAN, P.D., FLANIGAN, S., FLYNN, J.P., KIM, C., and STEVENS, J.R. (1955-1956). Hippocampal functions : Tentative correlations of conditioning EEG; drug and radioautographic studies. *Yale J. Biol. and Med.*, 28, 380-395.

MADEW, L., SINGER, G., and MACINDOE, I. (1966). Treatment and rehabilitation in the therapeutic community : A progress report. *Med. J. Aust.*, 1112-1114.

MAGARO, P.A., TALBOTT, J.A. and GLICK, I. (1984). The patient are of chronic Schizophrenia. In A.S. Bellack (Ed.) *Schizophrenia*, Orlando, FL, Grune & Stratton.

MAHLER, M.S., PINE, F., and BERGMANN, A. (1975). The psychological birth of the human infant. New York, Basic.

MAIN, T.E. (1946). The hospital as a therapeutic institution. *Bull. Menninger Clinic*, 10, 66-70.

MAIN, T.E., BRIDGER, H., BION, W.R., DEWAR, M.C., FOLUKES, S.H. and DAVIDSON, S. (1946). The hospital as a therapeutic institution. *Bull. Menninger Clin.*, 10, 66.

MALAMUD, N. (1967). Psychiatric disorders with intracranial tumours of the limbic system. *Arch. Neurol.*, 17, 113-123.

MANDAL, M.K. (1987). Decoding facial emotions in terms of expressiveness, by schizophrenics and depressives. *Psychiat: Interpersonal and Biol. Process*, 50, 371-376.

MANDAL, M.K., BHUSHAN, H.S. and MISHRA, R.C. (2001). Cultural variation in hemifacial asymmetry of emotion expressions. *Brit. J. Soc. Psychol.*, 40, 385-398.

MANDAL, M.K., BRYDEN, M.P. and BULMAN-FLEMING, M.B. (1996). Similarities and variations in facial expressions of emotion : cross-cultural evidence. *Int. J. Psychol.*, 31, 49-58.

MANDAL, M.K. and GEWALI, H. (1989). Identification of brief presentations of facial expressions of affects in schizophrenics. *Int. J. Psychol.*, 24, 605-616.

MANDAL, M.K., HARIZUKA, S., BHUSHAN, B., and MISRA, R.C. (2001). Cultural variations in Hemifacial asymmetry of emotion expression. *Brit. J. Soc. Psychol.*, 40, 385-398.

MANDAL, M.K., JAIN, A., HAQUE-NIZAMIE, S., WEISS, V., and SCHNEIDER, F. (1999). Generality and specificity of emotion recognition deficit in schizophrenic patients with positive and negative symptoms. *Psychiat. Res.*, 87(1), 39-46.

MANDAL, M.K. and PALCHOUDHURY, S. (1989). Identifying the components of facial emotions and schizophrenia. *Psychopathol.*, 22, 295-300.

MANDAL, M.K., PANDEY, G., SINGH, S.K. and ASTHANA, S. (1992). Hand preference in India. *Int. J. Psychol.*, 27, 433-442.

MANDAL, M.K., PANDEY, R., and PRASAD, A.B. (1998). Facial expressions of emotions and schizophrenia : A review. *Schizo. Bull.*, 24, 399-412.

MANDAL, M.K. and RAI, A. (1987). Responses to facial expressions of emotion in depression. *Psychol. Reports*, 56, 653-654.

MANDAL, M.K. and SINGH, S.K. (1993). Lateral hand performance in self-classified right handed schizophrenics. *Human Movt. Sci.*, 12, 507-514.

MANDAL, S.K., SINGH, S.K., ASTHANA, H.S., and SRIVASTAVA, P. (1992). Bilateral transfer deficit in schizophrenia. *Comp. Psychiat.*, 33, 319-324.

MANDELBROTE, B. and FOLKARD, S. (1963). The outcome of Schizophrenia in relation to a developing community psychiatric service. *Ment. Hyg.*, 47, 43.

MANOACH, D.S. (1994). Handedness is related to formal thought disorder and language dysfunction in schizophrenia. *J. Clin. Exptl. Neuropsychol.*, 16, 2-14.

MANOACH, D.S., MAHER, B.A. and MANSCHRECK, T.C. (1988). Left handedness and thought disorder in schizophrenia. *J. Abn. Psychol.*, 97, 97-99.

MARDER, R., WIRSHING, W.G., MINIZ, J., McKENZIE, J. *et al.* (1996). Two-year outcome of social skills training and group psychotherapy for out patients with schizophrenia. *Amer. J. Psychiat.*, 153, 1585-1592.

MARDER, S.R., JOHNSON-CRONK, K., WIRSHING, W.C., and ECKMAN, T. (1991). Schizophrenia and behavioural skill training. In : B. Beitman, and G.L. Klerman (Eds.), *Integrating Pharmacotherapy and Psychotherapy,* Washington, D.C., American Psychiatric Association.

MARGOLIS, R.R. and SHEMBERG, K.M. (1976). Cognitive instruction in process and reactive Schizophrenia : A failure to replicate. *Beha. Ther.*, 7, 668-671.

MARICQ, H.R. (1969). Nailfield capillary bed in Schizophrenics and the influence of institutional life. *Acta. Psychiat. Scand.*, 45, 355-366.

MARTIN, J.A. and LAGULLI, D.M. (1974). Elimination of middle of the night tantamus in a blind retarded child. *Beha. Ther.*, 5, 420-422.

MARTIN, P.L., and FOXX, R.M. (1973). Victim control of the aggression of an institutionalised retardate. *J. Beha. Ther. And Exptl. Psychiat.*, 4, 161-165.

MASROOR, J., HAQUE-NIZAMIE, S., NIZAMIE, A., and KHALIQUE, A. (2002). Efficacy of Luria-Nebrassca Neuropsychological Battery in identifying cognitive deficits in epileptic patients. *Ind. J. Clin. Psychol.*, 29(2), 130-135.

MATSON, J.L. and LaGRAW, S.J. (1983). Developmental and physical liabilities. In : M. Hersen, V.B. Vanhasselt, and J.L. Matson (Eds.), *Behaviour therapy for the developmentally and physically disabled* (pp. 3-24), New York, Academic Press.

MATSON, J.L. and STEPHENS, R.M. (1977). Overcorrection of aggressive behaviour in a chronic psychiatric patient. *Beha. Modification*, 1, 559-564.

MAY, P.R.A. (1968). *Treatment of Schizophrenia* : A comparative study of five treatment methods. New York : Science House.

MAYER, W. (1921). "Uber paraphrene psychosen", *Z. Ges. Neurol. Psychiat.*, 71, 187.

MAYER-GROSS, W. (1924). Self-descriptions from confusional states. The Oneiroid Experience. *Berlin*, 215, 299.

MAYER-GROSS, W., SLATER, E., and ROTH, M. (1974). *Clinical Psychiatry*, Cassell, London.

McCARTNEY, J.R. (1989). Thesis of Schizophrenia and autism : Issue in diagnosis assessment of psychological treatment. In Matson, J.L. (Ed.), *Chronic Schizophrenia and Adult Autism*, Springer Publishing Company, New York.

McCONAGHY, N. (1959). The use of an object-sorting test in elucidating the hereditary factors in Schizophrenia. *J. Neurol. Neurosurg. Psychiat.* 22, 243, 246.

McCORMICK, D.J. and BROEKEMA, W.J. (1978). Size estimation, perceptual recognition and cardiac rate response in acute paranoid and non-paranoid Schizophrenics. *J. Abn. Psychol.*, 87, 385-398.

McEWEN B.S., WEISS, J.M. and SCHWARTZ, L.S. (1968). Selective retention of corticosterone by limbic structure in rat brain. *Nature*, 220, 911-912.

McGHIE, A. (1961). A comparative study of the mother-child relationship in Schizophrenia. I. The interview. II. Psychological stating. *Brit. J. Med. Psychol.*, 34, 195.209.

McGHIE, A. (1969). *Pathology of Attention*, Harmondsworth : Penguin.

McGHIE, A. and CHAPMAN, J. (1961). Disorders of attention and perception in early Schizophrenia. *Brit. J. Med. Psy.*, 34, 103-115.

McJLASHEN, T.H. (1983). Intensive individual psychotherapy of schizophrenia. *Arch. Gen. Psychiat.*, 40, 909-920.

McJLASHEN, T.H. (1988). A selective review of recent North American Follow-up : Studies of Schizophrenia. *Schizo. Bull.*, 14, 567-581.

McJLASHEN, T.H., and CARPENTER, W.T. (1976). An investigation of the post-psychotic depressive syndrome. *Amer. J. Pscyhiat.*, 133, 14-19.

McNEIL, E.B. (1970). *The psychoses.* Englewood Cliffs, NJ : Prentice Hall.

MEASEL, C.J., and ALFIERI, P.A. (1976). Treatment of self-injurious behaviour by a combination of reinforcement for incompatible behaviour and overcorrection. *Amer. J. Ment. Self.*, 81, 147-153.

MEDNICK, S.A. (1970). Breendonen in individual at high risk for Schizophrenia: Possible predispositional perinatal factors. *Mental Hygiene*, 54, 50-63.

MEDNICK, S.A. (1978). Berusen's fallacy and high-rise research. In L.C. Wynne, R.L. Cromwell, and L. Mathysse (Eds.), *The nature of Schizophrenia*: New approaches to research and treatment. John Wiley: New York.

MEDNICK, S.A. and SCHULSINGER, F. (1968a). Some premorbid characteristics related to break down in children with Schizophrenic mothers. In Rosenthal, D., and Ketty, S.S. (eds.) *Transmission of Schizophrenia*, Pergamon Press, pp. 267-291.

MEDNICK, S.A., SCHULSINGER, F. (1968b). Some premorbid characteristics related by breakdown in children with Schizophrenic mothers. *J. Psychiat. Res.*, 6, 267-291 (Suppl. No.1).

MEDNICK, S.A. and SCHULSINGER, F. (1973). A learning theory of Schizophrenia: Thirteen years latest. In : Hammer, M., Salzinger, K., and Sutton, S. (Eds.) *Psychopathology*, Ch.18, John Wiley & Sons, New York, London.

MEDNICK, S.A. and SCHULESINGER, P. (1974a). Nature – Nurture aspects of Schizophrenia. In Lader, M.H. (Ed.) *Studies of Schizophrenia*, Royal College of Psychiat., London, pp. 36-41.

MEDNICK, S.A. and SCHULSINGER, F. (1974b). Some premorbid characteristics related to break-down in children with Schizophrenic mothers. In : S.A. Mednick, F. Schulsinger, J. Higgins, and B. Bell (Eds.), *Genetics, Environment and Psychopathology* North Holland, Amsterdam.

MEDNICK, S.A., SCHULSINGER, F., TEASDALE, T.W., SCHULSINGER, H., VENABALES, P.H. and ROCK, D.R. (1977). Schizophrenia in high-risk children: Sex differences and predisposing factors. *Presented to the kittary scientific foundation*, 5th International Symposium, New York.

MEDOW, W. (1922). A group of depressive psychoses in involutional age with unfavourable prognosis. *Arch. Psychiat. Nervenkar*, 64, 480.

MEICHENBAUM, D.H. and CAMERON, R. (1973). Training Schizophrenics to talk to themselves: A means of developing attentional controls. *Beha. Ther.*, 4, 515-534.

MELTEZER, H.Y. (1985). Dopamine and negative symptoms in Schizophrenia: Critique of the type I-II hypothesis. In M. Alport (Ed.) *Controversies in Schizophrenia*, New York, Guildford.

MELTEZER, H.Y., SACHAR, E.J., and FRANTZ, A.C. (1974). Serum prolactin level in unmedicated schizophrenic patients. *Arch. Gen. Psychiat.*, 31, 564-569.

MENDIS, N. (1986). The outcome of Schizophrenia in Sri Lanka : a ten-year follow-up study. *Cylon. Med.* J., 31, 119-134.

MENDOW, W. (1922). A group of depressive psychosis in involutional age with unfavourable prognosis. *Arch. Psychiat. Nervenkr.*, 64, 480. 297.

MENNINGER, K. (1958). *Theory of psychoanalytic technique.* New York : Basic Books.

MERRIN, E.L. (1984). Motor and sighting dominance in schizophrenia and affective disorders. *Brit. J. Psychiat.*, 146, 539-544.

MESIBOV, G.B. (1983). Current perspective and issues in autism and adolescence. In E. Schopler and G.B. Mesibov (Eds.) *Autism in Adolescents and Adults*, New York, Plenum.

MESIBOV, G.B., SCHOPLER, E., and SOLAN, J.L. (1983). Service development for adolescents and adults in North Carolina's Teach Program. In E. Schopler and G.B. Mesibov (Eds.), *Autism in Adolescents and Adults*, New York : Plenum.

MEYER, A. (1910). The nature and conception of Dementia Praecox. *J. Abnorm. (Soc) Psychol.*, 5, 274.

MEYER, A. (1944). The Wenick Syndrome. *J. Neurol. Psychiat.*, 7, 66-527.

MEYER, A. (1951). The collected papers of Adolf Meyer, vol.II, Psychiatry, Baltimore, Johns Hopkins Press.

MICHELS, R. (1969). Research design and training programme training. *Int. J. Psychiat.*, 8(4), 740-743.

MILSTEIN, V., STEVENS, J. and SACHDEV, K. (1969). Habituation of the alpha alternation response in children and adults with psychiatric disorders. *Electroencephs. Clin. Neurophysiol.*, 26, 12-18.

MIROWSKY, J. (1985). Disorder and its content : Paranoid beliefs and thematic elements of thought problems, hallucinations, and delusions under threatening social conditions. *Res. Comm. Ment. Health*, 5, 185-204.

MIRSKY, A.F., and DUNCAN, C.C. (1986). Etiology and expression of schizophrenia: Neurological and psychological factors. *Annu. Rev. Psychol.*, 37, 291-319.

MISCHAEL, A., MIRZA, K.A.H., MUKUNDAN, C.R., and CHANNABASAVANNA, S.M. (1995). Interhemispheric electroencephalographic coherence as a biological marker in alcoholism. *Acta. Psychiat. Scand.*, 87, 213-217.

MISHRA, S. and SHARMA, S. (1995). Cardiovascular changes in schizophrenic patients, their first degree relatives and controls. *Ind. J. Clin. Psychol.*, 22(1), 14-19.

MISRA, G., SAHOO, F.M., and PUHAN, B.N. (1999). Cultural bias in testing in India. *Rev. Appl. Psychol.*, 47(4), 309-316.

MITRA, T., BANDYOPADHYAY, G.K. and CHATTOPADHYAY, P.K. (2002). Variability issues in anxiety ratings in a double-blind drug study. *Ind. J. Clin. Psychol.*, 29(2), 136-143.

MITRA, T. and CHATTOPADHYAY, P.K. (2001). Drug induced behavioural changes in Panic and Mixed anxiety patients. *Psychol. Studies*, 46, 52-57.

MITRA, T. and CHATTOPADHYAY, P.K. (2003). Attribution of variables as predictions in drug treatment outcome of anxiety. *Soc. Sci. Int.*, 19, 21-26.

MOFFSON, A. (1954). Schizophrenia in male Bantee admissions to West Koppies Hospital; *South Africa Med.*, 7(28), 662.

MOHAMAD, S., PAULSON, J.S., O'LEARY, D., ARNDT, S., and ANDREASEN, N.C. (1999). Generalised cognitive deficits in schizophrenia : A study of first-episode patients. *Arch. Gen. Psychiat.*, 56, 749-754.

MOHANTY, A., DAS, B.S., MUKUNDAN, C.R., and JAMUNA, N. (1993a). Cognitive outcome and quality of life after aneurismal subarachnoid haemorrhage. Part I : Cognitive Outcome. *NIMHANS, J.*, 11, 107-111.

MOHANTY, A., DAS, B.S., MUKUNDAN, C.R. and JAMUNA, N. (1993b). Cognitive outcome and quality of life after aneurismal subarachnoid haemorrhage. Part II : Quality of Life. *NIMHANS, J.*, 11, 119-124.

MOREL, B.A. (1852). Traite des degenerescences physiques, intellectualies it morales. Paris: Bailliere.

MOREL, B.A. (1957). Traité des degenerescences physiques, intellectuelles of morales, Paris : Bailliere.

MORENO, J.L. (1959). Psychodrama : In, Ariets, S. (ed.) *American Handbook of Psychiatry* (vol.2), New York : Basil Books.

MORGAN, R. (1974). Industrial Therapy. *Brit. J. Hosp. Med.*, 11, 231.

MORRISON, J., WINOKUR, G., CROWE, R., and CLANCY, J. (1973). The IOWA 500: The first follow-up. *Arch. Gen. Psychiat.*, 29, 678-682.

MORRISON, R.L.M. and BELLACK, A.S. (1967). The social functioning of Schizophrenic patients : Clinical and Research Issues. *Schze. Bull.*, 13, 715-725.

MOSHER, L.R., and BURTI, L. (1992). Relationship in rehabilitation : When technology fails. *Psychoc. Rehab. J.*, 15, 11-17.

MUESER, K.T., and BELLACK, A.S. (1989). Social learning treament for chronic Schizophrenia and autism. In Matson, J.L. (Ed.). *Chronic Schizophrenia and adult autism*, issues in diagnosis, assessment, and psychological treatment. Springer Publishing Company, New York.

MUIJEN, M., MARKS, I.M., CONNOLLY, J., AUDIMI, B., and McNAMES, G. (1992). The daily living programme : Preliminary comparison of community vs hospital based treatment for the seriously mentally ill functioning emergency admission. *Brit. J. Psychiat.*, 160, 372-378.

MUKHERJEE, P., CHATTOPADHYAY, P.K., PAL, S.K. and GHOSH, K.K. (1982). Hormone profile and Trait anxiety in female infertility. *IRCS Med. Sc. (Lond)*., 10, 228.

MUKHOPADHYAY, P., BASU, S. and CHATTOPADHYAY, P.K. (1994). Biofeed back as a therapeutic intervention technique in the treatment of muscular disorders. *Ind. J. Physiol. & Allied Sciences*, 41(1), 14-20.

MUKHOPADHYAY, P., and CHATTOPADHYAY, P.K. (1995). LIV in psycho-physiological research : The concept revisited. *Soc. Sci. Int.*, 11 (1 & 2), 1-9.

MUKHOPADHYAY, P., and CHATTOPADHYAY, P.K. (2000). Menstrual distress and self-regulation : An experimental approach. *Ind. J. Clin. Psychol.*, 27(1), 104-111.

MUKHOPADHYAY, P. and DAS, S. (2003). Problem solving ability in psychiatric patients : A neuropsychological approach. *Psychol. Res. Jr.*, 26 (1 & 2), 26-34.

MUKHOPADHYAY, P., DE, S., CHATTOPADHYAY, P.K., and BISWAS, D. (1996). Deprivation : Its impact on arousal modulation and adjustment : A psychophysiological approach. *Ind. J. Clin. Psychol.*, 23(2), 161-169.

MUKHOPADHYAY, P., MUKHERJEE, S., CHOWDHURY, M., GUPTA, S., BASU, P. and DUTTA, A. (1999). Determination of lobe function in brain-damaged and psychiatric patients : Role of Bender-Visual Motor Gestalt Test. *Ind. J. Clin. Psychol.*, 26(2), 225-228.

MURPHY, G.H. and WILSON, B. (1981). *Long-term outcome of contingent shock treatment frontiers of knowledge in mental retardation.* London, IASSMD.

MURPHY, H.B.M. (1973). History and evolution of syndromes : The striking case of natal and amek. In : *Psychopathology : Contributions from the Social, Behavioural and Biological Sciences* (Eds.) M. Hammer, K. Salzinger and Selton, Wiley, New York.

MURPHY, H.B.M., and RAHMAN, A.C. (1971). The clonicity of Schizophrenia in indigenous tropical peoples. *Brit. J. Psychiat.*, 118, 489-4987.

MUSSER, K.T., and BERENBAUM, H. (1990). Psychodynamic treatment of schizophrenia : Is there a future? *Psychol. Med.*, 20, 253-262.

MYERSON, A. (1941). Review of Faris and Demlian. *Amer. J. Psychiat.*, 895, 995-997.

MYSLOBODSKY, M. (1976). Pharmacologic implications of hemisopheric asymmetry. *Life Science*, 19, 1467-1478.

NANDI, D.N., BANERJEE, G., SAHA, H., SEN, B. and BHATTACHARYA, A. (1992). An epidemic of Jhin-Jhini – A strange contagious psychogenic disorder in a village in West Bengal. *Ind. J. Psychiat.*, 34, 366-367.

NASRALLAH, H.A., JACOBY, C.G., McCALLEY-WHITTERS, M., and KUPOMAN, S. (1982). Cerebral ventricular enlargement in sub-types of chronic schizophrenia. *Arch. Gen. Psychiat.*, 39, 774-777.

NATIONAL INSTITUTE OF MENTAL HEALTH (1964). Collaborative study group (1964). Phenothiazine treatment in acute Schizophrenia : Effectiveness. *Arch. Gen. Psychiat.*, 10, 246-261.

NDETEI, D.M., and SINGH, A. (1983). Study of delusions in Kenyan schizophrenic patients diagnosed using a set of research diagnostic criteria. *Acta. Psychiat. Scandinevican*, 66, 208-215.

NDETEI, D.M., and VADHER, A. (1984). Frequency and clinical significance of delusions across cultures. *Acta. Psychiat. Scandinevican*, 70, 545-549.

NEDELMAN, D., and SULZBACHER, S.I. (1972). Dicky at thirteen years of age: A long term success following early application of operant conditioning procedures. In G. Semb (Ed.) *Behaviour analysis and education*, Lawrence, Kansas.

NEISSER, U. (1967). *Cognitive psychology*, New York, Appleton-Century Crofts.

NEKI, J.S. (1973). Guru-Chela Relationship: The possibility of a therapeutic paradigm. *Amer. J. Orthopsychiat.*, 43, 755-766.

NEKI, J.S. (1976). Aculturation of cultural relativism of dependence as a dynamic of social and therapeutic relationships. *Brit. J. Med. Psychol.*, 22, 14-26.

NORMAN, D.A. (1960). Toward a theory of memory and attention. *Psychol. Rev.*, 75, 522-536.

NOYES, A.P., and KOLB, L.C. (1963). Modern clinical psychiatry (6th ed), W.B. Saunders, Philadelphia.

O'BRIEN, F., AZRIN, N.H., HENSON, K. (1969). Increased communications of chronic mental patients by reinforcement and response priming. *J. Appl. Beh. Analysis*, 2, 23-29.

O'CONNOR, N., HERON, A., and CARSTAIRS, G.M. (1956). Work performance of chronic Schizophrenics. *Occup. Psychol.*, 30, 153-164.

O'LEARY, K.D. and WILSON, G.T. (1975). *Behaviour Therapy : Application and outcome.* Single Wood Cliffs, NJ : Prentice Hall.

O'NEAL, P., and ROBINS, L.N. (1958). Childhood patterns predictive of adult Schizophrenia : a 30 year follow-up study. *Amer. J. Psychiat.*, 115, 385-391.

OPLER, M.K. (1956). *Culture, psychiatry and human values.* Springfield, III : Thomas.

OPLER, M.K. (1959). Cultural differences in mental disorders : an Italian and Irish contrast in the Schizophrenias – U.S.A. In Opler, M.K. (ed.), *Cultures and Mental Health : Cross-Cultural Studies*, New York : MacMillan, pp. 425-442.

OSMOND, H. (1957). Review of the clinical effects of psychotomimetic agents. *Amer. N.Y. Acad. Sco.*, 66, 418.

OSMOND, H. and SMYTHIES (1952). Schizophrenia : A new approach. *J. Ment. Sci.*, 98, 309-315.

OSTOW, M. (1979). The psychodynamic approach to drug therapy. Toronto, Van Nostrand Reinhold.

OSWALD, L. (1962). Induction of illusionary and hallucinating voices with consideration of behaviour therapy. *J. Ment. Sci.*, 108, 106.

OVESEY, L. (1962). Fear of vocational success : A phobic extension of the paranoid reaction. *Arch. Gen. Psychiat.*, 7, 88-92.

PAASONEN, M.K., MacLEAN, P.D., and GIARMAN, N.J. (1957). 5-hydroxytrypt-amine (serotonin, enteramine) content of structures of the limbic system. *J. Neurochem.*, 1, 326-333.

PANSE, F. (1942). *Die Erb Chorea*, Leipzig – 301. 624.

PASTORE, N. (1949). Genetics of Schizophrenia : A special review. *Psychol. Bull.*, 46, 285.

PATEL, V. (1996). Recognizing common mental disorders in primary care in African countries – should "Mental" be dropped? *Lancet*, 347, 742-744.

PATEL, V. (2000). The need for treatment evidence for common mental disorders in developing countries. *Psychol. Med.*, 28, 135-145.

PATEL, V, PEREIRA, J., CONTINHO, Z., FERNANDEZ, R., FERNANDEZ, J. and MANN, A. (1998). Poverty, psychological disorder and disability in primary care attenders in Goa. *British Journal of Psychiatry*, 171, 533-536.

PATTERSON, R.L. and TEIGEN, J.R. (1973). Conditioning and post-generalisation of non-delusional responses in a chronic psychiatric patient. *J. Appl. Beha. Analysis*, 6, 65-70.

PATTERSON, T. (1976a). Skin conductance recovery and pupillometrices in chronic Schizophrenia. *Psychophysiol.*, 13, 189-193.

PATTERSON, T. (1976b). Skin conductance responding / non responding and pupillometrices in chronic Schizophrenia : A confirmation of Gruzelier and Venables. *J. Nerv. Ment. Dis.*, 163, 200-209.

PATTERSON, T.E. and VENABLES, P.H. (1978). Bilateral skin conductance and skin potential in Schizophrenic and normal subjects. The identification of the fat habituator group of Schizophrenics. *Psychophysiol.*, 15, 556-560.

PAUL, G.L. and LENTZ, R. (1977). *Psychosocial treatment of chronic mental patients.* London, Harvard University Press.

PAULEIKHOFF, B. (1957). *Atypische Psychosen* (atypical psychoses). Basle : Karger.

PAVLOV, I. (1927). Conditioned reflex. New York, Oxford University Press.

PAYKEL, E.S. and ULENHUTH (1972). Rating the magnitude of life stress. *Can. Psychiat. Asson. J.*, SS93-SS100.

PAYNE, R.W. (1962). An object classification test as a measure of ever-inclusive thinking in Schizophrenic patients. *Brit.J. Soc. Clin. Psychol.*, 1, 213.

PAYNE, R.W. and HIRST, H. (1957). Over-inclusive thinking in a depressive and control group. *J. Consul. Psychol.*, 21, 186-188.

PENN, D.L. and MUESER, K.T. (1996). Research update on the psychological treatment of schizophrenia. *Amer.J. Psychiat.*, 153, 607-617.

PERRIS, C. (1974). Averaged evoked responses (AER) in patients with affective disorders In : Perris, C., and Mattsson, G., eds. *Clinical Research from the Department of Psychiatry*, University of Umea, vol.II, Copenbagh. *Acta. Scandinarica*, pp. 89-98.

PERRIS, C., and SKAGERLIND, L. (1994). Cognitive therapy with schizophrenic patients. *Acta. Psychiat. Scand.*, 89 (Suppl. 382), 65-70.

PETRILOWITSCH, N. (1958). *Beitrage Zu einer Struktur– Psychopathologie* (contributions to a structure psychopathology), Basle : Karger.

PHILLIPS, L. (1966). Social competence, the process-reactive distinction and the nature of mental disorder. In Hoch, P.H. and Zubin, J. (Eds.) *Psychopathology of Schizophrenia* New York : Grune and Stratton.

PICKERING, D., and MORGAN, S.B. (1985). Parental ratings of treatments of self-injurious behaviour. *J. Autism and Dertl. Disorders.*, 15, 303-314.

POLLIN, W., CARDON, P.V., and KETTY, S.S. (1961). Effects of amino acid feedings in Schizophrenic patients treated with iproniazid. *Science*, 133, 104-105.

POST, F. (1966). *Persistent perscentory states of the elderly.* Oxford; Pergamon.

POST, R.M., FINK, E. and CARPENTER, W.I. (1975). Cerebrospinal fluid amine-metabolites in acute Schizophrenia. *Arch. Gen. Psychiat.*, 32, 1063.

PRABHU, G.G. (1987). Child and adolescent mental health research in India : An overview. *NIMHANS* J., 5, 79-89.

PRASADRAO, P.S.D.V. (2000). Cognitive behaviour in hallucinations. *Ind. J. Clin. Psychol.*, 27(2), 189-201.

PRATT, R.T.C. (1951). An investigation of the psychiatric aspects of discriminated salerosis. *J. Neurol. Neurosur. Psychiat.*, 14, 526.

PRESLEY, A.S., GRUBB, A.B., and SEMPLE, D. (1982). Predictors of successful rehabilitation in long story patients. *Acta. Psychiat. Scandinavica*, 66, 83-88.

PUHAN, B.N. (1995). Projective inventory : An indigenous approach to personality assessment. *Psychl. & Devl. Soc.*, 7, 115-131.

PUMPIAN-MINDIAN, E. (1953). Considerations in the situation of patients for short term therapy. *Amer.J. Psychother.*, 7, 641-652.

RACHLIN, H.L. (1935). A follow-up study of Hoch's benign stupor case. *Amer.J. Psychiat.*, 92, 531-319.

RACHMAN, S.J., and WILSON, G.T. (1983). *The effects of psychological therapy* (2nd edition), New York, Pergamon Press.

RAGAIN, R.D., and ANSON, J.E. (1976). The control of self-mutating behaviour with positive reinforcement. *Ment. Retd.*, 14, 22-25.

RAHMAN, A. (1992). Psychological factors in criminality. *J. Persona. Indi. Diff.*, 483-485.

RAMPRASAD, D. (2003). Integrating Indian mental health principles of life into psychotherapy. *Ind. J. Clin. Psychol.*, 30(1&2), 62-68.

RANGANATHAN, M., CHANNABASAVANNA, S.M., MURALI, T., BHARATHI, B.K., and PADANKATTI, B.S. (1996). An exploratory study of the participation of the community in psychiatric rehabilitation. *Ind. J. Clin. Psychol.*, 23(1), 57-61.

RANGANATHAN, M., and PARTHASWARATHY, R. (1982). Psychiatric rehabilitation programme and community involvement. *Jr. Rehab. Asia.*, 23, 20-21.

RANGANATHAN, M., REDDY, N., SHERIFF, I.H., PARTHASWARATHY, R., and KALIAPERUMAL, V.G. (1991). College student volunteers in mental hospital programme. *Ind. J. Soc. Work*, 11(2), 150-160.

RANGASWAMI, K. (1996). Indian system of psychotherapy. *Ind. J. Clin. Psychol.*, 23(1), 62-75.

RANGASWAMI, K. (2000). Psychosocial treatment for the first episode schizophrenia to prevent progression and relapse. *Ind. J. Clin. Psychol.*, 27(2), 209-213.

RAO, A.V. (1978a). Bhagvad Gita and Psychotherapy I, *Bhavan's Journal*, 2, 20-23.

RAO, A.V. (1978b). Bhagvad Gita and Psychotherapy II, *Bhavan's Journal*, 16, 36-38.

RAO, S. (1966). Culture and mental disorders : A study in an Indian mental hospital. *Int. J. Soc. Psychiat.*, 12, 2-3.

RAPOFF, M.A., ALTMAN, K.D. and CHRISTOPHERSEN, E.R. (1980). Suppression of self-injurious behaviour : Determining the least restrictive alternative. *J. Ment. Def. Res.*, 24, 37.

RAVINDRAN, O.S., and RANGASWAMI, K. (2004). A study of Frontal Obe Cognitive Dysfunctions in chronic schizophrenics. *Ind. J. Clin. Psychol.*, 31(1), 68-71.

REDDY, M.V., CHANNABASAVANNA, S.M., GOURI-DEVI, M., DOSS, B.S., PRABHU, G.G., SHERIFF, I.A., KALIAPERUMAL, V.G., and REDDAMMA, K. (1986). Extension of mental services by Satellite clinics – a model. *NIMHANS Jl.*, 4, 71-75.

REPP, A.C., and DEITZ, S.M. (1974). Reducing aggressive and self-injurious behaviour in institutionalised retarded children through reinforcement of other behaviours. *J. Appl. Beha. Anal.*, 7, 313-325.

REVITCH, E. (1954). The problem of conjugal paranoia. *Dis. Nerv. Spt.*, 15, 271-277.

RICKELS, D. (1981). Benzodiazepins : Use and misuse. In : D.F. Klein and J.G. Rabkin (eds.) *Anxiety, new research and changing concepts.* Ravens, New York.

RILEY, E.M., McGOVERN, D., MOCKER, D. *et al.* (1999). Neuropsychological functioning in first-episode psychosis : evidence of specific deficits. *Scizo. Res.*, 43(1), 47-56.

RIN, H. (1963). "Koro" : a consideration on Chinese concept of illness and case illustration. *Transcultural Psychiatric Research Review*, 15, 23-30.

ROBINSON, H.B. and ROBINSON, N.M. (1965). *The mentally retarded child : A psychological approach.* New York : McGraw Hill.

ROEMER, R.A., SHAGASS, C., STRAUMANIS, J.J. and AMADEO, M.P. (1978). Evoked potential measurements suggesting literalised hemispheric dysfunction in chronic Schizophrenics. *Biol. Psychiat.*, 13, 185-202.

ROGERS, C. (1951). *Client centered therapy : its current practices, implications, and theory.* Boster, Hougaton, Mifflin.

ROGERS, C. (1961). On becoming a person : a client's view of psychotherapy. Boston: Hougaton, Mifflin.

ROGERS, C. (1969). Freedom to learn : A view of what education might become. Columbia, Ohio : Charles and Merrill Company.

ROGERS, C.R., GENDLIN, E.T., KIESSLER, C. and TURAX, C.B. (1967). *The therapeutic relationship and its impact : A study of psychotherapy with Schizophrenics.* Madison : University Wisemsis Press.

ROMAN, P.M. and RICE, H.M. (1967). Schizophrenia and the poor Ithaca, N.Y. Cornell University Press.

ROSEN, J.N. (1947). The treatment of Schizophrenic psychoses by direct analytic therapy. *Psychiat. Qrmtay.*, 21, 3-37, 117-119.

ROSEN, J.N. (1953). *Direct analysis*: Selected Papers. New York, Grune and Stratton.

ROSEN, J. N. (1969). Psychotherapy and Schizophrenia. *Int. J. Psychiat.*, 8(4), 748-752.

ROTH, M. (1955). The natural history of mental disorder in old age. *J. Ment. Sci.*, 101, 281-301, 549, 580, 585.

ROTH, W.T. (1977). Late event-related potentials and psychopathology. *Schizo. Bull.*, 3, 105-120.

ROTH, W.T., and CANNON, E.H. (1972). Some features of the auditory evoked responses in Schizophrenics. *Arch. Gen. Psychiat.*, 27, 466-471.

ROTROSEN, J., ANGRIST, B., CLARK, C., GERSHON, S., HALPERN, F.S., and SECHER, E.J. (1978). Suppression of polaction by dopamine agonists in Schizophrenia and controls. *Amer. J. Psychiat.*, 7, 93-98.

ROY, A.R. (1981). Habituation of physiological responses in psychiatric patients and normal subjects. Unpublished *Ph.D. Thesis, Calcutta University.*

ROY, R. (1984). Role of medication in inducing psychological changes in psychiatric patients. Unpublished *Ph.D. thesis, Calcutta University.*

RUESCH, J., BRODSKY, C. and FISCHER, A. (1963). The acute nervous bracandmen. *Arch. Gen. Psychiat.*, 8, 197.

RUFFIN, J.E. (1984). The anxiety of meaninglessness. *J. Counsel and Development*, 63, 40-42.

RUSH, A.J., KUPFER, D.J. (1995). Strategies and tactics in treatment of depression. In : G.D. Gobbard (Ed.), *Treatment of Psychiatric Disorders*, Washington, D.C., American Psychiatric Association.

RUSSELL, J.A. (1994). Is there universal recognition of emotion from facial expression? A review of cross-cultural studies. *Psychol. Bull.*, 115, 102-141.

RUTTER, D.R. (1985). Language in Schizophrenia : The structure of monologous and conversation. *Brit. J. Psychiat.*, 146, 399-404.

SAHA, S., SAHA, S., MUKHOPADHYAY, P., and CHATTOPADHYAY, P.K. (2001). Nature of skin conductance orienting activity in high soccer performers. *Beng. J. Sports Sci.*, 1(1), 55-56.

SAHOO, D., GILLS, J.S. and MISRA, S.K. (2002). The selected client variables as predictors of response to behaviour therapy in obsessive-compulsive neurosis. *Ind. J. Clin. Psychol.*, 29(2), 110-117.

SAKEL, M. (1933). Neue Behandlung der Morphin Sucht. *J. Neurol. Psychiat.*, 143, 506.

SALETU, B., ITIL, T.M. and SALETU, M. (1971). Auditory evoked responses, EEG and thought processes in Schizophrenics. *Amer. J. Psychiat.*, 128, 330-344.

SALETU, B., SALETU, M., ITIL, T.M., and HSU, W. (1971a). Changes in somato-sensory evoked potentials during fluphenazine treatment. *Pharmakopsychiatric and Neuropsychophermakologie*, 4, 158-168.

SALETU, B., SALETU, M., ITIL, T. and JONES, J. (1971b). Somatosensory evoked potential changes during thiothixene treatment in Schizophrenic patients. *Psychopherm-cologia* (Berlin), 20, 242-253.

SALINGER, J.D. (1951). *A catcher in the rye.* Hamish Hamilton, London.

SANDERS, R., SMITH, R.S. and WEINMAN, B.S. (1967). Chronic psychosis and recovery, San Francisco, Jossey-Bass.

SANTOS, A.B. (1996). Assertive community treatment. In S. Soreff (ed.) *Handbook for the treatment of seriously mentally ill.* Toronto, Hogrefe and Huber.

SANYAL, S., CHATTOPADHYAY, P.K., and BISWAS, D. (1998). Electrodermal arousal and self-appraisal in patients with somatoform disorder. *Ind. J. Clin. Psychol.*, 25(2), 144-148.

SARBADHIKARY, D. (1999). Culture-bound psychiatric syndromes in South-East *Asia. Psychol. Res. J.*, 25, 15-20.

SARTÔTIUS, N., JABLENSKY, S., KORTEN, A., EMBERG, G., ANKER, M., COOPER, G.E., and DAYIR (1986). Early manifestations and first contact incidence of Schizophrenia in different cultures: A preliminary report of the initial evaluation phase of the WHO Study of determinants of outcome of severe mental disorder. *Psychol. Med.*, 16, 909-928.

SARTRE, J.P. (1957). Being and Nothingness (Trans. Barnes, H.E.) London, Mathuen.

SARVIS, M.A., DEWEES, S., and JOHNSON, R.F. (1958). A concept of ego-oriented psychotherapy. *Psychiat.*, 22, 277-287.

SATHYAVATHI, K. (1974). Perception of parents by schizophrenics : A consideration of Instrumentality-Expressivity Role. *Psychiat.*, 37, 261-266.

SATHYAVATHI, K. (1977). Perception of parents by male and female schizophrenics. *Ind. J. Clin. Psychol.*, 4(2), 115-121.

SATZ, P. (1972). Pathological left-handedness : An explanatory model. *Cortex*, 8, 121-137.

SCHAFFER, H.H., and MARTIN, P.L. (1975). Behavioural therapy. New York, McGraw Hill.

SCHEIDLINGER, S. (1969). Innovative group approaches, in Bellak, I.S., and Barten, H.H. (eds.) *Progress in Community Mental Health*, vol.1, Grune and Stratten, New York.

SCHNEIDER, C. (1925). Contribution to the problem of Schizophrenia : 4th Communication. On a general theory of Schizophrenic symptoms. *Z. Ges. Neurol. Psychiat.*, 96, 572.

SCHNEIDER, C. (1930). Die psychologie der Schizophrenen (the psychology of Schizophrenics) Leipzig : Thiems.

SCHNEIDER, C. (1942). Die Schizophrenen Symptomverbande (The Schizophrenic Symptom Complexes), Berlin : Springer.

SCHNEIDER, K. (1942). Mental symptoms and psychiatric diagnosis. Leipzig: Thieme.

SCHNEIDER, K. (1957). Primare Und Sekundare Symptomen bei Schizophrenia (Primary and Secondary Symptoms in Schizophrenia), *Fortscher, Neurol. Psychiat.*, 25, 487.

SCHOLLER, N.R., KEITH, S.J., SEVER, J.B. and MATHEWS, S.M. (1995). Maintenance treatment of schizophrenia : A review of dose reduction of family treatment strategies. *Psychiat. Quarterly.*, 66, 279-292.

SCHOOLER, C., and SPOHN, H. (1982). Social dysfunction and treatment failure in Schizophrenia. *Schizo. Bull.*, 8, 85-98.

SCHREBER, D.P. (1955). Memories of my nervous illness (Trans. Macalpine, L., and Hunter, R.A.), London : Dawson.

SCHREIBMAN, L. and KOEGEL, R.L. (1980). A guideline for planning behaviour modification programme for children : In S. TURNER, K. CALHOUN, and H. ADAMS (Eds.) *Handbook of Clinical Behaviour Therapy*, New York, John Wiley.

SCHROEDER, P. (1922). Degenerations psychosen; Dementia Praecox. *Arch. Psychiat. Nervenkr.*, 66, 1-298.

SCHROEDER, P. (1926). "Uber Degenerations Psychosen (Metabolische Enkrankun gen)" (On degeneration psychoses, Metabolic Illness), *Z. Ges. Neurol. Psychiat.*, 101, 539.

SCHUHAM, A. (1967). The double blind hypothesis : a decade later. *Psychol. Bull.*, 68: 409-416.

SCHULZ, B. and LEONHARD, K. (1940). Erbielegischklinische Untersuchungen an insgesant 99 iw Sinne Leonhards typischen bzw atypischen Schizophrenian. *Z. Ges. Neurol. Psychiat.*, 168, 587-243, 302.

SCHWARTZ-PLACE, E.J. and GILMORE, G.C. (1980). Perceptual organisation in Schizophrenia. *J. Abn. Psychol.*, 89, 409-418.

SCHWENT, V.L., SNYDER, E. and HILLYARD, S.A. (1976). Auditory evoked potential during multichannel selective bearing ones. *J. Expt. Psychol.*, 2, 313-325.

SEARLES, H.F. (1967). The Schizophrenic individual's experience of the world. *Psychiuat.*, 30, 119-131.

SECHEHAYE, M. (1954). Introduction a Une Psychotherapie des Schizophrenes. Paris, Presses Universiteires, 262.

SEEMAN, P. (1980). Brain Dopamine Receptors. *Pharmacol. Rev.*, 32, 229.

SEEMAN, P. (1985). Brain dopamine receptors in Schizophrenia. In M.N. Menuek and M.V. Seeman (Eds.) *New Perspectives in Schizophrenia*, pp. 71-80, New York, Macmillan.

SEN, G., and BOSE, K.C. (1931). Rauwelfia Serpentine, a new Indian drug for insanity and high blood pressure. *Ind. Med. Wld.*, 2, 194-201.

SERGEANT, J. (1988). Some theoretical and methodological issues in neuropsychological research . In : F. Boller and J. Grafman (Eds.), *Handbook of Neuropsychology*, vol.1, pp. 69-81 : Elseiver, North Holland.

SEROK, S. and ZEMET, R.M. (1983). An experiment on Gestalt group therapy with hospitalised Schizophrenics. *Psychother. Theor. Res. Pract.*, 20(4), 417-424.

SETHI, B.B. (1982). Editorial : Problems of adolescence. *Ind. J. Psychiat.*, 24, 1.

SETHI, B.B., GUPTA, S.C., RAJ, A.S., and NATHAWAT, S.S. (1971). Rorschach as a measure of psychopathology in murder. *Ind. J. Psychiat.*, 13, 243-247.

SHAGASS, C. (1972). Evoked brain potentials in psychiatry. New York, Plenum Press.

SHAGASS, C. (1977). Early evoked potentials, *Schizo. Bull.*, 3, 80-92.

SHAGASS, C. (1978). *Event related potentials in adult psychiatric disorders.* Report to NIMH, Grant MH, 12507.

SHAGASS, C., OVERTON, D.A. and STRAUMENTS, J.J. (1974). Evoked potentials in Schizophrenia. In MITSUDA, H., and FUKUDA, T., eds., *Biological Mechanisms of Schizophrenia and Schizophrenia – like Psychoses.* Tokyo; Igakushetn Ltd., pp. 214-234.

SHAGASS, C., ROEMER, R.A., STRAUMANIS, J.J. and AMADEO, M. (1978). Evoked potential correlates of psychosis. *Biol. Psychiat.*, 13, 108-184.

SHAILAJAKUMARI, K., and SATHYAVATHI, K. (1988). Interpersonal needs in schizophrenic patients. *Ind. J. Clin. Psychol.*, 15(2), 95-98.

SHAKOW, D. (1962). Segmented Set : A theory of the formal deficit in Schizophrenia. *Arch. Gen. Psychiat.*, 6, 1-17.

SHAKOW, D. (1963). Segmental Set : A theory of the formal psychological deficit in Schizophrenia. *Arch. Gen. Psychiat.*, 6, 1-17.

SHAKOW, D. (1979). Adaptation in Schizophrenia: New York, John Wiley.

SHAPIRO, S.A. (1981). Contemporary thesis of Schizophrenia : Review and Synthesis, New York, McGraw-Hill.

SHARMA, I. and AGNIHOTRI, S.S. (1986). Socio-cultural aspects of Hallucinations. *Ind. J. Clin. Psychol.*, 13(1), 45-50.

SHARMA, T. and ANTONOVA, L. (2003). Cognitive function in Schizophrenia : deficits, functional consequences, and future treatment. *Psychiat. Clinics of North America*, 26, 25-40.

SHELDON, W.H. (1954). *Atlas of man*, New York : Harper & Row.

SHERWOOD, S.L. (1955). Intraventicular administration of drugs. *Lancet*, 900-901.

SHIBATA, H., JOO, A., FUJII, Y., TANI, A., MAKINO C., HIRATA, NM., KIKUTA, R., NINOMIYA, H., TASHIRO, . and FUKUMAKI, Y. (2001). Association study of polymorphisms in the GluR5 Kainate receptor gene (GR1K1) with Schizophrenia. *Psychiat. Genet.*, 11(3), 139-144.

SHIRALI, K.A., and BHARTI, S.P. (1993). Hysteria in Hill Women : Life stress and personality, *Ind. J. Clin. Psychol.*, 20(2), 93-102.

SHIELDS, J., and SLATER, E.T.O. (1967). Genetic aspects of Schizophrenia. *Hospital Med.*, 1, 579-584.

SHUKLA, V., BEHERE, P.B. and MANDAL, M.K. (1993). The right ear advantage in Schizophrenia. *Brit. J. Clin. Psychol.*, 32, 221-223.

SHUKLA, V., BEHERE, P.B. and SAMANT, H.C. (1989). A study of cerebral dominance by laterality score and order of reporting in dichotic – *listening test. Ind. J. Psychiat.*, 31, 73-77.

SIFNEOS, P.E. (1967). Two different kinds of psychotherapy of brief duration. *Arch. J. Psychiat.*, 123, 1069-1074.

SILVERMAN, J. (1964). The problem of attention in research and theory in Schizophrenia. *Psychiat. Rev.*, 71, 352-379.

SILVERMAN, J. (1967). Variations in cognitive control and psychophysiological defence in the Schizophrenia. *Psychosm. Med.*, 29, 225-251.

SIMPSON, G.M., and LEE, J.H. (1978). A ten-year review of anti-psychotics. In M.A. LIPTON, A. DIMASICE, and D.F. KILLIAM (Eds.) *Psychopharmacology : A generation of progress.* New York, Raven Press.

SINGER, K. and CHENG, M.N. (1971). Thioprepazate hydrochloride in persistent dyskinesia. *Brit. Med.* J., 4, 22-25.

SINGH, A. (2002). Research methodological issues in clinical psychology. *Ind. J. Clin. Psychol.*, 29(2), 97-98.

SINGH, G. (1985). Dhat syndrome revisited. *Ind. J. Psychiat.*, 27, 119-122.

SINGH, G., KAUR, D., and KAUR, H. (1981). Stressful life events : development of 'A stressful life events scale for use in India. COMCO. *Mental Health Res. Monogr.* No.1 Patiala, India.

SINGH, N.N., WATSON, J.E., and WINTON, A.S.W. (1987). Parents' acceptability ratings of alternative treatments for use with mentally retarded children. *Beha. Modification.*, 11, 17-26.

SINHA, D., and HOLTZMAN, W.H. (1984). The impact of psychology on Third World development. *Int. J. Psychol.* (Suppl. Issue), 122, 15-20.

SITHOLEY, P., and CHAKRABORTY, S. (1992). Child psychiatric research in India : Epidemiology, assessment, and treatment. In S. Malhotra, A. Malhotra, and V.K. Verma (Eds.), *Child Mental Health in India*, McMillan India, New Delhi.

SKALWEIT, W. (1934). *Contribution and progress in Schizophrenia* – Leipzig: Thieme, 317.

SLATER, E. (1947). Genetical causes of Schizophrenic symptoms. *Monatschr. Psychiat. U. Neurol.*, 113-150.

SLATER, E. and BEARD, A.W. (1963). The Schizophrenia – like psychoses of epilepsy 1. Psychiatric Aspects. *Brit. J. Psychiat.*, 109, 95-150.

SLAVSON, S.R. (1950). Analytic group therapy with children, adolescents, and adults. New York, Columbia University Press.

SLAZINGER, K. (1981). Remedying Schizophrenic Behaviour. In S.M. TURNER, K.S. CALHOUN and H.E. ADAMS (Eds.) *Handbook of Clinical Behaviour Therapy*, New York, John Wiley.

SLYPH, J.A., ROSS, H.E. and KEDWAOD, H.B. (1978). Social disability in chronic psychiatric patients. *Amer. J. Psychiat.*, 134, 1391-1394.

SMARTT, C.G.F. (1956). Mental adjustment in the East Africans. *J. Ment. Sc.*, 102, 441.

SMITH, E.E., NOLEN-HOEKSEMA, S., FREDRICKSON, B., and LOFTUS, G.R. (2003). Atkinson and Hilgard's Introduction to Psychology, 14th edition, Chap-15, Thompson,/Wardsworth, U.S.A.

SMITH, M.D. and COLEMAN, D. (1986). Managing the behaviour of adults with autism in the job setting. *J. Autism and Developmental Disorders*, 16, 145-154.

SOKOLOV, E.N. (1960). Neurol models and the orienting reflex. In M.A.B. BRAZIER (Ed.), *The Central Nervous System and Behaviour*, New York Josiah Macy, Jr. Foundation, pp. 187-276.

SORLE, L., LANGNER, T.S., MICHAEL, S.T., OPLER, M.K., and RENNIE, T.A.C. (1962). Mental health in the metropolis : The Midtown Manhattan Study, New York : McGraw Hill.

SOVANI, A. and THATTE, S. (1994). Interpersonal interaction in groups of Schizophrenics : A psychological intervention. *Ind. J. Clin. Psychol.*, 21, 33-37.

SPECTOR, R.G. (1965). Enzyme chemistry of anoxie brain injury. In C.W.M. Adams (Ed.) *Neurohisto Chemistry*, New York, Elsevier, pp. 547-557.

SPIELBERGER, C.D. (1972). Current trends in theory and research in anxiety. In C.D. Spielberger (Ed.), *Anxiety : Current Trends in Theory and Research*, vol.I, New York, Academic Press.

SPOHN, H.E., LACOURSIERE, R., THOMPSON, K. and COYNE, L. (1977). The effect of phenothiazines an psychological and psychophysiological dysfunction in chronic Schizophrenics. *Arch. Gen. Psychiat.*, 34, 633-644.

SPOHN, H.E., THETFORD, P.E., and CANCRO, R. (1971). The effects of phenotheazine medication on skin conductances and heart rates in Schizophrenic Patients. *J. Nerv. Ment. Dis.*, 152, 129-139.

SRIVASTAVA, A.K., and MISRA, G. (1996). Changing perspective in understanding intelligence : An appraisal. *Ind. J. Abs. & Rev.*, 3, 3-4.

SRIVASTAVA, A.K., TRIPATHI, A.M., and MISRA, G. (1996). The status of intelligence testing in India : A preliminary analysis. *Ind. Edu. Rev.*, 31(1), 1-10.

SROLE, L., LANGER, T.S., MICHAEL, S.T., OPLER, M.K., and RENNIE, T.A.C. (1962). *Mental health in the metropolis, the Midtown Manhattan Study.* New York, McGraw Hill.

SRIVASTAVA, N., BARTHWAL, M.K., DALAL, P.K., AGARWAL, A.K., NAG, D., SRIMAL, R.C. SETH, P.K. and DIKSHIT, M. (2001). Nitrite content and antioxidant enzyme levels in the blood of Schizophrenia patients. *Psychopharmacol.*, 158(2), 140-145.

SRIVASTAVA, P. and MANDAL, M.K. (1990). Proximal spacing to facial affect expressions in Schizophrenia. *Compr. Psychiat.*, 31(2), 119-124.

STABENAU, J.R. and POLLIN, W. (1968). Comparative life history differences of families of Schizophrenics, delinquents and "normals". *Amer. J. Psychiat.*, 124, 1526-1534.

STAINBROOK, E. (1952). Some characteristics of the psychopathology of Schizophrenics behaviour in Indian society. *Amer. J. Psychiat.*, 109, 330.

STAINBROOK, E. (1972). The hospital is a therapeutic community. In Freedman, A.M. and Kaplan, H.J. (Eds.), *Treating mental illness : aspects of modern therapy.* Atheneum, New York.

STAUDT, V. and ZUBIN, J. (1957). A biometric evaluation of the therapies in Schizophrenia : A critical review. *Psychol. Bull.*, 54, 171.

STEPHENS, J. and ASTRUP, C. (1965). Treatment outcome in "process" and "non-process" Schizophrenics by "A" and "B" types of therapist. *J. Nerv. Ment. Dis.*, 140, 449.

STERN, J.A. and McDONALD, D.G. (1965). Physiological correlates of mental disease. *Annual Rev. Psychol.*, 16, 225-264.

STERN, R.A., and PROHASKA, M.L. (1996). Neuropsychological evaluation of Executive functioning. In : Neuropsychiatry for Clinicians. *Rev. of Psychiat.*, 15, 243-266.

STEVENS, J.R. (1982). Neuropathology of Schizophrenia. *Arch. Gen. Psychiat.*, 39, 1131.

STRACHAN, A.M., LEFF, J.P., GOLDSTEIN, M.J., DOANE, J.A. and BURTT, C. (1986). Emotional attitudes and direct communication in the families of Schizophrenics: A cross-national replication. *Brit. J. Psychiat.*, 149, 279-287.

STRAKER, M. (1968). Brief psychotherapy in an outpatient clinic : Evolution and evaluation. *Amer. J. Psychiat.*, 124, 1219-1225.

STRANSKY, E. (1914). Schizophrenia and intra-psychiatric ataria. *J1. Psychiat. Neurol.* 36, 485-264.

STRAUSS, J.S., and CARPENTER, W.J. Jr. (1981). Prediction outcome in Schizophrenia : III, Five Year outcome and its predictions. A report from the international pilot study of Schizophrenia. *Arch. Gen. Psychiat.*, 34, 159-163.

STRELETZKI, F. (1961). Psychoses in the course of Huntington's Chorea with special reference to the formation of delusions. *Arch. Psychiat. Nervenkr.*, 202, 202.301.

STRNSKY, E. (1904). "Zur Lehre Ven der dementia Praecox" (A contribution to the theory of dementia praecox). *Zlel. Nervenhilk*, 21, 1.

STROMGREN, E. (1948). Psychiatric researches in heredity during recent years in the northern countries. Schweiz. *Arch. Neurol. Psychiat.*, 62, 378.

SUHAIL, K. (2000). A comparative study of delusions and hallucinations in Indian and White psychiatric patients. *Ind. J. Clin. Psychol.*, 27(2), 202-206.

SUINN, R.M. (1975). *Fundamentals of behaviour pathology.* John Wiley & Sons, New York, London.

SULLIVAN, H.S. (1976). Conceptions of modern psychiatry, Washington, D.C. : W.A. White Psychiatric Asson.

SULLIVAN, H.S. (1953). *The interpersonal theory of psychiatry.* New York, Norton.

SULLIVAN, H.S. (1956). *Clinical studies in psychiatry.* New York : Norton.

SILLIVAN, R.C. (1976). Current trends in services for antitic persons in the United States : An overview. In E.R. RITVO, B.J. FREEMAN, E.M. ORNITZ, and P.E. TANGUAY (Eds.) *Autism : Diagnosis, Current Research and Management*, New York; Spectrum.

SUTTONS, S., HAKEREM, G., ZUBIN, J., and PORTNOY, M. (1961). The effect of shifting of sensory modality on serial reaction time : A comparison of Schizophrenics and normals. *Amer. J. Psychol.*, 74, 224-232.

SYLPH, J.A., ROSS, H.E. and KEDWARD, H.B. (1978). Social disability in chronic psychiatric patients. *Amer. J. Psychiat.*, 134, 1391-1394.

TALBOTT, J.A. (1981). *The chronic mentally*, New York : Human Science Press.

TALEYAMA, M., ASAI, M., KAMISADA, M., HASHIMOTO, M., BARTELS, M., and HELMANN, H. (1993). Comparison of schizophrenic delusions between Japan and Germany. *Psychopathol.*, 26, 151-158.

TARAFDAR, S., MUKHOPADHYAY, P. and BASU, S. (2004). Personality profile of siblings of children with autism : A comparative study. *SIS Jr. Proj. Psychol. & Ment. Health*, 11(1), 52-58.

TARRIER, N., BECKETT, R., HARWOOD, S., BAKER, A., *et al.* (1993). A trial of two-cognitive behavioural methods of treating drug resistant residual psychotic symptoms in Schizophrenia patients. I : Outcome. *Brit. J. Psychiat.*, 162, 524-532.

TARRIER, N., COOKE, E.C. and LADER, M.H. (1978). Electrodermal and heart rate measurement in chronic and partially remitted Schizophrenic patients. *Acta. Psychiat. Scand.*, 57, 369-376.

TARRIER, N., HARWOOD, S., YUSOPOFF, L., BECKETT, R., and BAKER, A. (1990). Coping strategy enhancement (CSE) : A method of treating residual schizophrenic symptoms. *Behav. Psychother.*, 18, 283-293.

TATE, B.G., and BAROFF, G.S. (1966). Aversive control of self-injurious behaviour in psychotic bey. *Beha. Res. And Ther.*, 4, 281-287.

TAYLOR, D.C. (1975). Factors influencing the occurrence of Schizophrenia-like-psychosis in patients with temporal to be epilepsy. *Psychol. Med.*, 5, 249-254.

TAYLOR, P.J., ROSEMARY, D. and FLEMINGER, J.J. (1980). Handedness in Schizophrenia. *Brit. J. Psychiat.*, 136, 375-383.

TEACE, J.J. (1970). Attention and evoked potentials in man. In : Mostopsky, D.I. ed., *Attention : Contemporary theory and analysis.* Century Psychology Series, Academic Press, New York; pp. 331-365.

TEACE, J.J. (1971). Contingent negative variation and individual differences : A new approach in brain research. *Arch. Gen. Psychiat.*, 24, 1-10.

TEACE, J.J. (1972). Contingent negative variation (CNV) and psychological processes in man. *Psychol. Bull.*, 77, 73-108.

TEICHNER, W.H. (1968). Interaction of behavioural and physiological stress reactions. *Psychol. Rev.*, 75, 271-291.

TEJA, J.S. (1970). Possession states in Indian patients. *Ind. J. Psychiat.*, 12, 71.

TERKELSON, K.G. (1983). Schizophrenia and the family. II. Adverse effects of family therapy. *Family Process*, 22, 191-200.

THAPA, K. (2000). Clinical psychology in India : Dilemmas and Challenges. *Indian Psychological Abstracts and Reviews*, 7(2), 233-272.

THAYER, J., and SILBER, D.E. (1971). Relationship between levels of arousal and responsiveness among schizophrenic and normal subjects. *J. Abn. Psychol.*, 77, 162-173.

THORNDIKE, R.L. (1898). Animal intelligence : An experimental study of the associative processes in animals. *Psychol. Monogr.*, 2(8)

TIWARI, G. and MANDAL, M.K. (1998). Side bias in schizophrenia : Hand, Foot, Eye and Ear. *J. Gen-Psychol.*, 125, 39-46.

TIWARI, P.S.N., SRIVASTAVA, N., and TRIPATHI, V.M. (2002). A study of rural development and value preferences of the people of eastern Uttar Pradesh villages. *Journal of Community Guidance and Research*, 19(2), 155-165.

TOOTH, G. (1950). *Studies in mental illness in the gold coast. Colonial Res. Pub.* No.6, London, A.M.S.O.

TOOTH, G. (1950). *Studies in mental illness in the gold coast. Colonial research publication* No.6, London: H.M.S.O.

TORD, N. *et al.* (1982). Dopamine metabolism increases in post-mortem Schizophrenic basal ganglia. *J. Neurol. Transm.*, 54, 181.

TORRY, E.F., YOLKEN, R.H. and WINFREY, C.J. (1982). Cytomogalovirus antibody in cerebrospinal fluid of Schizophrenic patients detected by enzyme immunoassay. *Science*, 216, 892.

TREISMAN, A.M. (1969). Strategies and models and selective attention. *Psychol. Rev.*, 76, 282-299.

TRESS, K.H., CAUDREY, D.J., and MEHTA, B. (1983). Tactile-evoked potentials in Schizophrenia: Interhemispheric transfer and drug effects. *Brit. J. Psychiat.*, 143, 156-164.

TRIPATHI, R.K., and JAHAN, M. (2004). Personality characteristics of schizophrenic patient with criminal record. *Ind. J. Clin. Psychol.*, 31(2), 106-111.

TUCKER, D.M. (1981). Lateral brain function, emotion and conceptualisation. *Psychol. Bull.*, 89, 19-46.

TURNER, S.M., HERSEN, M. and BELLACK, A.S. (1977). Effects of social disruption, stimulus interference and aversive conditioning on auditory hallucinations. *Beha. Med.*, 1, 249-258.

ULLMANN, L.P. and KRASNER, L. (1969a). *A psychological approach to abnormal behaviour*, Englewood Cliffs, N.J. Prentice Hall.

ULLMANN, L.P. and KRASNER, L. (1969b). The sociopsychological formulation and treatment of Schizophrenia. In *A Psychological approach to abnormal behaviour*, Chap.20, New Jersey, Prentice Hall.

VAGREECHA, Y.S. and ASTHANA, A.S. (1987) (cited by Shirlai and Bharti, 1993). "Purvaj Syndrome". A culture bound reaction to stress and a psychotherapeutic device observed in a rural community. Department of Psychology, Sagar University, Sagar, M.P., India.

VAILLANT, G. (1966). The prediction of recovery in Schizophrenia. *Int. J. Psychiat.*, 2, 617.

VANPUTTERN, T., and MAY, P.R.A. (1978). Akinetic depression in Schizophrenia. *Arch. Gen. Psychiat.*, 35, 1101-1107.

VAUGHAN, C.E. and LEFF, J.P. (1976). The influence of family and social factors on the courses of psychiatric illness. *Brit. J. Psychiat.*, 129, 125-137.

VAUGHAN, C.E., SNYDER, K.S., JONES, S., FREEMAN, W.B., and FALLOON, I.R.H. (1984). Family factors in Schizophrenic relapse : A California replication of the British Research on expressed emotion. *Arch. Gen. Psychiat.*, 41, 1169-1177.

VENABLES, P.H. (1960). The effect of auditory and visual stimulation on the skin potential response of Schizophrenics. *Brain*, 83, 77.

VENABLES, P.H. (1964). Input dysfunction in Schizophrenia In B. Mahar (Ed.) *Progress in Experimental Personality Research*, vol.1, New York: Academic Press, pp. 1-47.

VENABLES, P.H. (1967). Partial failure of cortical subcortical integration as a factor underlying Schizophrenic behaviour. In J.J. ROMANO (Ed.) *The Origins of Schizophrenia, Amsterdam*, Exerpta Medica, pp. 42-53.

VENABLES, P.H. (1973). Input regulation and psychopathology. In : M. HAMMER, K. SALZINGER, and S. SUTTCH (Eds.) *Psychopathology. Contributions from the social, behavioural and biological sciences.* John Wiley & Sons, New York.

VANABLES, P.H. (1975a). The recovery limb of the skin conductance response in "high-rises" research. In : Mednick, S.A. Schulsinger, F., Higgins, J. and Bell, B., eds. *Genetics, Environment and Psychopathology*, Amsterdam, North-Holland / American Elsevier, pp. 117-134.

VENABLES, P.H. (1975b). Psychophysiological studies of Schizophrenics pathology. In P.H. Venables and M.J. Christie (Eds.) *Research in Psychophysiology*, John Wiley & Sons, London.

VENABLES, P.H. (1977). The electrodermal psychophysiology of Schizophrenics and children at high rise for Schizophrenia : Current controversies and developments. *Schizo. Bull.*, 3, 28-48.

VENABLES, P.H. and CHRISTIE, M.J. (1974). Mechanisms, instrumentation, recording techniques and quantification of responses. In : RROKASY, W.F. and RASKIN, D.C., eds., *Electrodermal activity in psychological research*, Academic Press, New York.

VENABLES, P.H. and CHRISTIE, M.J. (1980). Electrodermal activity. In Martin, I. and Venables, P.H. (Eds.), *Techniques in Psychophysiology*, Ch.1.

VENABLES, P.H. and MARTIN, I. (1964). A manual of psychophysiological methods. New York: John Wiley & Sons.

VENABLES, P.H. and WING, J.K. (1972). Level of arousal and the sub classification of Schizophrenia. *Arch. Gen. Psychiat.*, 7, 114-119.

VERGHESE, A., JOHN, J.K., RAJKUMAR, S., RICHARD, J., SETHI, B.B. and TRIVEDI, J.K. (1989). Factors associated with the course and outcome of Schizophrenia in India. *Brit. J. Psychiat.*, 154, 499-503.

VERGHESE, M., BHATTI, R.S., RAGHURAM, A., CHANDRA, P.S., UDAYKUMAR, S.S. and SHAH, A. (1994). Training in family therapy at NIMHANS. Paper presented at the *National Symposium on Training in Psychotherapy*, NIMHANS, Bangalore.

VERMA, L.P., SRIVASTAVA, D.K. and SAHAY, R.N. (1970). Possession Syndrome. *Ind. J. Psychiat.*, 1, 12.

VOELTZ, L.M., EVANS, I.M., DERER, K.R. and HANASHIRO, R. (1983). Targetting excess behaviour for change : A clinical decision model for selecting priority goals in educational contexts. *Child and Family Beha. Ther.*, 5, 17-35.

VOCCARO, M.V. (1967). Review of Rogers *et al.'s* The therapeutic relationship and its impact : A study of psychotherapy with Schizophrenics. *J. Albert Einstein Med. Centre* (October).

VRTUNSKI, P.B., SIMPSON, D.M., WEISS, K.M., and DAVIS, G.C. (1986). Abnormalities of the five motor control in Schizophrenia. *Psychiat. Res.*, 18, 275-284.

VUKELICH, R. and HAKE, D.F. (1971). Reduction of dangerously aggressive behaviour in a severally retarded resident through a combination of positive reinforcement procedures. *J. Appl. Beha. Anal.*, 4, 215-225.

WARDSWORTH, M.V., WELLS, B.W.P. and SCOTT, R.F. (1962). Quantity and quality of industrial therapy. *Lancet*, 2, 1375-1376.

WALKER, C.E. (1981). Continuing professional development : In : C.E. Walker (ed.) *Clinical practice of psychology : A guide for mental health professionals.* Pergaman, New York.

WALKER, E. and McGUIRE, M. (1982). Intra and interhemispheric information processing in Schizophrenia. *Psychol. Bull.*, 92, 701-725.

WALLACE, C.J. and LIBERMAN, R.F. (1985). Social skill training for patients with Schizophrenia: A controlled clinical trial. *Psychiat. Res.*, 14, 239-247.

WALLERSTEIN, J.S., and BLAKESLEE, S. (1989). Second chances : men, women, and children a decade after divorce. New York : Ticknor and Fields.

WALTON, D. (1960). The relevance of learning theory to the treatment of an obsessive – compulsive state. In H.J. Sysenck (Ed.) *Behaviour in the neuroses*, New York, Pargamon Press.

WARBURTON, D.M. (1972). The cholinergic control of internal inhibition. In : BOAKES, R.A. and HALLIDAY, M.S., eds. *Inhibition and learning*, Academic Press, London, pp. 431-460.

WARNER, R. (1983). Recovery from Schizophrenia in the Third World. *Psychiat.*, 46, 197-212.

WARNER, R. (1985). Recovery from Schizophrenia : Psychiatric and political economy. Routledge and Kagan Paul, London.

WARRINGTON, E.K. and JAMES, M. (1967). An experimental investigation of facial recognition in patients with unilateral cerebral lesions. *Cortex*, 3, 317-326.

WASYLENKI, D.A.(1992). Psychotherapy of Schizophrenia revisited. *Hospital and Comm. Psychiat.*, 43, 123-127.

WATTS, F.N. and BENNETT, D.H. (1983). *Theory and practice of psychiatric rehabilitation*, Chichester, John Wiley.

WAXLER, N.E. (1979). Is outcome for Schizophrenia better in non-industrial societies. The use of Sri Lanka. *J. Nerv. Ment. Dis.*, 167, 144-158.

WEIL, J.L. (1989a). Instinctual stimulation of children (Vol.I), Medison, CT: International Universities Press.

WEIL, J.L. (1989b). Instinctual stimulation of children (Vol.II), Medison, CT: International Universities Press.

WEIL, J.L. (1992). Early deprivation of empathic care. Medison, CT: International Universities Press.

WEINBERGER, D.R., ALOIA, M.S., GOLDBERG, T.E., *et al.* (1994). The frontal lobes and Schizophrenia. *J. Neuropsychiat. Clin. Neurosci.*, 6, 419-427.

WEISSMAN, M.M. (1984). The psychological treatment of depression. *Arch. Gen. Psychiat.*, 36, 1261-1269.

WENDER, P.H., ROSENTHAL, D. and KETY, S.S. (1968). A psychiatric assessment of the adoptive parents of Schizophrenics. In *Transmission of Schizophrenia*: Rosenthal Hermonds, D. and Kety, S.S. (Eds.) Worth : Penguin.

WENDER, P.H., ROSENTHAL, D., ZAHN, T.P., and KETY, S.S. (1971). The psychiatric adjustment of the adopting parents of Schizophrenics. *Amer. J. Psychiat.*, 227, 1013-1017.

WEXLER, M. (1968). One path to recovery lies in the development of some object relationships with someone in the outside world. In : MAY, P.R.A, *Treatment of Schizophrenia: A comparative study of five treatment methods.* New York, Science House.

WEYGANDT, W. (1907). "Kritische Bemerkungen Zur Psychologie der Dementia Praecox" (Critical observation on the psychology of dementia praecox). *Mschr. Psychiat. Neurol.*, 22, 289.

WIG, N.N. (1960). Problems of mental health in India. *J. Abn. Soc. Psychiat.*, 17, 48-53.

WIG, N.N. (2000). WHO and mental health: A review from developing countries. *Bull. Who*, 78, 502-503.

WIJESTINGHE, G.P., DISSANAYAKE, S.A.W., and MENDIS, N. (1976). Possession trance in a semi-urban community in Sri Lanka. *Aust. & New Zeal. J. Psychiat.*, 10, 136-139.

WING, J. (1979). Social influences on the course of Schizophrenia. In L.C. Wynne, R.L., Cromwell, and S. Mathysee (Eds.) *The nature of Schizophrenia : New approaches to research and treatment*: New York, John Wiley & Sons.

WING, J.K. (1966). Five-year outcome in early Schizophrenia. *Proc. R. Soc. Med.*, 59, 17-18.

WING, J.K., BENNETT, J.H. and DENHAM, J. (1964). The industrial rehabilitation of long-story Schizophrenic patients. *Med. Res. Coune. Memo (Lond),* No.42, London: H.M.S.O.

WING, J.K., and BROWN, G.W. (1961). Social treatment of chronic Schizophrenia: A comparative survey of three mental hospitals. *J. Ment. Sci.*, 107, 847-861.

WITTKOWER, E.D. and DUBREUIL, G. (1968). Cultural factors in mental illness. In NORBECK, E., PRICE WILLIAMS, D. and MCCORD, W.M. (eds.) *The study of personality : an interdisciplinary appraisal*, New York : Holt, Rinechart and Winston, pp. 279-295.

WOLBERG, L.R. (1965). *Short term psychotherapy.* Grune and Stratten.

WOLF, M.M. (1978). Social validity: A case for subjective measurement of how behavioural analysis is finding its heart. *J. Appl. Beha. Analysis*, 11, 302-314.

WOLF, M.M., RISLEY, T.R. and MEES, H. (1964). Application of operant conditioning procedures to the behaviour problems of an autistic child. *Beha. Res. and Ther.*, 1, 305-312.

WONG, S.E., and MASSED, H.K., MOSK, M.D. and LIBERMAN, N.P. (1986). Behavioural approach to the treatment of Schizophrenia. In G.D. BURROWS, T.R. NORMAN and G. RUBENSTEIN (Eds.), *Handbook of Studies on Schizophrenia*: 2. Management and Research, New York, Elsevier.

WOODS, T.S. (1984). Social validation : Its implications for practitioners of applied behaviour analysis serving the developmental disabled. *Scandinavian J. Beha. Ther.*, 13, 67-84.

WORLD HEALTH ORGANISATION (1968). International classification of diseases, 8th revision, Geneva.

WORLD HEALTH ORGANISATION (1979). Schizophrenia: An international follow-up study, John Wiley, New York.

WORLD HEALTH ORGANISATION (1992). International classification of diseases. 10th revision (ICD-10). Mental and Behavioural Disorders. Geneva, Oxford University Press.

WORLD HEALTH ORGANISATION (2001). World Health Report: 2000-2001, Mental Health: New Understanding and New Hope, Geneva.

WYNNE, L.C. (1968). Schizophrenics and their families: recent research findings and implications. *Mental Health Fund*, 6th Annual Lecture, London, p.317.

WYNNE, L.C., and SINGER, M.T. (1963). Thought disorder and family relations of Schizophrenics. *Arch. Gen. Psychiat.*, 9, 191-198.

WYNNE, L.C. and SINGER, M.T. (1965). Thought disorder and family relations of Schizophrenia. II. A classification of forms of thinking. *Arch. Gen. Psychiat.*, 9, 199-317.

WYRSON, J. (1942). On theory and clinical observations of paranoid Schizophrenia. *Mschr. Psychiat. Neurol.*, 172, 797-309.

YAP, P.M. (1951). Mental disease peculiar to certain cultures. A Survey of Comparative Psychiatry. *J. Ment. Sc.*, 97, 313.

YAP, P.M. (1952). The Latah Reaction : Its Pathodynamics and Nosological Position. *J. Ment. Sc.*, 98, 512.

YAP, P.M. (1966). Culture-bound reactive syndromes. *Presented at the Conference on Mental Health in Asia and the Pacific.* March 28, April 1, 1966, East West Centre, Honolulu, Hawaii.

YATES, B.T. (1985). Cost effectiveness analysis and cost-benefit analysis, An Introduction. *Behavioural Assessment*, 7, 207-234.

YEATON, W.H. (1982). A critique of the effectiveness of applied behaviour analysis research. *Advances in Behavior Res. & Ther.*, 4, 75-96.

ZAHN, T.P. (1976). On the bimodality of the distribution of electrodermal orienting responses in Schizophrenic patients. *J. Nerv. Ment. Dis.*, 162, 195-199 and LAWLOR, N.G. (1968). Electrodermal and heart rate orienting reactions in chronic Schizophrenia. *J. Psychiat. Res.*, 6, 117-134.

ZIGLER, E. and GLICK, M. (1986). *A developmental approach to adult psychopathology.* New York, John Wiley.

ZUBIN, J. (1970). Problems of attention in Schizophrenia. *J. Nerv. Ment. Dis.*, 5, 351-359.

ZUBIN, J. and SPRING, R. (1977). Vulnerability – a new view of Schizophrenia. *J. Abn. Psychiat.*, 86, 103-126.

ZUBIN, J. and STEINHAURT, S. (1981). How to break the legjim in Schizophrenia. *J. Nerv. Ment. Dis.*, 167, 477-492.

ZUTT, J. (1952). "Dev as thetische Erbbinsbereich and scine Krankhafte abwandlungen. Min Beitray Zum Wabnpreblem" (the nesthetic zone of experience and its morbid modifications). *Nervenarzt*, 23, 163.

ZUTT, J. and KUHLENKAMPF, C. (1958). Das paranoids syndrome in anthropolegi-scher Sticht (the paranoid syndrome from the anthropological point of view), Berlin: Springer.

SUBJECT INDEX

A

B

F

G

H

Q

R

S

AUTHOR INDEX

A

B

C

F

G

H

M

N

O

P

R

S

T

U

V

W

Y

Z